OCCUPATIONAL THERAPY
ASSISTANT

CHESS Publications, Inc.

OCCUPATIONAL THERAPY ASSISTANT:

A

PRIMER

HARU HIRAMA, Ed. D.,O.T.R./L., FAOTA

Library of Congress Catalog Card Number 86-070479

ISBN 0-935273-00-X

Published by CHESS Publications, Inc.
232 East University Parkway
Baltimore, MD 21218

TABLE OF CONTENTS

FOREWORD

I n *Occupational Therapy Assistant: A Primer*, we finally have a textbook written specifically for students seeking to become occupational therapy assistants. After many years of adapting texts and materials written for occupational therapy students, faculty teaching prospective occupational therapy assistants should find it a refreshing experience to read and use this text. As its name implies, it is designed to be a first text covering the profession of occupational therapy assistant.

Faculty will benefit from the considerable amount of preparatory work that Dr. Haru Hirama has done for them in conjunction with each chapter; there are learning objectives, chapter summaries, review questions and answers, additional learning activities, references, and a suggested reading list.

Students will benefit from the detailed table of contents, glossary, and index, as well as the clear writing style, all of which make this text easy to use and highly readable.

The occupational therapy profession will benefit from a textbook that repeatedly and specifically describes the assistant's role in relation to the therapist's role in a variety of situations, including direct patient care and associated activities.

Those of us who teach future occupational therapy assistants in the classroom and in the field have been waiting for such a textbook to be published. Our wait is over!

Celestine Hamant, M.S., O.T.R., FAOTA
Associate Professor and Director of Occupational Therapy
Indiana University Medical Center

PREFACE

My goal for this book was to include enough information to help students during their orientation to occupational therapy. My aim was to arouse students' curiosity and entice students to read other textbooks, visit various occupational therapy settings, and talk to occupational therapy practitioners to learn more about the discipline.

The chapters are organized with the following elements, in order of their appearance: an overview, learning objectives, the content of the chapter, a summary, review questions and answers, additional learning activities, references for the chapter, and references to additional readings and listening/viewing activities. The information the text presents will be more interesting and meaningful if students can combine classroom instruction with observations and experiences in settings where occupational therapy services are provided.

The first edition of *Occupational Therapy Assistant: A Primer* was published in 1986. Two sections were added in the 1990 revision. The first, on neurodevelopmental treatment (NDT), was included to orient students to a treatment approach often used by therapists. The NDT approach is not used by entry-level occupational therapy assistants; however, students return to class with many questions after observing NDT therapists treat patients. The second new section was a study guide with suggestions on how to be effective students. Open-ended questions were included to encourage students to formulate their own answers and search for information to confirm the correctness of those answers.

In this revision, I updated information and added a chapter on arthritis. I hope instructors and students will find the book useful. I welcome comments from readers.

ACKNOWLEDGEMENTS

Several individuals have helped me persevere with this text. George W. Elison, retired dean of instruction, Lehigh Carbon Community College, first suggested that I write a text for students seeking to become occupational therapy assistants and supported my efforts with the first edition. Dolores Blickley, COTA/L, and Monica Lemke Knott, O.T.R, former COTA, persuaded me to write the first edition. The illustrations in the chapters on spinal cord injuries and cerebral vascular accidents were suggested by Monica and drawn by David Cerulli, artist. Monica drew the illustrations in the chapter on arthritis. Susan Lemke, O.T.R, former COTA, gave suggestions for the chapter on the philosophy of occupational therapy. I thank them all for helping me with this project.

My children, Monica, John, Christopher, and Susan, are the prime motivating factors for my life pursuits. I thank them for always being available to help me and for pursuing their own life goals to make their contributions to society.

Finally, I thank the following people who granted me permission to include their material in this text:

F. A. Davis Company, Philadelphia, PA, for definitions from *Taber's Cyclopedic Medical Dictionary*, 17th edition, C. L. Thomas, editor, copyright 1993.

Maude H. Malick, Harmarville Rehabilitation Center, Pittsburgh, PA, for the illustrations of basic types of prehension and grasp, the position of function, and the position of rest of the hand from *Manual on Static Hand Splinting*, copyright 1972.

The American Association on Mental Deficiency, Washington, DC, for the definition of mental retardation from *Classification in Mental Retardation*, H.J. Grossman, editor, copyright 1983.

The American Occupational Therapy Association, Inc., for the definition of occupational therapy and selected terminology.

Haru Hirama, Ed.D., O.T.R/L, FAOTA

Section I

OVERVIEW OF OCCUPATIONAL THERAPY

Each profession gives special meaning to commonly used words and phrases. This section defines occupational therapy, introduces words basic to the discipline, and discusses the philosophy guiding the profession. The history of occupational therapy and the occupational therapy assistant shows how world events influence the profession. Who may benefit from occupational therapy services, where these services can be obtained, and the personnel who provide such services are introduced.

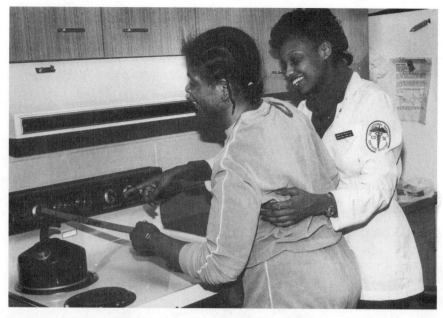
Jacqueline Young, COTA/L, teaches meal preparation skills.

1

DEFINING
OCCUPATIONAL THERAPY

This chapter provides an overview and definitions of occupational therapy and discusses the types of patients served, goals of treatment, and occupations used in treatment.

LEARNING OBJECTIVES

At the end of this chapter, you should be able to:

1. State a definition of occupational therapy.
2. Define and use the following words as they are used in occupational therapy: *occupational, therapy, activity, performance areas, performance components,* and *performance contexts.*
3. List at least five categories of disorders treated in occupational therapy.
4. State and give examples of the three occupational performance areas toward which occupational therapy intervention is directed.
5. Name and give examples of the three categories of performance components.
6. Identify a therapeutic activity, a therapeutic device, and a therapeutic exercise, and explain how they differ.

O ccupational therapy is an allied health service that uses purposeful activity to treat people who are limited in performing their daily living activities. Individuals affected by physical, cognitive, mental, or developmental impairment or disability are those most likely to benefit from occupational therapy. The goal of occupational therapy is to help the person function as independently as possible in all activities of daily living and to maintain a state of well-being.

Individuals of any age may be referred for occupational therapy.

An infant may need special sensorimotor stimulation because of a developmental delay or birth defect. A child may need a splint to prevent a joint from becoming deformed because of being burned. An adolescent may need to be taught to eat with special feeding devices because of quadriplegia resulting from a diving accident. An adult may need to be taught special dressing techniques because of hemiplegia following a stroke. A patient's family members may need education and training in the use of special techniques and devices to aid the patient during the entire treatment process. A person of any age may need to learn effective ways to relate to others because of mental illness or other psychosocial problems. Any of the above individuals may need diversional activities to cope with the effects of injury or conditions that result in dysfunction.

Occupational therapy practitioners work in a variety of settings, including general acute-care hospitals, subacute-care settings, rehabilitation centers, substance abuse treatment centers, schools, long-term care facilities, community day-care centers, and private homes.

Three major requirements to be met before the student studying to be an occupational therapy assistant can work as a qualified occupational therapy practitioner are (1) graduation from an accredited educational program for the occupational therapy assistant (AOTA, 1991b); (2) following graduation, successful completion of the national certification examination administered by the American Occupational Therapy Certification Board (AOTCB, 1994); and (3) licensure to practice occupational therapy in the regulated state where the certified practitioner plans to work. Some regulated states issue temporary licenses to individuals who can verify that they have completed all academic and fieldwork requirements and that they are eligible for graduation and admission to the certification examination.

Certification and licensure to practice occupational therapy are commonly designated by the letters COTA/L, following the individual's name. In most situations, the occupational therapy assistant is supervised by a certified occupational therapist who is a graduate of an accredited occupational therapy educational program (AOTA, 1991a) and has a baccalaureate or higher degree. The letters O.T.R designate that the occupational therapist is registered and certified by AOTCB. The letter L designates that the O.T.R is licensed by the regulated state in which he or she is employed.

The occupational therapy assistant may provide his or her services to patients of any age and any condition, as determined by the supervising occupational therapist. Patients may range in age from newly born to over 100 years or even older. Patients may reside at home, attend a day treatment program, be hospitalized in an acute-care or subacute-care setting, or reside in a long-term residential facility. The occupational therapist is primarily responsible for evaluating the patient's need for occupational therapy. The occupational therapy assistant is primarily responsible for providing direct treatment to the patient.

Therapeutic media and techniques used by occupational therapy practitioners vary, but can be categorized as activities, devices, or exercises (Ayres, 1972; Drake, 1992; Dutton, 1989; Pedretti & Zoltan, 1990; United States Department of the Army, 1980). Therapeutic activities include, but are not limited to, activities related to manual and creative arts, indoor and outdoor games, music, various aspects of self-care, tasks carried out with the aim of maintaining an appropriate home environment, and tasks related to vocational pursuits. Ideally, the occupations used in therapy interest and motivate the patient and provide the sensorimotor, cognitive, and psychosocial components that will enable the patient to function in the occupational performance area of concern.

Therapeutic devices range from orthotics, such as splints that prevent the deformity, protect, or enable the functional use of a body part, to the numerous items developed to allow an individual to be as independent as possible. Examples of therapeutic devices are transfer boards that enable a person to slide from a wheelchair to another chair without first standing, reachers that allow a seated person to grasp an object from the floor or from a high shelf, long-handled shoehorns and dressing sticks that enable an individual to dress independently in spite of decreased joint mobility, specially designed eating utensils such as spoons with bent handles and plates with built-up sides that enable a person to eat independently, and cutting boards with upright nails or corner rims that stabilize items placed on them and allow an individual to prepare food with one hand. When a patient cannot function independently, an appropriate device can still maximize the patient's independence.

Therapeutic exercises range from passive exercises for the patient who lacks muscle strength to active exercises with resistance for the patient whose goal is to increase his or her strength and endurance. An example of a passive therapeutic exercise is the occupational therapy practitioner moving a patient's elbow joint through the patient's available range of motion five times. An example of an active-resistive therapeutic exercise is the patient wearing a 5-pound wrist weight and actively moving the elbow joint through the available range of motion 10 times. The primary aim of occupational therapy is to enable the individual to function as independently as possible in all activities of daily living. Functioning as independently as possible may entail regaining lost skills, learning a different way of performing an activity, or using a special device. Other aims of occupational therapy are to educate individuals in the prevention of disabilities and to help individuals maintain their health and state of physical and emotional well-being.

The occupational therapy assistant is expected to have a background of diverse information and skills that are systematically acquired through formal occupational therapy assistant educational programs, typically 2 years in length. The formal curriculum should meet the essential requirements established by the American Occupational Therapy Association (AOTA, 1991b). Basic information includes information on human anatomy, physiology, psychology, sociology, and occupations. Knowledge of the characteristics of disabling conditions, interpersonal relationship skills, awareness of the precautions required when working with disabled individuals, and knowledge of therapeutic media and techniques used in occupational therapy are necessary to understand occupational therapy, its purpose, and its application.

DEFINITION OF OCCUPATIONAL THERAPY AND TERMINOLOGY

The American Occupational Therapy Association (AOTA, 1994b) recommends the following definition of occupational therapy as a guide for state regulation of occupational therapy practice:

> "Occupational therapy" is the use of purposeful activity or interventions designed to achieve functional outcomes which promote health, prevent injury or disability and which develop, improve, sustain, or restore the highest possible level of independence of any individual who has an injury, illness, cognitive impairment, psychosocial dysfunction, mental illness, developmental or learning disability, physical disability, or other disorder or condition. It includes assessment by means of skilled observation or evaluation through the administration and interpretation of standardized or nonstandardized tests and measurements. (pp. 1073)

Also, occupational therapy services include but are not limited to:

1. the assessment and provision of treatment in consultation with the individual, family or other appropriate persons; and
2. interventions directed toward developing, improving, sustaining or restoring daily living skills, including self-care skills and activities that involve interactions with others and the environment, work readiness or work performance, play skills or leisure capacities, or enhancing educational performance skills; and
3. developing, improving, sustaining or restoring sensory-motor, perceptual or neuromuscular functioning; or range of motion; or emotional, motivational, cognitive, or psychosocial components of performance; and
4. education of the individual, family or other appropriate persons in carrying out appropriate interventions.

These services may encompass assessment of need and the design, development, adaptation, application or training in the use of assistive technology devices; the design, fabrication, or application of rehabilitative technology such as selected orthotic devices; training in the use of orthotic or prosthetic devices; the application of physical agent modalities as an adjunct to or in preparation for purposeful activity; the application of ergonomic principles; the adaptation of environments and processes to enhance functional performance; or the promotion of health and wellness. (AOTA, 1994b, p. 1073)

Variations of the above definition of occupational therapy can be found in other sources, such as the dictionary (Gove, 1966). Dictionary definitions, however, are concise and limit explanation, which can lead to misunderstandings about the profession. Occupational therapy service areas and methods have expanded greatly since the profession began during World War 1 (1914-1918), and the definition has been revised many times to include new developments. The following AOTA dictionary definition of occupational therapy was adopted by the Representative Assembly in 1986: "Occupational therapy: therapeutic use of self-care, work and play activities to increase independent function, enhance development, and prevent disability; may include adaptation of task or environment to achieve maximum independence and to enhance quality of life." (AOTA, 1986, p. 582).

DEFINING WORDS

A review of the meaning of the specific words, *occupational therapy*, will help to understand the discipline in a broad sense. *Occupational,* an adjective, means relating to or resulting from a particular occupation. *Occupation,* a noun, means that which occupies or engages one's time, employment, or vocation—in other words, an activity. *Activity,* a noun, means the state of being active or any specific action, and is often used instead of the word *occupation. Therapy,* a noun, means something of a therapeutic nature. *Therapeutic,* an adjective, means serving to cure or heal. Thus, *occupational therapy,* in its most basic form, means engaging the patient's time in an activity in order to effect a cure of some kind. However, engaging a patient in an occupation does not guarantee a cure, so the definition of *occupational therapy* still needs to be elaborated.

An examination of other words in AOTA's definition of the term will help to understand the purpose and process of occupational therapy. *Evaluation,* which includes screening and assessment, record reviews, interviews, and observations, identifies the nature, characteristics, and extent of the patient's problem. Usually, the problem relates to the individual's inability to function as well as he or she would like to function in some aspect of daily living. The occupational therapy profession has identified three major occupational performance areas for intervention by practitioners: *activities of daily living, work and productive activities,* and *play or leisure activities.* These areas are described in detail in "Uniform Terminology for Occupational Therapy—Third Edition" (AOTA, 1994a). *Activities of daily living* are those activities related to self-care (e.g., bathing and brushing one's teeth), maintaining health (e.g., eating and taking one's medication), and maintaining oneself in the community (through functional communication and mobility). *Work and productive activities* relate to productive occupations, whether paid or unpaid. Examples include activities required to manage a home (e.g., preparing meals, cleaning the home, and managing money), all activities related to work done by a paid employee, activities done by a parent caring for a family, and any education-related activity performed by a student in school. *Play leisure activities* include active and passive recreational pursuits.

Intervention using selected therapeutic activities, devices, and exercises is directed at developing the performance components needed to achieve functional outcomes within the applicable context. Performance components are of four varieties: sensorimotor, cognitive, psychosocial, and psychological. The context in which intervention takes place consists of the temporal and environmental features that influence functional performance. The occupational performance areas, components, and contexts are described in detail in "Uniform Terminology for Occupational Therapy—Third Edition" (AOTA, 1994a).

Occupational therapy uses purposeful activity (occupations) to engage the patient's time and energy in specific movements, tasks, and behaviors in order to achieve previously identified functional outcomes and thus maximize the independence of the patient. The purposefulness of the activity is determined by the patient, not the occupational therapy practitioner. Therefore, effective occupational therapy requires not only extensive knowledge and application of the information required in the occupational therapy curriculum, but the added ability of the occupational therapy practitioner to work in concert with the patient to achieve the patient's desired goals. A complete explanation of the term *purposeful activity* is given in a position paper approved by AOTA's Representative Assembly (AOTA, 1993).

CONSUMERS OF OCCUPATIONAL THERAPY

Occupational therapy consumers are those who have difficulty performing their daily life tasks or activities, be they self-care, work, or leisure activities. A person's inability to function satisfactorily may be the result of a developmental or learning disability, a medical condition, an injury, a mental or physical illness, a cognitive impairment, or an environmental condition. Consumers can be of any age and from any socioeconomic background. Potential consumers with limitations that interfere with their normal performance can be assessed to determine whether they need occupational therapy.

AIM OF OCCUPATIONAL THERAPY

The principle aim of occupational therapy stated in AOTA's definition is to achieve functional outcomes. To help the patient achieve those outcomes, the result of occupational therapy intervention should maximize the independence of the patient. Independence in daily living may be maximized by teaching the individual different ways of performing a task. It may be possible to perform the task by using body parts in different ways or by changing the position of the body or objects to be used. It may be possible to adapt the objects or equipment in such a manner as to enable the patient to perform the task. Special equipment and devices may be selected to allow for maximum independence.

An individual's ability to function is dependent on his or her well-being. The physical, mental and social well-being of the patient is a general goal of occupational therapy. Special techniques for maintaining health are included in occupational therapy intervention. Preventing injury and disability can help to maintain health. Disability may be prevented by the use of special therapeutic activities or exercises. Correct positioning of the body may also prevent disability, as may splints and other orthotic devices and equipment adapted to the patient's level of functioning. An appropriate balance of life activities can aid in the maintenance of health. Therapy includes helping the patient adapt to an inevitable dysfunction or disability and to cope with daily stresses. Emotional and physical stress may be prevented by practicing appropriate behaviors and seeking help from special professionals.

OCCUPATIONS USED

Occupational therapy makes use of a wide variety of *occupations*—that is, activities that occupy the patient. Definitions of occupational therapy earlier than AOTA's state that occupations could be any physical or mental activities which aid in the patient's recovery from disease or injury.

Occupations that are familiar to the patient—that the patient considers appropriate and interesting—are preferred. The choice of occupations depend upon the patient's therapeutic needs, as well as certain safety factors associated with the performance of the task. The creativity, imagination, and ability of the occupational therapist and assistant, the community resources attainable, the treatment space, and the available funds can influence the choice of occupations used.

For approximately the first 40 years of the profession, the occupations most frequently used were work assignments and educational, recreational, manual, and creative activities (Brainerd, 1967; Drake, 1992). These occupations were usually available within the facility or in the nearby community. They could be easily adapted to meet the patient's needs. Expectations in the performance of such occupations were therapeutically graded to be more or less demanding of the patient's abilities, time, and energy. The variety of occupations provided choices and motivation for the patient.

Work assignments varied from delivering departmental messages within the facility to working in service areas, such as the kitchen, library, laundry, storeroom, or building grounds. Some large institutions grew their own food, and patients were assigned work on the institutional farm or dairy. Educational activities ranged from reading and individual studies to vocational preparation and classroom attendance. Sports, games, dances, and parties were also part of early occupational therapy programs. Woodworking, metalwork, leathercraft, graphic arts, ceramics (United States Department of the Army, 1980), needlecraft, cooking, sewing, photography, little theater groups, and patient-produced newspapers are examples of manual and creative occupations.

Additional methods of providing occupational therapy developed. The needs of patients with physical injuries and disabilities led occupational therapists to use equipment and exercise to provide specific treatment. Equipment such as skateboards and tilted tabletops were used to increase muscle strength and the range of motion of joints in the upper extremities. Therapeutic equipment and exercise began to be more prominently used during and after World War II (Dutton, 1989; Pedretti & Zoltan, 1990).

Therapeutic exercise became an important feature of occupational therapy as the need to measure the effects of therapy objectively became important. When therapeutic exercises were used, it was easier to measure changes by counting the number of times the movement was made, the number of pounds the patient was able to move, or the length of time the patient could exercise. Additional occupational therapy techniques were developed as the profession evolved. These techniques are described in detail in other texts (Ayres, 1972; Pedretti & Zoltan, 1990).

The basis of occupational therapy is the use of therapeutic occupations. Dutton (1989) proposed that exercise prepares the client for purposeful activity. Exercise (preparation) and purposeful activity (application) are two ends of a continuum in occupational therapy. Research to study the effectiveness of exercise and purposeful activity, separately and in combination, will contribute greatly to the efficacy of occupational therapy (Dutton, 1989).

SUMMARY

Occupational therapy is the process of engaging individuals who have limitations in purposeful activity in order to improve, enhance, or maintain functional performance in their daily life tasks and activities. A limitation may be due to a physical injury or illness, a cognitive impairment, a psychosocial dysfunction, mental illness, a developmental or learning disability, or an environmental condition. Purposeful activities include those normally engaged in during self-care, work, and leisure time. Such activities are carefully analyzed and used therapeutically to meet the needs of the particular individual.

REVIEW QUESTIONS

1. Define occupational therapy in your own words.
2. Define, in your own words, occupational, activity, therapy, performance areas, performance components, and performance contexts.
3. Name five categories of conditions often treated in occupational therapy.
4. In front of each phrase listed below, write ADL for activity of daily living, W/P for work and productive activity, and P/L for play or leisure activity, as the terms are used in the occupational therapy profession.

   1) _ADL_ Dressing to attend a play
   2) _PL_ Taking a noncredit photography class
   3) _WP_ Studying high school English
   4) _WP_ Preparing a meal for the family
   5) _ADL_ Sending e-mail to one's son
   6) _ADL_ Brushing teeth after dinner
   7) _ADL_ Taking medication after lunch
   8) _PL_ Painting a picture for a gift
   9) _WP_ Bathing a 6-month-old son
   10) _WP_ Reading to a 2-year-old child

5. In front of each word or phrase below, identify the category of performance component by writing SM for sensorimotor, C for cognitive, and P for psychosocial component.

   1) _P_ Voting no when friends vote yes.
   2) _C_ Focusing on an instructor's lengthy lecture.
   3) _P_ Thanking a person who helps clear snow off your car.
   4) _P_ Removing your large hat while in a theater audience.
   5) _SM_ Carrying your own textbooks.
   6) _SM_ Closing a zipper in the back of a garment.
   7) _C_ Correctly repeating seven numbers after hearing them.
   8) _C_ Applying classroom information during fieldwork.
   9) _SM_ Chewing with your mouth closed during a family dinner.
   10) _SM_ Identifying the shoe for your right foot in a dark room.

6. Identify each word or phrase below by writing A for therapeutic activity, D for therapeutic device, and E for therapeutic exercise in front of the word.

1) _E_ Move the extended upper extremities forward and back 10 times.
2) _A_ Play checkers.
3) _D_ Transfer board.
4) _A_ Shape a ceramic bowl.
5) _E_ Flex and extend a patient's elbow joint five times (for the therapist).
6) _A_ Play hopscotch.
7) _D_ Adapted cutting board.
8) _E_ Extend and flex the fingers 10 times.
9) _E_ Ascend and descend 11 steps for 5 minutes.
10) _A_ Plan a picnic with a group.

ANSWERS

1. Refer to the text. Include in the definition the unique feature of occupational therapy, the process and goal of occupational therapy, the population served, and the means of achieving set goals.
2. Refer to the text. State your definitions to another person to test their clarity.
3. Physical injury or illness
   Cognitive impairment
   Developmental or learning disability
   Psychosocial dysfunction
   Mental illness
   Limitations due to adverse environmental conditions
4. 1) ADL 2) P/L 3) W 4) W 5) ADL 6) ADL 7) ADL 8) P/L 9) W 10) W
5. 1) P; social self-expression 2) C; attention span 3) P; social conduct 4) P; self-management, self-control 5) SM; strength 6) SM; range of motion plus gross- and fine-motor coordination 7) C; memory 8) C; generalization of learning 9) SM; oral-motor control 10) SM; perceptual stereognosis.
6. 1) E 2) A 3) D 4) A 5) E 6) A 7) D 8) E 9) E 10) A

ADDITIONAL LEARNING ACTIVITIES

1. Ask a high school student the meaning of occupational therapy. If the student does not know, give an interesting, correct explanation.
2. After meeting new members at a district occupational therapy meeting, ask an occupational therapist or assistant what kinds of occupations he or she uses during therapy sessions. Relate your information to classmates during an appropriate class discussion.
3. Ask an occupational therapist or assistant what occupational performance areas are most often the focus of his or her intervention.

REFERENCES

American Occupational Therapy Association, Inc. (1986). Representative Assembly: Summary of minutes. *American Journal of Occupational Therapy, 40*(12), 851-853.

American Occupational Therapy Association, Inc. (1991a). Essentials and guidelines for an accredited educational program for the occupational therapist. *American Journal of Occupational Therapy, 45*(12), 1077-1084.

American Occupational Therapy Association, Inc. (1991b). Essentials and guidelines for an accredited educational program for the occupational therapy assistant. *American Journal of Occupational Therapy, 45*(12), 1085-1092.

American Occupational Therapy Association, Inc. (1993). Position paper: Purposeful activity. *American Journal of Occupational Therapy, 47*(12), 1081-1082.

American Occupational Therapy Association, Inc. (1994a). Uniform terminology for occupational therapy—third edition. *American Journal of Occupational Therapy, 48*(11), 1047-1054.

American Occupational Therapy Association, Inc. (1994b). Representative Assembly, Policy 5.3.1. Definition of occupational therapy practice for state regulation. Revised/amended 7/94. *American Journal of Occupational Therapy, 48*(11), 1072-1073.

American Occupational Therapy Certification Board, Inc. (1994). *Certification examination for occupational therapist, registered and certified occupational therapy assistant: Program directors reference manual.* Gaithersburg, MD: Author.

Ayres, A. J. (1972). *Sensory integration and learning disorders.* Los Angeles: Western Psychological Service.

Brainerd, W. (1967). OT and me: Early days at the sanitarium, Clifton Springs, New York. *American Journal of Occupational Therapy, 21*(5), 278-280.

Drake, M. (1992). *Crafts in therapy and rehabilitation.* Thorofare, NJ: Slack, Inc.

Dutton, R. (1989). Guidelines for using both activity and exercise. *American Journal of Occupational Therapy, 43*(9), 573-580.

Gove, P. B. (Editor-in-chief). (1976). *Webster's third new international dictionary of the English language, unabridged.* Springfield, MA: G. & C. Merriam Company.

Pedretti, L. W., and Zoltan, B. (1990). *Occupational therapy: Practice skills for physical dysfunction.* St. Louis: C.V. Mosby Company.

Random House dictionary of the English language. (1981). New York: Random House.

United States Department of the Army. (1980). *Craft techniques in occupational therapy.* FM8-1. Washington: Superintendent of Documents, U.S. Government Printing Office.

SUGGESTED READINGS

Engelhardt, H. T., Jr. (1977). Defining occupational therapy: The meaning of therapy and the virtues of occupation. *American Journal of Occupational Therapy, 31*(10), 666-672.

Reilly, M. (1977). A response to: Defining occupational therapy: The meaning of therapy and the virtues of occupation. *American Journal of Occupational Therapy, 31*(10), 673.

SUGGESTED LISTENING/VIEWING

The following videocassettes were produced by the American Occupational Therapy Association, Inc., 4720 Montgomery Lane, Bethesda, MD 21264:

1. *Occupational therapy: A commitment to caring.* (1991). (7 min.).
2. *Occupational therapy: A great career.* (1987). (11 min.).
3. *Occupational therapy: The quiet cure.* (1990). (12 min.).
4. *Success stories.* (1992). (8 min.).
5. *The human resource—occupational therapy.* (1980). (17 min.)
6. *The richness of activities.* (1980). (17 min.)
7. *Ben Vereen: 1994 CAN-AM keynote address.* (1994). (30 min.)

2

PHILOSOPHY OF OCCUPATIONAL THERAPY

This chapter discusses the meaning of philosophy and the philosophical base of occupational therapy. Occupational therapy is based on the philosophy that individuals are motivated to participate actively in their own development and well-being. Individuals adapt to environmental influences in order to survive and gain satisfaction from life's activities. Engaging in purposeful activity aids the individual's adaptive process, development, functioning, and well-being. Potential occupational therapy practitioners should examine their attitudes and values to see whether their philosophy is compatible with that of the philosophical base of occupational therapy.

LEARNING OBJECTIVES

At the end of this chapter, you should be able to:

1. State the meaning of philosophy.
2. State three questions that are considered when developing a philosophy.
3. State the belief regarding human beings upon which the philosophy of occupational therapy is based.
4. State the belief regarding purposeful activity upon which the philosophy of occupational therapy is based.
5. Identify values that influenced your choice of an occupational therapy career.
6. Identify what you value about individuals.

Values, which are beliefs or ideals, provide the foundation for a profession. The American Occupational Therapy Association's values and attitudes are presented in a discussion of the concepts of altruism, equality, freedom, justice, dignity, truth, and prudence as they relate to the practice of occupational therapy (AOTA, 1993b). It is assumed that members of the profession are committed to these values and attitudes.

Occupational therapy practitioners are confronted each day with issues that require decisions based on personal and professional beliefs about the concepts mentioned in the above paragraph. Conflicts can arise when patients or other individuals involved in the delivery of occupational therapy services present beliefs that differ from those of the practitioner. For example, how much freedom of choice is to be given to the patient if the practitioner views that choice as destructive to the patient or others? Is the practitioner in fact limiting the patient's freedom of choice through any words or actions? Is the practitioner objective and truthful in relating information to the patient? Is the practitioner following the AOTA code of ethics (AOTA, 1994) and local, state, and federal laws as they relate to occupational therapy?

The philosophical base for the practice of occupational therapy was adopted by the Representative Assembly of the American Occupational Therapy Association in 1979. The practice of occupational therapy views individuals as being active and inherently motivated to interact with and manipulate their environment. Independently functioning individuals are seen as continuously adapting to their environmental influences. The interaction, manipulation, and adaptation they exhibit enable those individuals to survive in their environment and seek self-fulfillment. Factors that interfere with the adaptation process may cause dysfunction in the individual. Purposeful activities are believed to have value in preventing and correcting dysfunction (AOTA, 1979).

The basic tenet of occupational therapy is that individuals engage in purposeful activity as part of their daily life routine. An activity is purposeful when the individual actively and voluntarily participates in it and when it is directed at a goal the individual views as meaningful. Such activities, used by occupational therapy practitioners, have therapeutic value. Purposeful activities are seen as important to the biological, psychological, and sociological well-being of individuals (AOTA, 1993a).

THE DEVELOPMENT OF PHILOSOPHY

Philosophy can be thought of as the very general ideals, principles, or laws in which a person believes. Philosophy is the core—the underlying code—governing a thing and the sum of all values individuals use to guide their lives.

In developing a philosophy concerning a specific idea, you may question basic assumptions of that idea and attempt to organize systematically the logical answers to the questions raised.

There are three basic categories of questions to be answered in developing a philosophy. Assumptions within these categories must be consistent with each other in the overall philosophical framework in order for your philosophy to be rational and coherent.

THREE QUESTIONS

The three categories of questions needing answers in order to develop a philosophy are 1) ontological questions, which deal with what is real; 2) epistemological questions, which examine what is true; and 3) axiological questions, which treat goodness and beauty.

In attempting to answer these questions, one soon realizes that there are no universal answers, but only a limitless range of possibilities.

As you develop your philosophy of occupational therapy, you will first consider the nature of the individual. You might ask such questions as What is the reality of human beings? How does an individual relate to the world? What does one consider real? Does the world, and thus the individual, exist? Or does the individual, and thus the world, exist? Is an individual governed by a supreme, orderly law of the universe? Or is the individual a free agent? What is the nature of human beings? Is the individual basically a biological being? Or is the individual ultimately formed through the mediation of his or her own thought processes? And if thoughts are the essence of the individual, what happens to those thoughts that are only thought and cannot be expressed verbally or in writing?

The second area of consideration regards knowledge. How do people come to know things? Is it because individuals are the source of knowledge? Then what are the limits of the mind? Or are people only seekers of knowledge, which exists outside their minds? If individuals are seekers of knowledge, what is the origin of knowledge? Is it possible for us to know all that is to be known? Again, what are the limits of the mind? Can it come to know the range of possibilities of knowledge?

Finally, what is good? What has value? Is beauty to be valued for beauty's sake, or because of its practical usefulness? Are beauty and goodness subjectively determined, or can they be determined objectively?

Many more questions can be raised in each of these areas. And answers usually lead to more questions. But posing the questions will help you clarify your own philosophical beliefs.

It will be helpful to consider what the words *altruism, equality, freedom, justice, dignity, truth,* and *prudence* mean and how they are viewed, especially by the person who will receive occupational therapy. Conflicts of varying magnitude related to attitudes and values arise almost daily for the occupational therapy practitioner. Resolving these conflicts can be made easier by examining one's attitudes and values, setting priorities, and making decisions based on those fundamental attitudes and values.

THE STUDENT'S PHILOSOPHY

As a student, you are encouraged to assess your own value system. Why? Because you must be aware of your basic assumptions before any rational order can be made in a larger framework such as occupational therapy. Consider issues such as the value of components basic to occupational therapy. Are self-care, work, and leisure skills of value? Is one set of skills more valuable than another? Does it matter whether a person cares for him- or herself or becomes dependent on a willing caretaker? Is work necessary for the psychological and physiological well-being of the individual or only as a means of obtaining goods and services?

Are leisure activities necessary for the psychological and physiological well-being of the individual? When does leisure activity become work? Does work ever become leisure? For a person who enjoys working, leisure may be a short walk and a snack. For a person who values leisure, work may serve merely as a way to accumulate money for the next leisure activity. How do you assess your work time and play time? Do you work to play, or do you play to work? When we clarify the value we place on leisure activities, it aids us in helping patients incorporate leisure and play activities into their lives. Those of us who value work more than play may need to make a greater effort to remember the leisure portion of occupational therapy.

What do you value about an individual? Is a person with superior intellectual ability valued more than a person with mental retardation? Are you repelled by a person who does not have the physical characteristics familiar to you? Do you value persons of your own age range more than others? Should a young adult receive more health care than an elderly person? Is it more valuable to provide treatment to a dysfunctional child than to a dysfunctional 90-year-old adult? Is it acceptable to you that a prominent person or a person with more wealth will receive services from the most expert individual, while persons without funds receive services from the least qualified individual? Is it more valuable to provide treatment to a verbal, intellectual person with a spinal cord injury than to a person who is nonverbal, nonambulatory, and profoundly mentally retarded? Ethically, we are bound to provide services equally to all who seek occupational therapy, to respect their rights to privacy and confidentiality, and to maintain competency to assure that patients are receiving services from qualified practitioners.

The questions raised above cannot be answered here, and your answers may change over your lifetime, but will be influenced by core values that you hold. As you learn more about occupational therapy, it will be useful to return to these questions. Your understanding of your belief system is essential to carry out occupational therapy effectively.

SUMMARY

Occupational therapy is based on the philosophy that individuals are motivated to be active participants in their own development and well-being. Individuals adapt to environmental influences in order to survive and gain satisfaction from life's activities. Engaging in purposeful activity aids the individual's adaptive process, development, functioning, and well-being. Periodically reviewing our attitudes and values to see whether our philosophy is compatible with the philosophical base of occupational therapy helps us to be effective occupational therapy practitioners.

REVIEW QUESTIONS

1. Philosophy can be thought of as the_____, principles, or laws governing a person. A philosophy has a set of principles or beliefs organized in a_____ and _____ manner.
2. In philosophy, ontological questions consider what is _____, epistemological questions deal with what is_____, and axiological questions examine_____ and _____.
3. The practice of occupational therapy is based on the belief that individuals are _____ beings whose _____ _____ is influenced by the use of_____ _____.
4. Name two activities you consider purposeful. Name two activities that were purposeful 2 years ago, but that are no longer purposeful to you.
5. Occupational therapy students often say, "I want to help people." Interpret this statement, and discuss how the help given by lawyers, teachers, physical therapists, and psychologists differs from or is the same as the help given by occupational therapy practitioners.
6. Have you ever heard or made the statement, "I don't want to work with old people" (or any other groups of individuals with limitations)? Discuss this statement in relation to *dignity*, one of the core concepts of the profession, which emphasizes the importance of valuing the inherent worth and uniqueness of each individual.

ANSWERS

1. ideals   systematic   logical
2. real   true   goodness   beauty
3. active   ability to function   purposeful activity
4., 5., and 6. Write out your individualized answers. Discuss your answers with classmates, family members, or other appropriate persons.

REFERENCES

American Occupational Therapy Association, Inc. (1979). Resolution C, 531-79: The philosophical base of occupational therapy. *American Journal of Occupational Therapy, 33*(11), 785.

American Occupational Therapy Association, Inc. (1993a). Position paper: Purposeful activity. *American Journal of Occupational Therapy, 47*(12), 1081-1082.

American Occupational Therapy Association, Inc. (1993b). Core values and attitudes of occupational therapy practice. *American Journal of Occupational Therapy, 47*(12), 1085-1086.

American Occupational Therapy Association, Inc. (1994). Occupational therapy code of ethics. *American Journal of Occupational Therapy, 48*(11), 1037-1038.

SUGGESTED READINGS

Englehardt, H. T., Jr. (1977). Defining occupational therapy: The meaning of therapy and the virtues of occupation. *American Journal of Occupational Therapy, 31*(10), 666-672.

Meyer, A. (1922). The philosophy of occupational therapy. *Archives of Occupational Therapy, 1*, 1-10.

Wells, C. (1976). Ethics in conflict: Yesterday's standards—outdated guide for tomorrow? *American Journal of Occupational Therapy, 30*(1), 44-47.

Yerxa, E. (1979). The philosophical base of occupational therapy. In *Occupational therapy: 2001 ad. Papers presented at the special session of the Representative Assembly, November 1978* (pp. 26-30). Bethesda, MD, American Occupational Therapy Association.

3

History of Occupational Therapy

The origin of occupational therapy is presented. Changes made over the years in practice and education are summarized.

LEARNING OBJECTIVES

At the end of this chapter, you should be able to:

1. State the period in history when the occupational therapy profession began.
2. Name at least two people who worked to establish the profession.
3. Name five kinds of occupations used in the early years of the profession.
4. Describe physicians' attitudes about occupational therapy during the early years of the profession.
5. Discuss the effect of national and world events upon the profession.
6. State the year the profession's organization was named the American Occupational Therapy Association, Inc.
7. Summarize the changes that have taken place in occupational therapy education.
8. Name at least three practice models of occupational therapy, and for each, state for what dysfunction it was originally used.
9. Name at least three occupational therapists who have formulated and published a theory about the practice of occupational therapy.

The occupational therapy profession was founded with the basic belief that human beings have a capacity to change. Individuals are valued, regardless of their level of functional ability. The profession values the unique qualities of individuals and aims to provide occupational therapy services for all those in need of such services. People are viewed as intrinsically motivated to interact actively with their environment and adapt in such manner as to influence their development. Patients are believed to have the potential to participate actively in affecting their state of wellness. All individuals are viewed as having responsibilities toward other individuals.

VALUE OF OCCUPATIONS EXPLORED

Adolph Meyer (1977/1922), a psychiatrist, stated that the first medical paper he ever presented, in 1892 or 1893, was about occupations. He felt that the proper use of an individual's time in a gratifying activity was a fundamental issue in the treatment of neuropsychiatric patients. He referred to an 1822 report signed by Dr. Henry M. Hurd of a visit by a committee from Michigan institutions to European institutions for the insane in which a physician described successful results in hiring the insane as employees. Apparently, some European institutions were engaging patients in occupations instead of using restraints on them.

In U.S. institutions, patients were commonly given work assignments during the 1900s to relieve the workload of employees. The observed therapeutic effect of work led these institutions to engage patients in other activities that were both pleasant and profitable to them. Patients who were uncontrollably excited or who were mischievous troublemakers were able to remain calm and productive while engaged in activities such as "picking the hairs of mattresses," weaving, bookbinding, and creating objects with raffia, reeds, metal, and leather (Meyer, 1977/1922).

The ability to manage patients with mental illness by having them expend energy through work or creative and recreational activities was remarked by workers in psychiatric hospitals in the 1900s. Drug therapy, common in current treatment, was seldom used before the 1950s.

Two major events were taking place during the time Meyer and other psychiatrists were observing the therapeutic effects of systematically planned activities. One was the rebirth of moral treatment. Moral treatment in mental hospitals, which began in the early 19th century, was based on the philosophy of "the law of love." There was a new respect for the human individual and the rights of individuals. Attitudes about the treatment of mental illness changed. It was believed that individuals with mental disorders were more likely to recover in the company of persons who were kind and mentally healthy.

The second major event was World War I. Many soldiers remained hospitalized after the war because of mental and physical disabilities that resulted from it (Brokoven, 1971).

The philosophy of moral treatment advocated by prominent psychiatrists and the need for rehabilitation programs to aid those who were physically injured during World War I were major influences in the development of occupational therapy as an independent profession. The early concept of occupational therapy was related to its value in vocational training. It was thought that crafts and other planned activities could reactivate the mind and motivate the mentally ill and physically disabled to take an interest in some area of vocational training (Woodside, 1971).

The people who taught and supervised patients in these manual, creative, and work activities were doctors, nurses, craftspersons, and volunteers. The changed behaviors in the patients convinced the people supervising them that the activities gave the patients a feeling of productivity and self-worth. The work activities and group interactions resulted in improved social relations and increased the patients' sense of responsibility for themselves and others (Woodside, 1971).

During World War I, Dr. Frankwood Williams, associate director of the National Committee for Mental Hygiene, requested that occupational workers go to Base Hospital 117 in La Fauche, France. The military authorities denied his request. The explanations he gave for using occupations for therapy were misunderstood to mean that they would be used for vocational training. The authorities reasoned that no one could make a living doing craft work after the war; therefore, sending workers to the base hospital to teach the wounded soldiers such work was futile (Myers, 1948).

The prospects of including the therapeutic occupational program at Base Hospital 117 were dim. As the unit prepared to sail for France, it was learned that civilian aides were needed to work as scrubwomen. Mrs. C. M. Myers began recruiting women who were willing to be classified as aides, without military rank or privileges, to provide the treatment that Dr. Williams felt was essential for military patients (Myers, 1948).

In March 1918, a group of women composed of nurses, a physiotherapist, a dietician, and civilian aides was given three lectures on neuropsychiatry and sent abroad. Eventually, the members of the group were given the title "reconstruction aide" (Myers, 1948; Woodside, 1971).

At the base hospital, the women who were prepared to teach occupations to the patients set up a workshop in part of a barracks. They cleaned, built worktables, and salvaged surplus and discarded items for supplies. Patients voluntarily joined them and helped to make the workshop functional for building furniture. Gradually, the patients were taught to make candlesticks, jewelry, rugs, and other useful and ornamental items. The patients' involvement and physical and mental improvement caused hospital staff to show interest in the work being done by the foreign civilian aides.

Results of the work by the civilian aides prompted Colonel Salmon, Chief of the U.S. Army Psychiatric Division in France, to ask for 1 thousand civilian aides to be sent to that country. He stated that the women were worth their weight in gold (Myers, 1948).

THE NATIONAL SOCIETY

George Barton, an architect with tuberculosis, read Dr. William Rush Dunton's *Occupational Therapy, a Manual for Nurses*, published in 1915. Convinced of the therapeutic value of occupations for patients, Barton contacted Dr. Dunton about establishing a national society for occupational therapy (Licht, 1967).

On March 15, 1917, the National Society for the Promotion of Occupational Therapy held its first meeting in Clifton Spring, New York. The founders were Barton, Dunton, Susan C. Johnson, Thomas B. Kidner, Isabel G. Newton, and Eleanor Clarke Slagle. The intent was to incorporate the Society in New York; however, the secretary of the state of New York could not decide whether the application should be considered under the heading of industry or education, so the Society was finally incorporated in Washington, DC (Licht, 1967).

The first annual meeting of the Society was held at the Russell Sage Foundation Building in New York City on Labor Day, 1917. Twenty-six persons in attendance heard reports and papers presented by committee chairpersons and participants. The treasurer's report indicated that the Society had a balance of 51 cents. Slagle asked that the day's meeting conclude with dinner. Because many people had already made plans for the holiday evening, only eight people attended the profession's first annual banquet (Licht, 1967).

Physicians served as president of the new organization for most of its first 30 years, because the early members felt that the organization needed the support of the medical profession. Barton was the first president. Then Slagle served as president from 1919 to 1920. Practitioners from the mental health field, the military, and people doing similar work joined the new organization. By 1921, 4 years after its first meeting, the Society had 450 members. In 1923, the name of the organization was changed to the American Occupational Therapy Association, Inc. (AOTA) (Licht, 1967).

Federal legislation influenced the growth and development of the AOTA. The Public Health Service, established in 1912, considered the protection of health and provision of health care a human right. The 1920 Smith-Bankhead Bill emphasized vocational rehabilitation (Woodside, 1971). These early actions were followed by many health-related laws that increased the need for occupational therapy services.

The need for occupational therapy services increased as new knowledge and technology provided means for keeping alive those who became seriously ill or injured during wars, work, and daily life activities, as well as many who previously would not have survived during the birth process. Members of the AOTA pondered ways to solve the shortage of occupational therapists.

In 1958, plans were completed for a training program for occupational therapy assistants. It was thought that assistants would help alleviate the shortage of occupational therapists. In 1959, a year after the program for occupational therapy assistants began, the AOTA established a procedure for recognizing and certifying assistants (AOTA, 1959).

EDUCATION

Before the formal establishment of a professional organization, occupational therapy programs were supervised by physicians and carried out by craftspersons, volunteers, or aides. In 1911, Susan E. Tracy, a nurse, began a course called "invalid occupations" for student nurses at Massachusetts General Hospital. Nurses gradually replaced craftspersons in teaching activities to patients. In 1913, Milwaukee-Downer College began a similar course. Dr. Dunton started the first instruction for nurses at Sheppard and Enoch Pratt Hospital in Baltimore, Maryland. He titled his course "occupational therapy" (Woodside, 1971). Slagle is credited with creating the first official school for occupational therapy, the Henry P. Favill School of Occupation in Chicago, Illinois, in 1915 (Christensen, 1991).

In 1918, Milwaukee-Downer College began the first occupational therapy school within an academic institution. Other schools that began occupational therapy education the same year were the Philadelphia School of Occupational Therapy, the St. Louis School for Reconstruction Aides, and the Boston School of Occupational Therapy. The first teachers were craftspersons, and the curriculum stressed handiwork for rehabilitation and recreation. The early educational programs were 4 months long and included 30 hours of lecture and at least 1 half day a week of hospital practice (Woodside, 1971).

As the need for occupational therapy services expanded, so did the need for improved and expanded occupational therapy education. In 1922, a chairman for the education committee of the national society was appointed. In 1923, minimum standards for educational courses were published, as the "Essentials for Professional Education." Passage of an examination administered by the AOTA was required for registration as an occupational therapist. In 1929, a method of national registration began. The educational standards and the examination helped to define the qualifications and knowledge of occupational therapists (Woodside, 1971).

The "Essentials and Guidelines for an Accredited Educational Program for the Occupational Therapist" ("Essentials"), by the American Occupational Therapy Association and the Council on Medical Education of the American Medical Association (AOTA & AMA, 1991), was initially adopted by these two organizations in 1935. Educational programs continued to be accredited by the Committee on Allied Health Education and Accreditation (CAHEA) of the AMA upon recommendation by the Accreditation Committee of the AOTA until 1994. The "Essentials" are revised periodically as the requirements of the profession change the educational needs of future practitioners. The revised "Essentials" are usually published in the archival issue of the *American Journal of Occupational Therapy* the year the revisions are approved.

In 1994, the new Accreditation Council for Occupational Therapy Education (ACOTE) of the AOTA replaced the AMA/CAHEA and began the accreditation process for all occupational therapy educational programs. Currently, there are more than 200 programs in the process (Graves, 1994; AOTA Accreditation Department, 1995).

CERTIFICATION

In 1931, the AOTA began to register qualified occupational therapists as a means of protecting the public from unqualified practitioners. The first national registry listed 318 occupational therapists (AOTA, 1980). In 1938, an earlier ruling to register only graduates of AMA-approved schools of occupational therapy was changed to admit successful test takers who were otherwise not eligible for the registry. The first test for occupational therapists was given in 1939 (Baum & Gray, 1988).

In 1986, in order to protect the public interest and avoid a potential conflict of interest, the AOTA established an independent board to set policies and procedures regarding qualification for certification. In November 1988, the American Occupational Therapy Certification Board, Inc. (AOTCB), was legally incorporated as a national agency that certified qualified persons as "Occupational Therapist, Registered" (OTR) and "Certified Occupational Therapy Assistant" (COTA). The AOTCB is independent of the AOTA. The AOTCB develops and implements all policies related to the certification of occupational therapy personnel. Certification by the AOTCB means that the OTR or COTA has graduated from an accredited occupational therapy program, has completed all field work requirements, and has successfully completed the AOTCB examination. Certification by the AOTCB is permanent, but can be revoked or suspended as a disciplinary action (Baum & Gray, 1988).

MODELS FOR TREATMENT

By the 1930s, treatment with a humanistic and holistic view of the individual and health, which influenced the development of the profession in the early 1900s, no longer satisfied the growing need for scientific accountability. In the 1940s and 1950s, the profession was under pressure from the medical profession to develop a scientific base for treatment. By the end of the 1950s, occupational therapy developed its theoretical framework for treatment based on psychoanalysis, kinesiology, and neurology (Johnson, 1981; Kielhofner & Burke, 1977).

The *psychoanalytic* model of occupational therapy, for psychiatric patients, perceived those patients as having intrapsychic conflicts that were not consciously understood. The premise was that occupational therapy techniques using crafts would alleviate tension-producing conflicts and provide gratifying, successful experiences. The crafts were analyzed for their ability to provide the patient with the opportunity to express or sublimate his or her feelings. The therapeutic therapist-patient relationship was essential to the treatment. The goals of treatment were psychosexual maturation, effective communication, and the expression and reduction of psychiatric symptoms (Kielhofner & Burke, 1977; Miller & Walker, 1993).

The *kinesiological model* of occupational therapy for the physically disabled patient sought to make the patient as independent as possible despite the pathology. The occupational therapy techniques used were exercises, constructive activities, adaptive equipment, bracing of affected body parts, retraining in activities of daily living, and prevocational training. The goals of treatment were to regain or increase motion, strength, endurance, and coordination in order to enable the patient to perform necessary daily living activities. If the person's physical limitations could not be changed, the patient was taught to adjust cognitively to his or her changed body (Huss, 1981; Kielhofner & Burke, 1977). The term *biomechanical model* is often used instead of the term *kinesiological model.*

The *neurological model* of occupational therapy, for the treatment of children with perceptual motor dysfunction, sought to reduce the dysfunction and provide opportunities for adaptive responses by controlling sensory input and eliciting more appropriate motor output. Therapists using these techniques worked with the premise that sensory integration was essential for a child to make appropriate adaptive responses to environmental stimuli (Kielhofner & Burke, 1977).

Fundamental to all of these models of practice is the active involvement of the patient in normal, purposeful, goal-directed activities during occupational therapy. The use of activities, whether with crafts, exercise, games, music, recreation, or other familiar or unfamiliar modalities, cannot be considered occupational therapy unless the activities meet the unique criteria of purposefulness with respect to both the patient and the treatment (Huss, 1981).

In the 1960s and 1970s, occupational therapists expressed their concern over the narrow view many had of the profession based on the medical model. The expanding need to provide services for the chronically disabled could not be met by the occupational therapy models of the previous decades. Occupational therapists pointed out the need to describe what the discipline was and what it should be. The profession lacked a philosophical base (Kielhofner & Burke, 1977), as well as a theoretical base for practice, yet the treatment arena continued to expand in several directions without apparent boundaries (Huss, 1981; Johnson, 1981; Kielhofner & Burke, 1977).

Since the late 1970s, the Association has increased its effort to define and clarify the profession's role, its beliefs, and the changing services delivered to its consumers, the general public, and members of the profession. Occupational therapy will continue to change and define its areas of practice as societal changes and new knowledge demand revisions in the profession's position on numerous issues. Statements, position papers, and official documents are published in Association publications as they are approved or rescinded, and it behooves the student to keep abreast of changes within the profession.

Since the 1970s, greater numbers of occupational therapists have articulated their theories, researched the efficacy of various interventions, and published the results of such interventions as the profession came under greater scrutiny. Consumers, federal laws, and funding identified occupational therapy as a needed service, increasing the exigency to document and provide accountability for the services offered. Research, graduate education programs, and professional publications increased as the public need for occupational therapy validated the profession as a valued service.

THE THEORETICAL BASE OF OCCUPATIONAL THERAPY

Every occupational therapy practitioner contributes to the information upon which the discipline is based. Increasing numbers of practitioners, researchers, educators, and students contribute to the literature on occupational therapy. This section briefly highlights five individuals whose writings the reader is most likely to encounter upon being introduced to the profession. The reader is encouraged to study each researcher's current publications and professional presentations.

Claudia Allen focused on evaluating the cognitive level of individuals in order to plan interventions intended to alleviate their psychosocial dysfunction. She described the performance she expected at six cognitive levels. She used specific craft activities to evaluate the patient's performance. A test she devised for the six levels of expected performance was named the Allen Cognitive Levels (ACL) test. She continues to add to her research findings that corroborated the reliability and validity of the test. Since developing a more comprehensive evaluation called the Routine Task Inventory (RTI), she now refers to the ACL as a screening test. Allen emphasizes that the goal of treatment is to enable the patient to engage safely in everyday activities. She has used crafts in the ACL test and in the intervention process, with the belief that patients' performance in specific activities can identify their cognitive deficits, as well as help them learn to function safely and more appropriately in the community. She feels that the ACL and RTI evaluations and the Allen treatment methods apply to the individual with physical disabilities, in addition to the individual with mental illness or psychosocial dysfunction, and continues to research her theory (Allen, Earhart & Blue, 1992; Miller & Walker, 1993).

A. Jean Ayres hypothesized a neurological dysfunction that interfered with the ability of the child to integrate sensory input and use the information obtained thereby for appropriate motor, cognitive, and psychosocial behavior. The lack of sensory integration was believed to result in hypersensitivity to sensory stimuli, inattention, hyperactivity, learning disabilities, deficits in visual perceptual and fine- and gross-motor performance, and other problems that interfered with the normal development of children. Ayres spent most of her professional career researching her theories. She developed the Southern California Sensory Integration Tests in the early 1970s and continued to study their reliability and validity (Ayres, 1980). When her research showed a need to revise her early battery of tests, she developed the *Sensory Integration and Praxis Tests* (Ayres, 1989). Her tests require users to be certified. The interventions she applies to correct various dysfunctions include a variety of equipment and activities fashioned specifically to her concepts of how to help the child integrate sensory input and make an appropriate motor response. A torso-sized scooter board, a net swing, a platform and bolster swing, and equipment covered with textured materials are examples of the equipment she used in therapy for children with sensory integrative dysfunctions (Ayres, 1972, 1979; Fisher, Murray, & Bundy, 1991; Miller & Walker, 1993).

Gary Kielhofner developed the Model of Human Occupation as a basis for what he hopes will be the theoretical foundation for the occupational therapy profession. Kielhofner and his colleagues continue to research occupational therapy evaluations and interventions from the perspective of this basic concept. The model is based on a general systems theory, and a general understanding of the theory is needed to understand the model. The model of human occupation identifies three subsystems—volition, habituation, and performance—that influence human beings. The subsystems are conceptualized in a hierarchy in which the higher systems organize the lower ones. The systems are open and self-maintaining in their interaction with the environment, which involves input to the system from the environment, processing of the input (referred to as throughput), and the resultant action on the environment (referred to as output). The action on the environment provides feedback to the system and influences future input, throughput, and output. The entire process is believed not only to result in the development of habits in human beings, but also to permit increasingly complex behaviors. Kielhofner and his colleagues continue to apply and study various test instruments to determine their usefulness with the model of human occupation. The instruments include, but are not limited to, the Role Checklist, the Assessment of Occupational Functioning, the Preschool Play Scale, and the Occupational Performance History Interview (Kielhofner, 1995; Miller & Walker, 1993).

Prior to holding the position of director of an occupational therapy educational program, Lela A. Llorens was an occupational therapist in a facility serving children with psychosocial dysfunction. She based her occupational therapy evaluation and treatment of children with psychosocial dysfunction on concepts of normal development. She believes that mastery of skills is an expectation of normal growth and development, and also is needed for satisfactory coping behavior and adaptive relationships. Disease, injury, and environmental factors can interfere with the normal developmental process and thus make the child vulnerable to maladaptive behaviors. Llorens developed a schematic outline of the occupational therapy process based on developmental theory. In her Developmental Analysis Evaluation and Intervention Schedule (DAEIS), she also provided practitioners with an applicable framework for using developmental theory for evaluation and intervention with patients of all ages (Llorens, 1976; Miller & Walker, 1993).

Anne Cronin Mosey has focused on identifying a foundation for occupational therapy that unifies the various areas of the profession from which areas of specialization can emerge. In this effort, she has described what constitutes a profession and what are the characteristics of a model of a profession. She has also contributed to practice, offering occupational therapy evaluation and treatment for individuals with psychosocial dysfunction. Her evaluation and treatment concepts are developmentally based. Mosey believes that changing psychological and physical needs and environmental demands can create a state of disequilibrium. Individuals are able to function adequately in their environment when they are in a state of equilibrium and can adapt to the various changing needs and demands. She formulated an outline of seven adaptive skills, each with subskills that she said were sequentially acquired during normal development. Dysfunction results when necessary skill components are not acquired. The patient is evaluated by observing him or her in roles and activities that will identify whether particular skill components are present or absent. The seven adaptive skills are perceptual-motor, cognitive, drive object, dyadic interaction, primary group interaction, self-identity, and sexual identity interaction skills. The goal of treatment is to move the patient from a dysfunctional state to a state that will enable the patient to function in his or her community. The intervention process engages the patient in therapeutic activities and group interactions that will develop the absent adaptive skill(s) (Miller & Walker, 1993; Mosey, 1970, 1973).

Schultz and Schkade (1992) presented a practice Model of Occupational Adaptation. They believe that the patient's internal processing is of prime importance during therapeutic intervention and that the effectiveness of the intervention is seen by the change in the patient's internally driven occupational adaptation. In the process of achieving relative mastery of a given occupation, the internal effect is believed to be the key to helping the patient adapt to his or her condition and to the environmental demands placed on the patient. In the Model of Occupational Adaptation, environment is as important as the patient's mental and physical condition. For a particular patient, the occupational environment is the combination of physical, social, and cultural influences on that patient. Schultz and Schkade believe that the Occupational Adaptation Model reflects the uniqueness of occupational therapy by its holistic view. The model emphasizes the creation of a therapeutic climate, the use of occupational activities, and the importance of relative mastery of the activity. The model needs to be tested, but the authors believe that it is applicable to many settings and is an appropriate practice model for a variety of conditions (Schultz & Schkade, 1992).

SUMMARY

Occupational therapy as a profession began during World War I (1914-1918). Craftspersons, volunteers, nurses, and aides were first trained by physicians to provide occupational therapy. College-level courses in occupational therapy were first offered in 1918. The profession's official association was renamed in 1923. The profession developed the technically trained assistant in an effort to meet the rising demand for occupational therapy services. Occupational therapy practitioners increased their efforts to validate the profession through more precise documentation, publications, the articulation of theories, and research.

REVIEW QUESTIONS

1. The occupational therapy profession began around 19____ - 19____.
2. Physicians, nurses, and craftspersons were members of the original occupational therapy organization. Which two of the following members served as president?
   a. George Barton and Eleanor Clarke Slagle.
   b. Sigmund Freud and C. M. Myers.
   c. Dr. Frankwood Williams and Isabel Newton.
   d. Dr. Frankwood Williams and Dr. John Adams.
   e. Dr. George White and Marjorie Taylor.
3. Name at least three types of activities used during the early years of the profession.

4. Discuss the changing attitude toward occupational therapy of physicians who treated individuals with mental illness during World War I and the early 1900s.
5. Name at least three national events that influenced the growth of occupational therapy.
6. When did the National Society for the Promotion of Occupational Therapy become the American Occupational Therapy Association, Inc.?
7. Briefly describe the educational requirements at the beginning of the profession and compare them with current educational requirements.
8. Identify early models for treatment used by occupational therapists, and describe the emphasis of each.
9. Name at least three occupational therapists who developed a treatment model or theory for the profession, and state how each evaluates dysfunction in the patient.

ANSWERS

1. 1914-1918.
2. a.
3. Work, vocational training, recreation, manual activities, gardening, crafts.
4. Physicians in the military service initially thought that the purpose of occupational therapy was to train soldiers who were mentally ill to be employed doing craft work and did not believe that the therapy was worthwhile. After seeing the behavioral changes in the patients, the doctors began to accept the use of activities as a therapeutic modality. Physicians who accepted the moral treatment concept also accepted the use of occupations as therapy.
5. World War I, World War II, other wars, the 1920 Smith-Bankhead Bill, the industrial era.
6. The National Society for the Promotion of Occupational Therapy became the American Occupational Therapy Association, Inc, in 1923.
7. The first educational programs for occupational therapists were 4 months long and included 30 hours of lecture and at least one half-day a week of hospital practice. Current educational programs for occupational therapists require liberal arts and professional courses, fieldwork experiences, and graduation with a baccalaureate or higher degree from an accredited program of occupational therapy.
8. The models were titled the psychoanalytic model, the kinesiological or biomechanical model, and the neurological model.
   1) The psychoanalytic model was used for patients with psychiatric diagnoses. Occupational therapy provided opportunities for the patients to express or sublimate their feelings and develop acceptable behaviors through engaging in crafts and other normal activities.

2) The kinesiological or biomechanical model was used for patients with physical disabilities. Occupational therapy provided opportunities for these patients to become as independent as possible through the use of exercise and mechanical and adaptive devices.

3) The neurological model was used for patients with perceptual motor and neurological dysfunction. Occupational therapy provided these patients with opportunities to experience appropriate responses by controlling their sensory input and facilitating normal responses.

9. 1) Claudia Allen. Cognitive disabilities model. Cognitive disability is evaluated by the Allen Cognitive Level screening test and the comprehensive Routine Task Inventory.

2) A. Jean Ayres. Sensory integration. Sensory integrative dysfunction is evaluated by the Sensory Integration and Praxis Test.

3) Gary Kielhofner. Model of Human Occupation. Numerous tests, such as the Role Checklist, the Assessment of Occupational Functioning, the Preschool Play Scale, and the Occupational Questionnaire, are being researched for use with the Model of Human Occupation.

4) Lela A. Llorens. Developmental model. The Developmental Analysis Evaluation and Intervention Schedule is used to evaluate areas of disruption in development and to plan intervention to treat dysfunction.

5) Anne Cronin Mosey. Developmental model. Evaluation of the levels of seven adaptive skills, with subskills, includes tests for perceptual-motor, cognitive, drive object, dyadic interaction, primary group interaction, self-identity, and sexual identity interaction skills.

ADDITIONAL LEARNING ACTIVITIES

1. Scan some occupational therapy journals published 20 or more years ago. What differences do you notice in the content of the articles and advertisements in those journals, compared with that of current issues of the *American Journal of Occupational Therapy*?

2. See the occupational therapy exhibit at the Smithsonian museums when you next visit Washington, DC.

3. Review library material on the history of occupational therapy.

REFERENCES

Allen, C. K., Earhart, C. A., & Blue, T. (1992). *Occupational therapy treatment goals for the physically and cognitively disabled.* Bethesda, MD: American Occupational Therapy Association.

American Occupational Therapy Association. (1959). Annual reports. *American Journal of Occupational Therapy, 13*(1), 27-50.

American Occupational Therapy Association. (1980). *Member handbook.* Bethesda, MD: Author.

American Occupational Therapy Association, Inc., Accrediatation Department. (1995). ACOTE takes accreditation action. *OT Week, 9*(33), 11.

American Occupational Therapy Association and American Medical Association. (1991). Essentials and guidelines for an accredited educational program for the occupational therapist. *American Journal of Occupational Therapy, 45*(12), 1077-1084.

Ayres, A. J. (1972). *Sensory integration and learning disorders.* Los Angeles: Western Psychological Services.

Ayres, A. J. (1979). *Sensory integration and the child.* Los Angeles: Western Psychological Services.

Ayres, A. J. (1980). *Southern California Sensory Integration Tests—revised 1980.* Los Angeles: Western Psychological Services.

Ayres, A. J. (1988). *Sensory Integration and Praxis Tests.* Los Angeles, CA: Western Psychological Services.

Baum, C. M., & Gray, M. S. (1988). Certification: Serving the public interest. *American Journal of Occupational Therapy, 42*(2), 77-79.

Brokoven, J. S. (1971). Legacy of moral treatment, 1800s to 1919. *American Journal of Occupational Therapy, 25*(5), 223-225.

Christensen, E. (1991). *A proud heritage: The American Occupational Therapy Association at seventy-five.* Bethesda, MD: American Occupational Therapy Association, Inc.

Fisher, A. G., Murray, E. A., & Bundy, A. C. (1991). *Sensory integration: Theory and practice.* Philadelphia: F. A. Davis Company.

Graves, S. (1994). ACOTE's first accreditation actions. *OT Week, 8*(28), 9.

Huss, A. J. (1981). From kinesiology to adaptation. *American Journal of Occupational Therapy, 35*(9), 574-580.

Johnson, J. (1981). Old values—new directions: Competence, adaptation, integration. *American Journal of Occupational Therapy, 35*(9), 589-598.

Kielhofner, G. (Ed.). (1995). *A model of human occupation: Theory and application.* Baltimore: Williams & Wilkins.

Kielhofner, G., & Burke, J. P. (1977). Occupational therapy after 60 years: An account of changing identity and knowledge. *American Journal of Occupational Therapy, 31*(10), 675-689.

Licht, S. (1967). The founding and founders of the American Occupational Therapy Association. *American Journal of Occupational Therapy, 21*(5), 269-277.

Llorens, L. A. (1976). *Application of a developmental theory for health and rehabilitation.* Bethesda, MD: American Occupational Therapy Association, Inc.

Meyer, A. (1922). The philosophy of occupational therapy. *Archives of*

Occupational Therapy, 1, 1-10. (Reprinted in *American Journal of Occupational Therapy,* 1977, *31*(10), 639-642)

Miller, R. J., & Walker, K. F. (1993). *Perspectives on theory for the practice of occupational therapy.* Gaithersburg, MD: Aspen Publishers, Inc.

Mosey, A. C. (1970). *Three frames of reference for mental health.* Thorofare, NJ: Charles B. Slack.

Mosey, A. C. (1973). *Activities therapy.* New York: Raven Press.

Myers, C. M. (1948). Pioneer occupational therapists in World War I. *American Journal of Occupational Therapy, 2,* 208-215.

Schultz, S., & Schkade, J. K. (1992). Occupational adaptation: Toward a holistic approach for contemporary practice, part 2. *American Journal of Occupational Therapy, 46*(10), 917-925.

Woodside, H. H. (1971). The development of occupational therapy, 1910-1929. *American Journal of Occupational Therapy, 25*(5), 226-230.

SUGGESTED READINGS

Bing, R. K. (1992). Point of departure (a play about founding the profession). *American Journal of Occupational Therapy, 46*(1), 27-32.

Reitz, S. M. (1992). A historical review of occupational therapy's role in preventive health and wellness. *American Journal of Occupational Therapy, 46*(1), 50-55.

West, W. L. (1992). Ten milestone issues in AOTA history. *American Journal of Occupational Therapy, 46*(12), 1066-1074.

Yerxa, E. J. (1992). Some implications of occupational therapy's history for its epistemology, values, and relation to medicine. *American Journal of Occupational Therapy, 46*(1), 79-83.

SUGGESTED LISTENING/VIEWING

1. AOTA. (1979). *Visual History Series: The early years* (videocassette). (41 min.) The AOTA Distribution Center, 4720 Montgomery Lane, Bethesda MD, 21264.

History of the Certified Occupational Therapy Assistant

The development of the certified occupational therapy assistant (COTA) is presented. Changes in education, certification, employment, and role of the COTA are discussed.

LEARNING OBJECTIVES

At the end of this chapter, you should be able to:

1. State the main reason that the COTA position was developed.
2. State the year that the first education program for COTAs began.
3. Compare the current educational program for COTAs with that of the 1960s.
4. Compare the current responsibilities of the COTA with those of the 1960s.
5. Compare the current certification process for COTAs with that of the 1960s.
6. Compare the current employment settings for COTAs with those of the 1960s.
7. Name 10 ways that COTAs can be involved with occupational therapy associations.
8. Name AOTA awards that COTAs may be eligible to receive.

World War II and medical technology expanded the need for rehabilitation services. The lives of many who were injured or ill were saved by new knowledge and techniques. The need for occupational therapy services increased as the number of people with war-related and industrial injuries grew, as the needs of infants and children with developmental delays became apparent, as the population increased in age and number, and as new laws were enacted to assist in the rehabilitation of all these individuals.

ORIGIN OF THE COTA

The shortage of registered occupational therapists (OTRs) prompted a proposal at the 1949 American Occupational Therapy Association (AOTA) conference to provide a 1-year educational program for occupational therapy aides working in psychiatric hospitals. The program would prepare aides to carry out routine departmental tasks and allow OTRs more time to provide treatment. In 1958, plans for the proposed certified occupational therapy assistant program to alleviate the shortage of occupational therapists were completed. AOTA members voted to authorize the expenditure of any funds needed to implement the plan. The plan included establishing a curriculum, a faculty-to-student ratio, and qualifications of individuals to be admitted to the program, acquiring needed space and support from AOTA, and designing an insignia with the words, *Certified Occupational Therapy Assistant*, to identify the COTA (AOTA, 1958).

EDUCATION

Training sites for the new students were in psychiatric hospitals. Graduates were prepared to work only in psychiatric facilities. One instructor was required for every 15 students. Admission requirements included high school graduation or the equivalent, good physical and emotional health, age between 18 and 55 years, intelligence, maturity, emotional stability, flexibility, cooperativeness, ability to establish and maintain effective interpersonal relationships, and recommendation by a qualified person. The curriculum required 460 hours within a 12-week period, including a minimum of 140 hours of didactic content, emphasizing specialty skills, and supervised experience (AOTA, 1959).

The effectiveness of COTAs in psychiatric facilities spawned discussions about training COTAs for positions in other types of facilities. In 1960, the first curriculum to prepare COTAs for general practice was implemented in Maryland. The early occupational therapy assistant programs were operated by a variety of organizations, such as the Senior Centers of Metropolitan Chicago, rather than in higher education systems. All programs were surveyed by AOTA to gain and maintain the Association's approval (Cromwell, 1968; Schwagmeyer, 1969).

In 1965, changes in occupational therapy assistant educational programs were implemented. The changes included 1) establishing programs that combined psychiatry and general practice curricula; 2) establishing programs in educational institutions based on geographical area of need; 3) establishing programs in junior or community colleges that would be longer than 18 weeks; and 4) reinterpreting the AOTA policy that occupational therapy assistant programs would not be in institutions where occupational therapy curricula were conducted. All specialty occupational therapy assistant programs that prepared the graduate only in psychiatry or only in general practice were scheduled to be terminated by December 31, 1972 (AOTA, 1965, 1966, 1970). In the 1960s, the number of junior and community colleges in the United States increased significantly, and many such colleges included occupational therapy assistant programs in their degree offerings. By 1994, there were 2,103 graduates from 94 occupational therapy assistant educational programs (AOTA, 1995), making that year the first that graduates numbered over 2 thousand. The number of graduates is expected to rise with the rapid increase in the numbers of educational programs and students.

The *Essentials of an Approved Educational Program for the Occupational Therapy Assistant* (*Essentials*) was adopted by AOTA in April 1975 as the minimum requirements for an educational program. The *Essentials* were revised for the sixth time in 1991 (AOTA, 1991a). They require that COTAs graduate from an accredited educational program based in a degree-granting college or university. They also require a minimum of 12 weeks of supervised fieldwork experience. The first Fieldwork Evaluation Form for occupational therapy assistants was adopted by AOTA in 1983 (AOTA, 1983).

CERTIFICATION

From 1959 to 1977, occupational therapy assistants were certified upon graduation from an approved occupational therapy assistant program without additional tests after graduation. Occupational therapy aides who worked in one disability area for at least 2 years prior to the establishment of occupational therapy assistant education programs were permitted to be certified without a formal education in occupational therapy until 1962. Military occupational therapy technicians were permitted to apply for certification in January 1971. Seventeen Army, 14 Air Force, and 11 Navy technicians became COTAs through this plan (AOTA, 1970; Schwagmeyer, 1969).

The first nationally administered occupational therapy assistant certification examination was given in June 1977 (AOTA, 1977). Since 1978, the examination has been scheduled twice annually in designated locations throughout the United States.

In 1986, the American Occupational Therapy Certification Board (AOTCB) was established. An individual who has successfully completed all academic and fieldwork requirements of an accredited educational program for an occupational therapy assistant is eligible to apply to sit for the certification examination. Upon payment of all required fees and successful completion of the examination, the individual is certified as an occupational therapy assistant. Certification by the AOTCB is permanent, unless disciplinary action is taken against the COTA and the certification is suspended or revoked (AOTCB, 1993). In 1960, 336 occupational therapy aides were certified under the grandfather clause, making a total of 863 COTAs by 1964 (AOTA, 1964). In 1995, an estimated 13,087 COTAs were in the U.S. work force (Burchman, 1995). Seven thousand of these were members of AOTA.

EMPLOYMENT

Initially, COTAs were employed only in psychiatric facilities. The shortage of OTRs led to the preparation of assistants for general practice. At first, the role of COTAs was to prepare crafts and other projects used for treatment, to transport patients, and to maintain work areas. Some COTAs were assigned to provide diversional activities for 15 to 20 patients per day. Other assignments included ordering and maintaining supplies, adapting and maintaining equipment, and providing general care for the department (Adamson & Anderson, 1966).

A 10th-anniversary survey of COTAs (Schwagmeyer, 1969) revealed that they were used cautiously and were often employed at the minimum wage. Many continued to be given responsibilities previously held by occupational therapy aides. The roles and responsibilities of COTAs were not clearly defined. They held a variety of titles, such as occupational therapy instructor and activity therapist, as well as director of occupational therapy. Many job descriptions delineated positions for which COTAs were not educationally prepared.

In 1967, the Social Security Administration certified 3,500 nursing homes as extended care facilities to render acute posthospital care to Medicare patients. Fifteen thousand occupational therapy positions were anticipated in these nursing homes. Nursing home administrators hired COTAs to provide activities and occupational therapy programs for their residents (Carr, 1967). The need for occupational therapy services in extended care facilities continued; however, by 1990, hospitals, rehabilitation centers for the physically disabled, and school systems were the three highest employment settings for COTAs due to the expanding role of COTAs in providing other services (AOTA, 1991b).

Increased demand for COTAs in the 1980s and 1990s resulted in unfilled positions and increased salaries. The shortage of COTAs estimated on a demand-based calculation was 17% in 1993, and on a need-based calculation it was 256%. Translated into numbers, this amounted to 28,700

COTAs needed in 1994 (Silvergleit, 1994). The need for occupational therapy services has continued to grow ever since the profession was founded.

ROLE

The role of the COTA has changed with that of the OTR. In the 1950s and early 1960s, OTRs included crafts, leisure activities, and work assignments in their treatment process. The major portion of the COTA's time was spent preparing craft materials for use by the patients and supervising patients in diversional activities. The COTA also assisted in routine paperwork such as ordering supplies, requesting maintenance for equipment, and recording attendance. Adaptations to equipment, furniture, play materials, and other items needed for occupational therapy were made by the COTA, depending upon his or her skills.

As the COTA gained experience in and knowledge about the work situation and performed effectively, the variety of his or her duties and responsibilities increased. This expansion prompted the Association to study the roles of the COTA and OTR more closely in an effort to define them more clearly. Data were collected in 1976 to learn what the COTA did in practice. In 1981, a delineation of the tasks of entry-level OTRs and COTAs (Shapiro & Brown, 1981) was adopted; however, a 1986 study showed that experienced COTAs and OTRs were performing the same functions in many of their direct-service areas (AOTA, 1988). The entry-level role of the COTA will continue to change as occupational therapy practitioners provide service in settings that are different from traditional hospital settings. The entry-level COTA will need to keep abreast of Association guidelines and federal and state regulations that govern practice.

TITLE AND INSIGNIA

Objections to the word "assistant" in the title of the COTA as not truly describing the role of these independent, highly responsible workers have resulted in proposals for a change in the title. Resolutions based on such proposals have failed to pass the AOTA Representative Assembly. Hirama (1994) and Schwagmeyer (1969) have suggested that inadequate communication in OTR-COTA relationships and misperceptions about each other's role, as well as their own roles, may be creating more of the dissatisfaction than does the title.

The original emblem for the COTA was replaced in 1984 and is now similar to that of the OTR (Jones, 1985). Emblems for the COTA and the OTR can be purchased only from the association and only by certified occupational therapists and certified occupational therapy assistants. The emblems are not to be worn by persons who are not certified occupational therapy practitioners.

CAREER MOBILITY

The continuing and increasing need for OTRs led to discussions on ways to help COTAs become OTRs. In 1973, the AOTA Executive Board endorsed a Career Mobility Plan to permit COTAs to sit for the OTR certification examination under established criteria that included letters of recommendation, experience working as a COTA, and additional field-work experience. The 1982 Representative Assembly voted to terminate the program, based on the large number of applications that required hours of review by committee members, the small numbers completing the program, the requirements of licensure laws that prohibited OTRs without formal degrees from becoming licensed to work in certain states, and the cost to the AOTA. All candidates who were accepted in the program were to complete it by 1988 (AOTA, 1973, 1982; Hightower-Vandamm, 1981).

COTA-OTR RELATIONSHIP

Early in the history of the COTA, cooperative, collaborative, or re-spectful working relationships between the COTA and the OTR were not common. Some OTRs were unaware of the existence of COTAs even 2 decades after the first COTAs were working in the field. Some OTRs praised the work of COTAs, but referred to the COTA as an aide. In 1963, a number of OTRs voiced their concern over the growing number of COTAs and expressed the desire to have occupational therapy be a pro-fessional, baccalaureate-, and graduate-degree-level discipline. The OTRs raised the possibility of assisting COTAs to achieve independence as a separate group. In 1967, the AOTA president described the OTR-COTA relationship as abrasive. She reminded AOTA members that both groups were part of the AOTA, each having distinct roles to fill (Brunyate, 1967b; Oliver, 1972; Paggen, 1972).

The continuing need for occupational therapy services and the short-age of OTRs demanded alternative ways to meet the need. The potential for other disciplines to try to provide what is occupational therapy ser-vices exists (Brunyate, 1967a). Some OTRs felt that COTAs, together with OTR consultants, could help fill the anticipated 15 thousand occupational therapy positions in nursing homes. The need to consider COTAs pro-viding direct treatment under OTR supervision was discussed again in 1968 when 50 OTRs met to find solutions to the shortage of OTRs. At that time, 1,213 COTAs and 8,905 OTRs were members of AOTA.

The COTA-OTR relationship gradually improved as COTAs and OTRs developed working relationships on treatment teams, on conference com-mittees, and during their education. At the 1990 annual AOTA confer-ence, the establishment of a new COTA-OTR collaborative award was announced. The award continues to be granted today.

THE COTA AND THE AOTA

Although the COTA role was developed, through a vote and with the support of the AOTA membership, to alleviate the shortage of occupational therapists needed to provide occupational therapy services, numerous questions and negative feelings surfaced as COTAs joined the work force. Perhaps the questions and feelings were due to a lack of long-range planning by AOTA. Perhaps they were due to the rapid increase in both OTRs and COTAS, without either group having a global view of occupational therapy in health care. Perhaps they were due to OTRs and COTAs not understanding each other's role, their own roles, or that they were to work together in providing their services. Whatever the reasons, the feelings and questions raised are part of COTA history.

The first COTAs had few privileges as members of AOTA. They could not vote, hold office, receive the *American Journal of Occupational Therapy*, or be nominated for any AOTA award (AOTA, 1964). A 1965 resolution to give COTAs proportional representation in state and national association affairs failed to pass the Delegate Assembly (AOTA, 1966). Twenty-nine of the 1,101 COTAs attended the 50th annual AOTA conference in 1969. During a session for COTAs, a survey asked whether they felt that they should take advantage of the member privileges outlined in the bylaws. It was revealed that COTAs were not provided a copy of the bylaws and therefore did not know what privileges they had. The bylaws were mailed for the first time to each COTA in 1970, together with the AOTA directory (AOTA, 1971). For the first time, the 1971 AOTA registry and directory listed OTRs and COTAs in the same volume. The bylaws were amended in 1973, making a COTA eligible for nomination and election to a position of member-at-large on the Executive Board of AOTA. In 1973, a motion to amend the bylaws to allow COTAs to receive the *American Journal of Occupational Therapy* failed (AOTA, 1973). Two years later, however, a resolution allowing COTAs to receive the journal as a regular membership benefit was passed at a special Delegate Assembly session (AOTA, 1976). In 1975, a resolution to confer eligibility on COTAs for the positions of delegate and alternate delegate failed. Finally, in 1983, the Representative Assembly passed a motion allowing the COTA member-at-large to the Assembly a voice and vote (AOTA, 1983).

The first COTA meeting at an annual AOTA conference was held in 1967. Forty-seven COTAs representing nine states attended (AOTA, 1968). Professional involvement and networking with colleagues at conferences increased gradually, and in 1983 11 COTAs presented formal sessions at the annual AOTA conference, held that year in Portland, Oregon.

By 1994, COTAs were eligible to be nominated for the COTA Award of Excellence, the highest honor the Association can award a COTA; the

Eleanor Clarke Slagle Lectureship Award, an honor established as a memorial to one of the outstanding pioneers in the profession; the Roster of Honor, which recognizes COTA members of the AOTA who made a significant contribution to the continuing education and professional development of members of the association; the Lindy Boggs Award, which recognizes the significant contributions made by an OTR or a COTA in promoting occupational therapy in the political arena; the Certificate of Appreciation, which expresses appreciation for extraordinary contributions to the advancement of occupational therapy; the Service Award, which recognizes individual members of AOTA who provided outstanding service to the association and profession; and the Terry Brittell COTA-OTR Partnership Award, which recognizes a COTA and an OTR who, through their collaborative efforts to promote the profession, exemplify the professional partnership (AOTA, 1975, 1978, 1994).

The AOTA funded a 2-year COTA advocacy position after noting in 1980 that COTAs had no formal means of communicating their needs to AOTA. In August 1980, a task force was formed to inventory COTA needs and to suggest ways that state associations and AOTA could respond to those needs.

The COTA Task Force (1981) developed a list of concerns on education, practice, and the profession. The educational concerns included refresher courses for COTAs reentering the field, affordable and relevant continuing education, means of pursuing the OTR level of competence, increased preparation at the entry level through more theoretical information, and information on program administration, on working within the system, and on how to be more assertive. The practice concerns included a clearer policy on supervision of the COTA, pay scales, and COTA representation on licensure boards. The professional concerns included advocacy at the national, state, and regional levels, more representation on association committees, more written material relevant to COTAs in AOTA professional publications, and public relations material to increase the visibility of COTAs.

AOTA continues to support the COTA level of practice at the same time that the profession sees a growing need for graduate-level practitioners. Just as the patient's involvement is essential in treatment, the practitioner's involvement in the professional organization is essential in the performance of service.

SUMMARY

The certified occupational therapy assistant (COTA) was developed by AOTA because of an increased need for occupational therapy services and a shortage of occupational therapists. The first COTAs graduated in 1959 and were certified upon completion of the approved educational program and recommendation by the program director. In 1977, a formal national certification examination process was initiated. COTAs have gradually been given more responsibility in all areas of the profession. They continue to gain the respect of consumers, employers, and health care professionals as their occupational therapy intervention helps the patient achieve treatment goals.

REVIEW QUESTIONS

Complete the following to make the best correct statements:

1. The main reason for establishing the COTA was:
   a) An increased number of injured military personnel.
   b) A shortage of occupational therapists and a need for services.
   c) An increase in head injuries from motor vehicle accidents.
   d) A shortage of occupational and activities therapists.
2. The original COTA education program was approved by AOTA in:
   a) 1949.
   b) 1958.
   c) 1965.
   d) 1977.
3. How does the current education of a COTA differ from that prior to 1972?
4. How does the current responsibility of a COTA differ from that of the early 1960s?
5. Describe the current process for becoming qualified to provide occupational therapy services as a COTA, and contrast it with the process that existed prior to 1977.
6. The first COTAs worked primarily in:
   a) School systems
   b) Nursing homes
   c) Rehabilitation centers
   d) Psychiatric hospitals
7. List at least five ways in which COTAs can be involved with AOTA.
8. Name the AOTA awards for which COTAs may be nominated.

ANSWERS

1. b.
2. b.
3. Prior to 1972, the curriculum for the COTA required 460 hours in a 12-week period of education that included 140 hours of didactic content and learning skills plus supervised experience. Currently, the COTA curriculum requires an associate's degree from an accredited educa-

tional program for an occupational therapy assistant. The curriculum includes liberal arts, science, and professional courses, as well as field-work experience.

4. In the early 1960s, the COTA worked only in psychiatric hospitals and prepared projects, maintained work areas and supply levels, and, on occasion, provided diversional activities for patients. Currently, COTAs are supervised by OTRs and provide direct therapy to patients in any setting where occupational therapy services are provided.

5. Before 1977, COTAs were certified by AOTA upon recommendation from the educational program director when they completed the educational program. Currently, before an individual receives credentials to provide occupational therapy services as a COTA, he or she must complete an accredited educational program for the OTA, receive an associate's degree, pass the AOTCB certification examination, and, in parts of the United States, be licensed to practice in regulated states.

6. d.

7. 1) Join the American Occupational Therapy Association.
   2) Represent the state occupational therapy association at AOTA meetings.
   3) Be a candidate for member-at-large of the Executive Board of AOTA.
   4) Be a candidate for member-at-large of the Representative Assembly.
   5) Submit a paper to present at the annual conference.
   6) Serve on conference committees.
   7) Volunteer to help at annual conferences.
   8) Voice opinions to the COTA representative.
   9) Write articles or book reviews for professional journals.
   10) Write to occupational therapy news magazines.
   11) Write opinions on annual resolutions to the state representative to AOTA's Representative Assembly.

8. 1) Roster of Honor
   2) COTA Award of Excellence
   3) Terry Brittell COTA/OTR Partnership Award
   4) Eleanor Clarke Slagle Award
   5) Service Awards
   6) OTR/COTA Collaborative Team Award

ADDITIONAL LEARNING ACTIVITIES

1. Speak to a COTA who became certified 10 or more years ago. What courses were in the educational program then? What textbooks did they use?

2. Read the history of occupational therapy in occupational therapy journals or textbooks. What mention is made of COTAs?

3. Look through *OT Week* for AOTA decisions on issues related to the COTA.
4. At a state or district meeting, try to learn what offices were held by COTAs, and try to meet and speak to those COTAs to learn about serving as an officer.

REFERENCES

Adamson, M.J., & Anderson, M. A. (1966). A study of the utilization of occupational therapy assistants and aides. *American Journal of Occupational Therapy, 20*(2), 75-79.

American Occupational Therapy Association, Inc. (1958). Abstracts of annual reports: Reports of special committees. *American Journal of Occupational Therapy, 12*(1), 37-49.

American Occupational Therapy Association, Inc. (1959). Annual reports: Executive director's report. *American Journal of Occupational Therapy, 13*(1), 27-50.

American Occupational Therapy Association, Inc. (1964). Board of Management. *American Journal of Occupational Therapy, 18*(1), 34-35, 45.

American Occupational Therapy Association, Inc. (1965). Board of Management: Report. *American Journal of Occupational Therapy, 19*(2), 93-106.

American Occupational Therapy Association, Inc. (1966). Delegate Assembly minutes. *American Journal of Occupational Therapy, 20*(1), 49-53.

American Occupational Therapy Association, Inc. (1968). Minutes of the annual business meeting. *American Journal of Occupational Therapy, 22*(2), 99-118.

American Occupational Therapy Association, Inc. (1970). Delegate Assembly: Minutes. *American Journal of Occupational Therapy, 24*(6), 438-443.

American Occupational Therapy Association, Inc. (1971). 50th Annual Conference: Minutes of the 1970 annual business meeting. *American Journal of Occupational Therapy, 25*(2), 112-132.

American Occupational Therapy Association, Inc. (1973). Statement on career mobility. *American Journal of Occupational Therapy, 27*(3), 157-158.

American Occupational Therapy Association, Inc. (1975). Guidelines for AOTA recognition. *American Journal of Occupational Therapy, 29*(10): 632-633.

American Occupational Therapy Association, Inc. (1976). Delegate Assembly: Minutes. *American Journal of Occupational Therapy, 30*(3), 168-180.

American Occupational Therapy Association, Inc. (1977). 1976 Delegate Assembly: Annual business meeting. *American Journal of Occupational Therapy, 31*(3), 177-194.

American Occupational Therapy Association, Inc. (1978). Annual business meeting. *American Journal of Occupational Therapy, 32*(10), 671-677.

American Occupational Therapy Association, Inc. (1982). 1982 Representative Assembly: 62nd annual conference. *American Journal of Occupational Therapy, 36*(12), 808-826.

American Oceupational Therapy Association, Inc. (1983). 1983 Representative Assembly minutes: 63rd annual conference. *American Journal of Occupational Therapy, 37*(12), 831-840.

American Occupational Therapy Association, Inc. (1988). *Professional and Technical Role Analysis Survey.* Bethesda, MD: Author.

American Occupational Therapy Association, Inc. (1991a). Essentials and guidelines for an accredited educational program for the occupational therapy assistant. *American Journal of Occupational Therapy,* 45(12), 1085-1092.

American Occupational Therapy Association, Inc. (1991b). Research information and evaluation division. *1990 Member data survey: Summary report.* Bethesda, MD: Author.

American Occupational Therapy Association, Inc. (1995). *1995 educational data survey final report: Survey of educational programs 1993-94 academic year.* Bethesda, MD: Author.

American Occupational Therapy Association, Inc. (1994). AOTA's 1995 award nominations. *OT Week, 8*(34), insert, A1-A32.

American Occupational Therapy Certification Board, Inc. (1993). *Certification examination for occupational therapist, registered and certified occupational therapy assistant: Program directors reference manual.* Gaithersburg, MD: Author.

Brunyate, R. (1967a). Nationally speaking: From the president. A modification of role for nursing home service. *American Journal of Occupational Therapy, 21*(5), 126-127.

Brunyate, R. (1967b). After fifty years, what status do we hold? *American Journal of Occupational Therapy, 21*(5), 262-267.

Burchman, P. (1995, December). Personal communication.

Carr, S. (1967). A modification of role for nursing home service. *American Journal of Occupational Therapy, 21*(3), 126-127.

COTA Task Force. (1981). Chart of COTA concerns. *Occupational Therapy Newspaper, 35*(4), 4.

Cromwell, F. (1968). The newest of our member category: The COTA. *American Journal of Occupational Therapy, 22*(5), 377-379.

Hightower-Vandamm, M. (1981). Soaring into the '80s—New directions. *American Journal of Occupational Therapy, 35*(12), 767-774.

Hirama, H. (1994). The issue is: Should certified occupational therapy assistants provide occupational therapy services independently? *American Journal of Occupational Therapy, 48*(9), 840-843.

Jones, R. (1985). New COTA patch available from AOTA products. *Occupational Therapy Newspaper, 39*(1), 3.

Oliver, R. (1972). To the editor. *American Journal of Occupational Therapy, 26*(4), 218.

Paggen, J. (1972). To the editor. *American Journal of Occupational Therapy, 26*(4), 219.

Schwagmeyer, M. (1969). The COTA today. *American Journal of Occupational Therapy, 23*(1), 69-74.

Shapiro, D., & Brown, D. (1981). The delineation of the role of entry-level occupational therapy personnel. *American Journal of Occupational Therapy, 35*(5), 306-311.

5

OCCUPATIONAL THERAPY SETTINGS

Settings where occupational therapy services are typically provided are presented. Organizational structures are discussed.

LEARNING OBJECTIVES

At the end of this section, you should be able to:

1. Name five types of settings where occupational therapy is usually provided.
2. Name four occupational therapy settings and state their primary source of funding.
3. Explain how the words *physical disability* and *psychosocial dysfunction* are generally used in occupational therapy.
4. Explain the terms *acute care facility* and *subacute care facility*.
5. Discuss how the philosophy of a given facility affects the staff.
6. State the general role of the board of directors of a facility.
7. State the general responsibility of the administrators of a facility.
8. Discuss how the structure of an organization affects employees of the organization.
9. State one reason an employee should carry liability insurance.

Patients receive occupational therapy in many different treatment settings. In any setting where an individual lacks the functional ability to be as independent as possible in daily self-care, work, or leisure activities, occupational therapy services may be needed. While such services are not always available on a full-time basis in many settings, they may be provided on a temporary, part-time, or consultative basis. In any setting where occupational therapy services are needed, a COTA can be the practitioner providing the services.

TREATMENT SETTINGS

Agencies providing occupational therapy services may have a variety of names, but can be classified as follows:

1. Day treatment centers
   - Associations for retarded citizens
   - Centers for clients with psychosocial dysfunctions
   - Community mental health centers
   - Day care centers for the elderly
   - Easter Seal Society
   - Outpatient rehabilitation centers for physical disabilities
   - Senior citizen centers
   - Sheltered workshops
   - United Cerebral Palsy Association
2. Home health agencies
   - Therapists in private practice
   - Visiting nurse associations
3. Hospitals
   - General
   - Pediatric
   - Psychiatric
   - Rehabilitation
4. Independent and semi-independent living facilities
   - Community homes for individuals with psychosocial dysfunctions
   - Community living arrangements for individuals with physical disabilities
   - Group homes for individuals with mental retardation
   - Halfway houses for patients with psychosocial dysfunctions
5. Long-term care
   - County nursing homes
   - Developmental centers
   - Private nursing homes
   - Retirement villages
6. School system
   - Home treatment
   - Private schools
   - Regular schools
   - Special classes in day settings

7. Other
- Community centers for psychosocial rehabilitation
- Correctional institutions
- Health maintenance organizations
- Hospices
- Private industry
- Private practice
- Industrial rehabilitation centers

Occupational therapy practitioners base their intervention on the belief that the patient's diagnosis is affected by all current and past influences. The individual is influenced by biological, neurophysiological, psychological, sociological, cultural, environmental, and economic factors. However, the patient who needs specialized medical or rehabilitative care is admitted to a setting that is most appropriate for treating primary complaints or conditions requiring special care. Other than general hospitals and private home settings, the name of the setting usually gives some clue as to the type of treatment it provides.

Two terms that are often used by occupational therapy practitioners to identify the type of treatment setting or the groups of patients who are being treated are *physical disability* and *psychosocial dysfunction*. Even though occupational therapy is based on treating the whole person, a general understanding of these terms will help the reader identify treatment settings and the patients in them.

The term *physical disability* is used to refer to that condition of the patient whose primary reason for seeking treatment is physical. The complaint usually relates to muscle weakness, loss of movement in the joints, pain in the joints, or loss of endurance. Patients with diagnoses such as arthritis, stroke, and hip replacement are classified as having physical disabilities. The term *psychosocial dysfunction* is used to refer to that condition of the patient whose primary reason for seeking treatment is a psychological or cognitive disorder that interferes with his or her functioning in society. Patients with diagnoses such as mental retardation, anxiety disorders, schizophrenia and bipolar disorders, major depression, and substance abuse or addiction disorders, are classified as having psychosocial dysfunctions. Using the broad terms is an attempt to simplify communication when specificity is not needed.

ACUTE CARE, SUBACUTE CARE, AND LONG-TERM CARE

The increase in the number of persons needing health care, the shortage of health care personnel, the cost of health care, and the various attempts to meet the health care needs of individuals in the United States result in ongoing changes to resolve issues related to health care. Over the years, health care has changed from treatment in the home or the general practitioner's office to treatment in a variety of settings.

The length of a given treatment or intervention affects the cost of health care. Medicare benefits for those on Social Security were believed to be in jeopardy because of an increasing number of persons eligible for benefits. In 1983, an amendment to the Social Security Act was signed into law according to which hospitals would receive payment for Medicare-eligible services, based on a preset rate. The payment was dependent upon the type of medical diagnosis and procedure. Each medical diagnosis was given a diagnosis-related group (DRG) number, and the hospital received a predetermined amount for each DRG. If the medical treatment cost more than the amount set by the prospective payment system (PPS), the hospital absorbed the cost. If the treatment cost less than the PPS amount, the hospital was allowed to keep the excess (Carlson & Oriol, 1985). To remain profitable and thus fiscally sound, hospital administrators had to contain costs and yet continue to provide needed services. It was during this period that hospitals began to focus on expenditure and profit. Increasingly, health care facilities had to be managed as businesses. Hospitals needed to be financially profitable in order to continue to provide health care. Accordingly, they began to discharge patients as soon as possible. Increased numbers of treatments and discharged patients became the desired end product. Many health care facilities became for-profit rather than nonprofit facilities.

Acute care refers to treatment that requires a short intervention period. A patient in need of acute care may require an examination, the administration of medication, and specialized procedures to resolve the medical problem in a few days or a few weeks. In 1993, the average length of hospital stay for the most frequently reported first-listed diagnosis of men and women aged 65 years and older was 7.5 days for males and 8.1 days for females (U.S. Bureau of the Census, 1995). Acute care is usually provided in the practitioner's office, a clinic, or a general hospital.

Subacute care is care that goes beyond the acute period, but without the intense monitoring or the number of specialized services and professionals needed for acute care. Subacute care was developed as a way to move Medicare patients out of the DRG beds and yet continue to provide managed care when those patients were not eligible to be accepted by acute rehabilitation providers or nursing homes. Prior to DRGs, PPSs, and other regulations that limited treatment in certain settings, such treatment was continued in the general hospital. Subacute programs can provide treatment at approximately half the cost of acute care. They also allow services to be delivered to a broader range of patients than Medicare allows. General hospitals, rehabilitation hospitals, and nursing homes began subacute care as a means of serving the health care needs of patients who could not receive care because of Medicare mandates. It soon became apparent that subacute care was cost effective in those facilities. The International Subacute Health Care Association estimates that there will be 10 thousand subacute care facilities by the year 2000 (Gill & Fowler, 1994; Munro, 1994).

Long-term care is for patients who require medical care or monitoring and social intervention over an extended time. When patients have a chronic condition, the need for care may extend over their lifetime. Such care traditionally was projected for individuals with severe mental retardation or chronic mental illness, as well as for elderly individuals. Long-term care facilities were nursing homes for elderly individuals and large institutions for the mentally retarded and the mentally ill. The increase in the general population, longer life spans, and a rise in the number of individuals who sustain severe injuries increase the incidence of chronic conditions in all ages and, thus, the need for long-term care.

The delivery of health care will continue to change rapidly. In an effort to control costs, many health care providers are reorganizing and merging with other such providers in order to be able to offer the full range of services. Independent and privately funded providers may become part of a larger organization, and closings, buy-outs, mergers, and new names for health care providers can be expected.

GENERAL, PSYCHIATRIC, AND REHABILITATION HOSPITALS

When the primary condition for which occupational therapy is prescribed is an acute medical problem, the patient is usually admitted and treated in a general hospital. The condition can be due to disease, injury, or a physical or psychosocial problem. Historically, general hospitals provided short-term care; currently, many provide all services, including acute care, subacute care, long-term skilled nursing care, rehabilitation services for physical or psychosocial conditions, inpatient and outpatient services, and residential and day services. If the acute condition for which the patient was admitted—-for example, an injury sustained in an auto accident—-is treated, and the patient still requires subacute or long-term care because of the condition—-for example, the existing head injury—-the patient may be discharged from acute care and be admitted to the hospital's subacute care facility or long-term care facility. If the general hospital has an outpatient rehabilitation facility, the patient may be an outpatient at the same hospital. If the general hospital does not have full services, the patient needing further treatment may be discharged to his or her home or to another setting that provides the treatment required.

Rehabilitation hospitals may be designated as providing care for patients with specific diagnoses, whether of physical disabilities or psychosocial dysfunctions, for designated age ranges, or for residential patients or outpatients (or both). Rehabilitation hospitals that specialize in the treatment of physical disabilities or psychosocial dysfunctions may further specialize in children or another age group.

General hospitals that have a psychiatric unit usually treat psychosocial dysfunctions on a short-term basis. Often, they provide inpatient psychiatric diagnostic services and treatment. The patient may be discharged without further treatment being recommended, or he or she may be discharged with a referral for another service. When further treatment is recommended, it may take place in the hospital's mental health day program. Community-based day programs for individuals with psychosocial dysfunctions are also available in most cities. Most such programs do not require the patient to attend regularly. Instead, individuals attend day programs on a voluntary basis, unless otherwise determined by a physician. When the psychiatric problem requires longer continued treatment, the patient is usually transferred to a hospital whose primary care is for psychiatric patients.

General hospitals frequently have detoxification units for patients with drug or alcohol abuse or addiction problems. These units are often separate from the hospital's mental health units serving patients with psychological and psychiatric problems. When the drug or alcohol problem requires a longer treatment period, the patient may be referred to a community-based outpatient or inpatient drug and alcohol rehabilitation center. There are facilities throughout the country that are specifically for drug-dependent and alcohol-dependent individuals.

NURSING HOMES AND RETIREMENT VILLAGES

Nursing homes provide the medical, physical, and psychosocial rehabilitation needed to sustain the life-style the patient who enters such facilities seeks. Nursing homes have added the word "rehabilitation" to their names, and rehabilitation and discharge are the goals for those admitted to such centers.

Many nursing homes include apartments for individuals who desire more space or for married couples who wish to reside together. Some nursing and rehabilitation centers provide full services, including freestanding cottages as well as luxury apartments. In nursing homes with expanded services and in retirement villages, the full range of health care is available. Acute care is provided in the centers' infirmaries or at the local hospital. If no health care is needed, the individual lives as independently as he or she desires.

CENTERS FOR THE DEVELOPMENTALLY DELAYED

Centers for the developmentally delayed usually provide intervention and residency for individuals 22 years of age and younger. Individuals with developmental delay may have physical disabilities or psychosocial dysfunctions as their primary problem. The centers that house them may be privately or state funded. If residential care is provided, the length of residency depends on the policy of the particular setting. Respite or short-term care, as well as long-term care, may be available.

Often, in state funded long-term residential settings, many elderly adults are among the population. In many of these centers, the individual has been a resident of the center from an early age and has remained a resident while receiving educational and therapeutic intervention there. Many residents of such settings are bussed to educational classes or vocational settings during the day. When the person previously classified as developmentally delayed is older and is given another classification requiring skilled care or intermediate care, and when the setting has areas designated to provide such care, the person is usually reassigned to reside in one of those areas.

Upon reaching adult age, some individuals are discharged from centers for the developmentally delayed to community group homes. The home with five or more individuals living together becomes the setting for learning community living skills. Staff members provide a rehabilitation program to integrate each person into the community.

Day treatment centers for individuals with developmental delay include those operated by the Easter Seal Society and United Cerebral Palsy centers. Children with developmental delay are enrolled in regular and special schools and in Head Start programs.

Children with medical or surgical conditions may be hospitalized in general or children's hospitals. If long-term treatment is required, referrals may be made to specialized treatment centers on an outpatient or residential basis.

ADMINISTRATION OF A FACILITY

Facilities are usually classified according to the funding they receive, as well as the type of patient they serve. Generally, funds are provided primarily by the federal government, by state or county governments, or by private citizens. Government-funded hospitals are Medical Centers of the Department of Veterans' Affairs, military hospitals, and hospitals on special government posts. State facilities are usually psychiatric hospitals and centers for the developmentally delayed, although some states fund both general and specialized hospitals. Many counties fund nursing homes, group homes for the mentally ill or mentally retarded, and day treatment centers. Private facilities range from general hospitals for acute care or subacute care to long-term residential nursing homes and retirement villages that include full health care services.

In the 1990s, for-profit corporations increased their holdings of health care facilities. Nursing homes, rehabilitation hospitals, and general hospitals continue to be added to the numbers that are funded and administered by large corporations and managed-care groups.

BOARD OF DIRECTORS

The board of directors or board of trustees of a facility is composed of those individuals selected to guide and advise the administrators of the facility. The board members volunteer their services in the interest of the facility and its consumers. The administrators of the facility meet regularly—usually once a month—with the board to discuss ongoing practices and issues of concern.

ADMINISTRATORS

The person in charge of the facility may be called the chief executive officer (CEO) or the president, or may have another title. Those individuals who are directly supervised by and report to the CEO make up the administrative staff and are called administrators or the executive committee. Most facilities delegate the responsibility for large categories of individuals to persons designated as vice-presidents, managers, or directors. Such individuals may have titles such as vice-president for business affairs, manager of therapeutic services, director of rehabilitation services, or medical director. The administrators usually determine policies that directly affect the personnel and consumers of the facility. The CEO meets regularly with his or her executive committee. Each member of the executive committee meets regularly with personnel under his or her direct supervision. These regularly held small-group meetings facilitate open communication. Appropriately channeled communication assists the CEO and all employees of the facility in striving to provide the highest quality of service possible.

The expectation on the part of consumers that they would receive quality services and products at a health care facility resulted in service providers seeking ways to evaluate and document the quality of services they offered. Among the methods used for performing this task are quality assurance, referred to as QA (Joe, 1991), and total quality management (TQM) (Dean & Evans, 1994). Today, health care facilities routinely conduct ongoing quality assurance reviews. The process usually involves all of a facility's employees. Each employee serves on a committee given responsibility for a designated area of service. The committee members evaluate the quality of the facility's services, identify existing and potential problems, develop plans for resolving the problems, put the plans into effect, systematically monitor changes made to correct problems in order to make sure that the desired results have been achieved, identify ways to improve services for patients, and document the entire evaluation process.

Accreditation by a recognized body is often used to confirm that the health care facility meets a designated standard. To achieve accreditation, the facility voluntarily requests an onsite evaluation from the accrediting body. Examples of accrediting organizations are the Joint Commission on Accreditation of Healthcare Organizations (JCAHO), the Commission for the Accreditation of Rehabilitation Facilities (CARF), and the Accreditation Council on Services for People with Developmental Disabilities (ACDD).

TABLE OF ORGANIZATION

A diagram of the organizational structure of a health care facility is referred to as a *table of organization*. Figures 5.1, 5.2, and 5.3 present tables of organization of some typical facilities.

Many settings use an interdisciplinary team approach when providing rehabilitation services. In such organizational structures, the COTA is supervised by an OTR, but the manager of the particular interdisciplinary team can be a physical therapist, speech therapist, psychologist, social worker, rehabilitation engineer, nurse, occupational therapist, or person from another discipline, depending on the composition of the team.

THE ASSISTANT AND THE ORGANIZATIONAL STRUCTURE

The COTA should know where his or her position fits in the total organizational structure in order to function effectively. In some situations, the COTA is supervised by a consultant for occupational therapy procedures and by a facility administrator for other aspects of employment. The COTA should know who his or her supervisor is and whom he or she supervises. Knowledge of the organizational structure of the facility enables the COTA to direct questions and comments to the appropriate supervisor. In the immediate supervisor's absence, the COTA should know to whom to report. If problems arise with the immediate supervisor and cannot be resolved, permission should be requested to discuss the problems with the supervisor's direct supervisor. Discussing the problem in the presence of both the immediate supervisor and the supervisor's supervisor may clarify the issues and prevent misperceptions. If the COTA supervises another employee or a volunteer, any problem that comes up with that person should be discussed with the COTA's direct supervisor. In some facilities, the COTA will belong to a union. If problems arise that cannot be resolved by discussing them with the COTA's supervisor, the union representative, usually employed at the same facility, may assist in resolving the problems.

Table of Organization: Facility

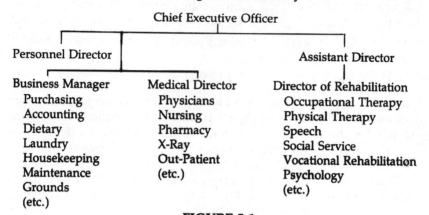

FIGURE 5.1

Table of Organization: Occupational Therapy Department

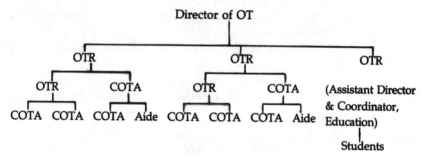

FIGURE 5.2

Table of Organization: Long-Term Care Facility

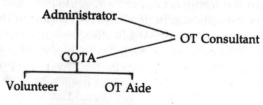

FIGURE 5.3

The COTA who uses information from the table of organization and who directs comments and questions to the appropriate person communicates more effectively with his or her coworkers and supervisors, and such communication can help reduce stress and create a more desirable work place. (Devereaux, 1992).

LIABILITY

Liability means anything for which one is legally responsible. *Malpractice* means incorrect or negligent treatment of a patient by persons responsible for the care of that patient, such as physicians, dentists, or nurses (Thomas, 1993). All health care practitioners and students of health care disciplines need to realize their legal responsibility in the health care setting. Even when all known precautions are taken and malpractice is not intended, an incident can occur that results in a legal investigation or litigation.

SUMMARY

Five major types of treatment settings in which occupational therapy services can be provided have been described. The availability of occupational therapy services is not limited to these types of settings; a COTA may be employed wherever occupational therapy services are provided. The organizational structure of the employment setting outlines the facility's supervisory levels and channels for communication. Appropriately directed communication with supervisors, coworkers, and patients can prevent and help resolve conflicts, reduce stress, and create a more desirable work place.

REVIEW QUESTIONS

1. Name five settings where occupational therapy services are provided.
2. Name four occupational therapy settings, and give the primary funding source of each.
3. Explain how the terms *physical disability* and *psychosocial dysfunction* are generally used when referring to patients.
4. Explain the terms *acute care, subacute care,* and *long-term care.*
5. How is the philosophy of a facility relevant to the staff of the facility?
6. What is the role of a board of directors of a facility?
7. What is one purpose of the administrators of a facility?
8. State one way that the table of organization relates to the COTA.
9. Give one reason a COTA should have liability coverage.

ANSWERS

1. General hospitals, psychiatric hospitals, rehabilitation centers, centers for children with developmental delay, nursing homes.

2. Medical Centers of the Department of Veterans' Affairs—federal; St. Luke's Hospital—private; state center for developmental delay—state; Fitzsimons Army Hospital—federal; Cedarbrook Nursing Home—county; Easter Seal Society—primarily private.

3. *Physical disability* is used to indicate that an individual's primary problem is a physical problem usually related to muscles, joints, strength, or endurance, or a pain related to physical movement.

   Psychosocial dysfunction indicates that the primary problem is an inability to function independently or appropriately in society. The cause may be related to mental, psychological, or cognitive factors.

4. *Acute care* means treatment that requires a short period of time and that is usually provided in a doctor's office, clinic, or general hospital. *Subacute care* means care that cannot be provided in the general hospital, acute care setting or in a rehabilitation setting, a long-term care facility, or the patient's home. *Long-term care* means care for a chronic condition that will require treatment or monitoring over an extended period—even over the patient's lifetime.

5. When the philosophy of the employee is compatible with the philosophical goals of the health care facility, the work situation is more likely to be a productive and pleasant. If the primary goal of the facility is to increase the number of persons treated as efficiently as possible, without concern for the quality of care provided, and the COTA's belief is that a high quality of care should be provided regardless of the time taken and the resources used, the COTA is likely to perceive the difference in goals and feel distressed, think negatively of the organization, and decrease his or her productivity.

6. The board of directors is a voluntary group that provides guidance and advice to the administrators of a facility.

7. Administrators are responsible for maintaining a facility that is productive, is fiscally sound, and provides the best care possible for its consumers. This includes objectively evaluating the facility's services to identify potential or existing problems, developing plans to resolve those problems, effecting and monitoring changes, and making good judgments in developing policies that affect all employees and consumers of the facility.

8. The table of organization diagrams the level of supervision and channels of communication in a facility. Using the table, the COTA will know from whom to expect supervision and will be able to direct communication appropriately.

9. Despite any number of precautions taken, accidents can happen. For example, during a cooking training session in the kitchen, a patient might fall and hit his head on the counter. The family may then decide to see an attorney to investigate the legal responsibility of the COTA who was supervising the session. Whether or not the investigation proceeds, the COTA will be in a more comfortable position if he or she has liability coverage.

ADDITIONAL LEARNING ACTIVITIES

1. Ask whether and how an OTR or a COTA is involved in the quality assurance process at his or her place of employment.
2. When visiting a health care facility, notice or ask whether the accreditation of the facility is from JCAHO, CARF, or some other designated source of accreditation.

REFERENCES

Carlson, E., & Oriol, W. (1985). Surviving Medicare's new obstacle course. *Modern Maturity, 28,* 25-27, 87-88, 94-103.

Dean, J., Jr., & Evans, J. (1994). *Total quality management, organization, and strategy.* St. Paul: West Publishing Company.

Devereaux, E. (1992). Principles of communication. In J. Bair & M. Gray (Eds.), *The occupational therapy manager.* (pp. 261-273). Bethesda, MD: American Occupational Therapy Association, Inc.

Gill, H., & Fowler, F. (1994). Putting together the pieces. *Rehab Management, 7*(4), 99, 108-109, 119.

Joe, B. (Ed.). (1991). *Quality assurance in occupational therapy: A practitioner's guide to setting up a quality assurance system using three models.* Bethesda, MD: American Occupational Therapy Association, Inc.

Munro, D. (1994). Subacute subtleties. *Rehabilitation Today, 4*(1), 18-21.

Thomas, C. (1993). *Taber's cyclopedic medical dictionary* (17th ed.). Philadelphia: F. A. Davis Company.

U.S. Bureau of the Census. (1995). *Statistical abstracts of the United States; 1995* (115th ed.). Washington, DC: Author.

Section II

GENERAL OCCUPATIONAL THERAPY ASSISTANT SKILLS

The knowledge and skills required of the certified occupational therapy assistant (COTA) may differ from setting to setting and are dependent upon the needs of the consumer, the aims of the supervising occupational therapist, sources of funding, and current regulations that affect occupational therapy practice, as well as other influences. The entry-level role of the COTA, as described by the American Occupational Therapy Association (AOTA), changes as the needs of consumers, the delivery of health care services, the role of the occupational therapist, and the educational standards for occupational therapy practitioners change. To keep up with all of these changes, the reader is referred to current official documents of the AOTA and regulations affecting federal, state, and local occupational therapy practice. Examples of the role of the experienced COTA are included in this section, as is basic information on interviewing skills, documentation, evaluation, planning treatment, and supervisory skills.

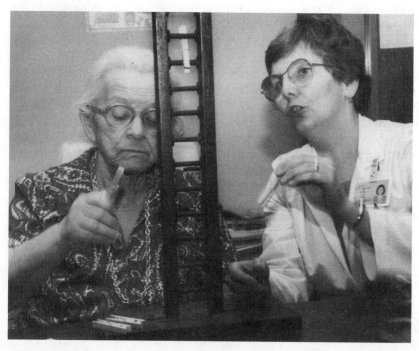

Judith Clark, COTA/L, and Beatrice Frankenfield work on upper extremity range of motion and fine motor coordination. Photo courtesy of Phoebe-Devitt Homes.

6

THE ASSISTANT'S ROLE

The role of the certified occupational therapy assistant (COTA) is summarized.

LEARNING OBJECTIVES

At the end of this chapter, you should be able to:

1. Explain what is meant by entry-level occupational therapy practice.
2. Discuss the supervision required of the entry-level COTA.
3. Name a situation when the supervision required is similar for an experienced COTA and the entry-level COTA.
4. Name at least eight occupational therapy service areas in which the COTA has a role.
5. Name two tasks an entry-level COTA is qualified to perform under each of six occupational therapy service areas.
6. State two sources from which the COTA can gather current professional information.

The following is the current, generally accepted entry-level role of the certified occupational therapy assistant (COTA), as described in AOTA documents and state regulations. The roles of the certified occupational therapist, registered (OTR), and the COTA change as consumers' needs change and as the delivery of health care services changes. The COTA must be aware of and adhere to federal, state, and local regulations as they apply to occupational therapy services.

PROFESSIONAL STANDING

Occupational therapy practitioners—that is, OTRs and COTAs—are required to have completed the minimum educational requirements for their level of practice, to have fulfilled the requirements for certification by the American Occupational Therapy Certification Board (AOTCB, 1993), and to maintain a current license or registration, as required by state law. Occupational therapy practitioners are expected to abide by the AOTA (1994b) "Occupational Therapy Code of Ethics," as well as the code of ethics governing the specific employment setting. COTAs are to receive supervision from qualified OTRs, in accordance with state laws and regulations. Occupational therapy practitioners are expected to keep their knowledge and skills current, in order to delivery their services effectively.

Guidelines and documents for occupational therapy practice and revisions of AOTA documents appear in AOTA publications. An efficient way to keep abreast of official documents that have been adopted and documents that have been rescinded by the AOTA Representative Assembly in a given year is to review the archival issue—usually the December issue—of the *American Journal of Occupational Therapy*. The last issue of a given year includes the annual index, in which guidelines, position papers, statements, and other official documents are indexed under the title "Association."

In most employment settings, the COTA functions as an assistant to the OTR in providing occupational therapy services. According to the AOTA (1994c) "Standards of Practice for Occupational Therapy," the COTA assists the OTR in procedures related to referrals, screening, assessment, planning interventions, the interventions themselves, transition services, discontinuation of service, continuous quality improvement, and management. The COTA may be requested to assist in research conducted at the setting and is expected to document his or her involvement in any occupational therapy procedure.

SUPERVISION

The OTR and COTA should jointly strive to promote optimum performance in providing occupational therapy services. The organizational structure of the employment setting usually illustrates the patterns of supervision used. For example, when the organization contracts with an OTR, and the COTA is employed by the organization, the COTA may receive supervision from an employee of the organization for carrying out those responsibilities and duties that are not related directly to occupational therapy and from the OTR under contract for carrying out those related directly to occupational therapy services.

Supervision may be categorized as 1) *close,* meaning that the OTR has direct contact with the COTA daily at the work site; 2) *routine,* meaning that the OTR is in direct contact with the COTA at least every 2 weeks at the work site and supervises the COTA by telephone or written communication at other times; 3) *general,* meaning that the OTR makes direct contact with the COTA at least once a month and is available to the COTA as needed by any method of contact; or 4) *minimal,* meaning that supervision is provided as needed by the COTA and may be less than monthly (AOTA, 1994d). Most state regulations require that OTRs supervise COTAs. Specific requirements, such as the number of hours of supervision and the amount and kind of supervision to be given during an extended absence by the OTR, are written in the laws regulating occupational therapy practice for individual states.

In the 10 service areas identified by AOTA, the amount of supervision the experienced COTA receives will vary. Although each COTA completes the minimum requirements of an accredited occupational therapy assistant educational program, the curriculum and requirements for graduation may vary from setting to setting. The background knowledge and experiences of each COTA are different. The effective supervisor is aware of these differences and helps the COTA use his or her own special skills, talents, educational background, and experiences that are relevant to occupational therapy practice. The effective COTA assumes responsibility for informing the supervisor about those relevant background experiences so that both can take advantage of the COTA's strengths and deal with the COTA's weaknesses.

Both the experienced and the entry-level COTA are required to be closely supervised by an experienced OTR when the patient's condition is complex or is expected to change rapidly. Examples of situations that require close supervision are acute injuries, such as a severe industrial injury to the hand or a traumatic head injury, recent cerebral vascular accidents, and recent psychotic episodes.

The experienced COTA may also require close supervision during the acute phase of treatment of a patient and then may function under routine, general, or minimal supervision when the patient's condition stabilizes and fewer changes in treatment procedures are required.

Although AOTA provides guidelines for practice, each state that regulates occupational therapy services has its own practice laws. The state laws supersede the AOTA guidelines. The COTA should refer to the regulations of the state in which he or she is employed. A copy of those regulations can be requested from the state licensure board.

THE ENTRY-LEVEL COTA AND THE EXPERIENCED COTA

The entry-level COTA is an individual who has worked as a COTA less than 12 months. An experienced COTA is a person who has worked longer than 12 months as a COTA. Thus, if a COTA begins his or her 13th month of employment in a new setting, where the age range and condition of the patients are quite different from those the COTA has seen for the previous 12 months, the COTA is still considered experienced.

The role assumed by an experienced COTA will depend upon the skills and knowledge the COTA has gained over the years, the state licensure laws, the amount of responsibility the COTA is willing to assume, and the kind and amount of responsibility that is delegated to the COTA. Because roles assumed by experienced COTAs differ from setting to setting and within settings, a job description and a mutual understanding of the expected performance will help to establish a positive working relationship between the OTR and the COTA.

The role of the experienced COTA normally is very different from that of the entry-level COTA. Indeed, casual observers of occupational therapy settings and interventions may find it difficult to distinguish between the experienced COTA and the OTR when both are providing treatment.

REFERRAL

A referral for occupational therapy services commonly originates from health care professionals—most frequently, a physician—from teachers or parents of students, or from the potential patient. Referrals are initiated before any screening or evaluation process begins. The OTR accepts and then acts upon the referrals (AOTA, 1994a). On occasion a verbal request for occupational therapy will be received. Informal as well as formal referrals received by the COTA should be relayed to the supervising OTR or the team manager, depending on the facility's routine procedures. The COTA should inform individuals who refer patients to him or her, rather than to the OTR, about the referral procedure used. Informing the supervising OTR when referrals are made to the COTA will enable the OTR to help individuals use the appropriate referral process and will help maintain an effective system.

SCREENING

Screening is a process used by the OTR to determine a person's need for occupational therapy. The COTA contributes to the screening process in a manner determined by the supervising OTR. When the COTA in fact carries out screening tasks, it means that the OTR has determined the competency of the COTA to perform such tasks.

Among the responsibilities that can be delegated to the experienced COTA are 1) gathering a general history and information from the patient and significant others, using routine forms and checklists or administering structured screening tests; 2) summarizing information gathered orally or in writing; and 3) communicating information about the screening orally or in writing.

The entry-level COTA may be requested to report factual data and to collect data and communicate information from the screening after his or her competency has been established.

ASSESSMENT

When screening indicates that a patient needs occupational therapy, the patient is referred for a comprehensive evaluation to determine the extent of his or her need for therapy and the kind of occupational therapy that will be required. Information gleaned from the evaluation enables the OTR to develop a logical intervention plan.

The extent of the COTA's participation in the evaluation process is determined by the supervising OTR. As in the screening process, the COTA's competency to administer tests or perform other evaluative tasks is established by the OTR. Among the responsibilities that may be delegated to the COTA are to 1) review the patient's record for relevant data; 2) educate the patient and his or her family about the purposes and procedures of the assessment; 3) interview the patient, family, and significant others to obtain information about the family history and the patient's self-care, abilities and disabilities, academic history, vocational history, leisure time history, and interests; 4) observe the patient while he or she is engaged in individual or group activities, in order to gather general information related to the patient's daily living, sensorimotor, cognitive, and psychosocial skills; and 5) administer standardized and criterion-referenced tests.

After the supervising OTR has determined that the entry-level COTA is competent, the COTA is able to collect data through reviews of records, interviews, and general observations, as well as by completing behavioral checklists, administering standardized and criterion-referenced tests, and scoring test protocols. The entry-level COTA contributes to the communication, to appropriate persons, of information related to the evaluation, within the boundaries of confidentiality. The entry-level COTA does not communicate any such information independently.

The OTR selects appropriate assessment methods, conducts assessments individually or with other professionals, analyzes and summarizes the data obtained from an assessment, documents results of the assessment in the patient's record, and refers the patient to appropriate services or requests additional consultations if the results indicate a need for intervention by other professionals.

INTERVENTION

Intervention refers to the implementation of the plans to achieve the goals and objectives agreed upon by the treatment team, which includes the patient. The OTR is responsible for formulating the intervention program, supervising the occupational therapy practitioner who implements the program, and making modifications to the program. The OTR is responsible for the outcome of the intervention and for delegating components of the intervention to the COTA. The particular components assigned to an experienced COTA will depend on the competency of the COTA to perform specific skills needed for the intervention.

The OTR develops and documents the intervention plan, based on data from the assessment and the goals the patient expects from occupational therapy. The COTA may contribute to the plan under the supervision of the OTR. The plan should include the patient's strengths and weaknesses, as well as the OTR's estimation of the patient's potential for rehabilitation. The documented plan should state goals that are measurable, behavioral, functional, and appropriate for the patient. The plan should include short-term and long-term goals; the methods, media, environment, and personnel needed to accomplish the goals; the frequency and estimated duration of the occupational therapy services; and the plan as to when to discharge the patient. A reevaluation plan is included in the intervention plan.

The experienced COTA engages the patient in purposeful activities, reports any changes that may affect the intervention plan, and may be able to alter the intervention plan without supervision following a discussion with the OTR. The COTA should be able to provide direct services related to the performance components of the intervention and also should be able to make necessary interpretations. The COTA may be responsible for monitoring aides, volunteers, and other persons making contributions to the intervention process and may in some instances be qualified to provide consultation on a case or to a colleague.

The entry-level COTA is qualified to engage the patient in purposeful activities, provide direct services related to the performance components that follow a generally accepted routine, and report changes in the patient or environment that may affect the intervention plan. After demonstrating his or her competency, the entry-level COTA provides direct services related to performance components that require ongoing interpretation. The entry-level COTA also contributes to monitoring non-occupational-therapy personnel—for example, volunteers—as they perform intervention-related tasks.

Reevaluation is the process of gathering information relevant to the patient's progress during intervention and interpreting the information to determine whether to continue, revise, or discontinue the intervention. Both the experienced and the entry-level COTA monitor the patient's progress during intervention and report changes to the supervising OTR, who determines whether there is a need for reevaluation. The OTR specifies any changes to be made in the intervention, as well as any referrals to another professional discipline for additional treatment. Some experienced COTAs may perform reevaluations independently when the OTR has determined their competency to do so. Entry-level COTAs contribute to the reevaluation process as determined by the OTR, but do not perform any reevaluations independently.

TRANSITION SERVICES

Transition services are actions needed to prepare the patient to make a change. The change may be from one functional level to another, from one life stage to another, from one program to another, or from one environment to another. An OTR conducts community-referenced assessments to identify a patient's occupational performance needs related to a transition, prepares a formal individualized transition plan based on the patient's needs, and facilitates the transition process in cooperation with the patient and team members. The OTR initiates referrals to appropriate community agencies to provide needed services for the transition. Either the OTR or a COTA whose competency for the task has been established evaluates the effectiveness of transition programs.

The patient's successful transition from one setting to another, be it from an acute care to a subacute care setting or from a psychosocial treatment setting to independent living in the community, results from the cooperative effort of a multidisciplinary team. Determining the patient's needs, abilities and disabilities, and level of independence in the performance of daily living, work, and play or leisure activities; evaluating community settings; documenting and reporting the information learned; and communicating with a variety of people are some of the occupational therapy services rendered in helping the patient make the transition from setting to setting. The COTA's involvement will depend upon his or her established competency in relevant knowledge and skills.

DISCONTINUATION OF SERVICES

The OTR discontinues occupational therapy services when the patient has achieved the specified goals, has obtained the maximum benefit from such services, or is transferred to another treatment agency. The OTR develops the discharge plan and documents the changes made during intervention and the patient's functional abilities and deficits in the various performance areas, components, and contexts. When appropriate, the OTR documents recommendations for follow-up or reevaluation of the patient.

The experienced COTA contributes to the discontinuation process by recognizing factors that warrant discontinuation of intervention and by communicating the information orally and in writing to the supervising OTR. In some settings and situations, the COTA contributes to the discharge plan and follow-up plan, submitting them to the supervising OTR or team manager, depending on the facility's usual procedures. In some settings and situations, the experienced COTA evaluates the environment to which the patient will be discharged and formulates the discharge and follow-up plans in collaboration with the patient, family members, staff, and others with the authority to do so.

The entry-level COTA, after demonstrating his or her competency, contributes to the discontinuation of occupational therapy by recognizing the factors that warrant such discontinuation and communicating those factors to the supervising OTR. The entry-level COTA contributes to the plan for discharge and the follow-up plan as determined by the supervising OTR.

DOCUMENTATION

Both experienced and entry-level COTAs should be competent to document their performance of occupational therapy processes when they begin employment. If a newly hired COTA is unfamiliar with a particular style of documentation, his or her competency should be established during the orientation period. If regulations require the OTR's countersignature on the COTA's documentation, the COTA should take the initiative to ensure that the OTR signs the documentation.

CONTINUOUS QUALITY IMPROVEMENT

In most facilities, a multidisciplinary team is responsible for the systematic, ongoing evaluation of the quality of services provided and for establishing strategies for improving said quality. An OTR systematically assesses the review process by means of which the occupational therapy services are evaluated, in order to determine the appropriateness and effectiveness of the process. When an occupational therapy intervention does not meet the established standards of care, it must be justified by appropriate means within the setting. Occupational therapy services are to be discontinued when the patient no longer needs them.

The COTA monitors and documents all aspects of his or her occupational therapy services for effectiveness and timeliness. The COTA's documentation is reviewed by the OTR responsible for monitoring occupational therapy services.

MANAGEMENT

The experienced COTA may assist in any management activity specified by, and under the supervision of, the OTR. Examples of management activities include educating physicians and other health care professionals about occupational therapy; conducting tours and explaining the purpose of occupational therapy; orienting, supervising, training, and evaluating volunteers and uncertified occupational therapy personnel; providing in-service training in the area of the COTA's expertise; participating in fieldwork education for occupational therapy assistant students; participating in continuous quality review and improvement; determining the supply and equipment needs of the occupational therapy department; coordinating a treatment program area, such as the home management area; and submitting news briefs about the occupational therapy department to the facility newsletter.

The entry-level COTA is qualified to plan and manage his or her own daily schedule and needs for space, equipment, and supplies, with an eye toward ensuring the safe use of program areas and equipment based on assignments and according to procedures established by the supervisor or agency. The entry-level COTA summarizes departmental data, participates in work-related meetings and accreditation reviews, provides in-service training, manages and supervises personnel and students as assigned, and adheres to relevant policies and procedures in support of the departmental function. After demonstrating his or her competency, the entry-level COTA manages the department's records and budget and implements evaluations of the occupational therapy program.

RESEARCH

Both the experienced COTA and the entry-level COTA should understand the importance of research. The competencies of the experienced COTA and the particular research project will determine his or her participation in research. Following a demonstration of competency for the task, the entry-level COTA participates in research by collecting data.

PROFESSIONAL COMPETENCY

The COTA and the OTR achieve and maintain professional competence through self-directed learning. The latter requires the COTA and OTR to identify their professional needs and learning resources and then select and implement appropriate measures to achieve professional competence.

Numerous opportunities are available for continuing education, through the setting in which the COTA is employed, through the occupational therapy associations, and through privately sponsored workshops. Formal education is also available to the COTA at local colleges and universities.

Professional journals, texts, and newsletters provide current information affecting the practice of occupational therapy. Among the professional occupational therapy journals are the *American Journal of Occupational Therapy* and the *Journal of Occupational Therapy Research. OT Week* and *ADVANCE for Occupational Therapists* are news magazines that contain current association-related information, a listing of available employment positions, and a calendar of available courses, as well as articles relevant to practitioners. *OSERS*, a publication of the U. S. Department of Education, provides current information on special education. There are numerous journals on physical rehabilitation, such as *Rehab Management*, which is an interdisciplinary journal. The rapid changes that affect health care require occupational therapy practitioners to keep abreast of research and legislative information from related professional journals. Professional newsletters include abstracts of such information and direct the practitioner to the original source.

PROMOTION OF THE PROFESSION

The COTA can promote the profession through activities such as recruiting potential OTRs and COTAs, public relations, marketing the profession, and participating in professional organizations.

Experienced COTAs and OTRs represent educational occupational therapy programs during high school career days to recruit students to the profession. They also explain the purpose and value of occupational therapy by making presentations to students in health-related courses and activities. During Occupational Therapy Month, COTAs and OTRs promote the profession by participating in activities organized at the place of employment or in the community. These activities may include a display in the lobby of a facility with literature and demonstrations of occupational therapy evaluations and intervention techniques, a program on occupational therapy on the local radio or television station, a display at a shopping mall, a newspaper article with photographs that explain occupational therapy, and a meeting with state representatives, the city mayor, or the state governor to proclaim National Occupational Therapy Month.

Occupational therapy news magazines annually publish interesting events that occurred throughout the nation to promote the profession during Occupational Therapy Month.

The entry-level COTA identifies and exploits opportunities to explain the purpose and value of occupational therapy, participates in professional organizations, and represents the profession to consumers, associates, and the community.

SUMMARY

The COTA assists the OTR in all service areas of occupational therapy. The role of one experienced COTA may differ significantly from that of another, depending upon their educational background and experiences, current service area, and relationship to the OTR. When state regulations and the AOTA guidelines on COTA and OTR roles differ, the state regulations supersede the guidelines of the AOTA. The rapid changes in health care delivery and occupational therapy require COTAs and OTRs to keep abreast of current information by reading professional journals and publications and by attending continuing education seminars and workshops.

REVIEW QUESTIONS

Circle the letter preceding the best answer.

1. The entry-level COTA has occupational therapy experience of
   a. zero to 12 years.
   b. zero to 18 months.
   c. zero to 24 months.
   d. zero to 36 months.
2. The entry-level COTA is required to have
   a. close supervision from an OTR.
   b. general supervision from an OTR.
   c. medical supervision from an OTR.
   d. a consultant OTR or administrator.
3. Name a situation in which an experienced COTA requires supervision similar to that of an entry-level COTA.
   a. A patient with a recent hand injury is new to the hand clinic.
   b. An 8-year-old student is receiving training in dressing herself.
   c. A group is engaged in leisure activities in a long-term care center.
   d. A student with a diagnosis of autism is learning work skills.
4. Name 10 occupational therapy services in which COTAs assist OTRs.
5. State the role of an entry-level COTA in each of six occupational therapy services.
6. State two sources from which the COTA can gather current professional information.

ANSWERS

1. a
2. a
3. a
4. Referral
   Screening
   Assessment
   Intervention plan
   Intervention

Transition services
Discontinuation of services
Continuous quality improvement
Documentation
Management
Research
5. 1) Screening: Report factual data, and after demonstrating competency, communicate results of screening.
   2) Intervention: Engage the patient in purposeful activities, and report changes in the patient or environment that may affect the intervention plan.
   3) Discontinuation: Recognize factors that warrant discontinuation of intervention, and report factual data at the time the patient is to be discharged.
   4) Documentation: Record occupational therapy services, and take the initiative to get a cosignature if required.
   5) Management: Plan a daily schedule compatible with the work assignment, and ensure the safety of program areas and equipment.
   6) Research: Recognize the importance of research, and collect data when competency is established.
   7) Promotion of the profession: Explain the purpose and value of occupational therapy, and join professional organizations.
6. The *American Journal of Occupational Therapy,* the *Journal of Occupational Therapy Research, OT Week,* AOTA Self-study series, AOTA and state association conferences, and continuing education courses.

ADDITIONAL LEARNING ACTIVITIES

1. Ask a COTA in a long-term care facility what duties and responsibilities he or she has. Are they similar to those listed in the COTA roles in the text?
2. Ask a COTA in an acute care hospital what duties and responsibilities he or she has. What type of supervision does the COTA receive? Is the COTA an experienced or entry-level COTA? How does the COTA feel about an entry-level COTA working in an acute care hospital?
3. Compare the differences and similarities in duties and responsibilities among COTA positions in school settings, day programs, rehabilitation centers for physical disabilities, and rehabilitation centers for substance addiction.

REFERENCES

American Occupational Therapy Association, Inc. (1994a). Statement of occupational therapy referral. *American Journal of Occupational Therapy, 48*(11), 1034.

American Occupational Therapy Association, Inc. (1994b). Occupational therapy code of ethics. *American Journal of Occupational Therapy, 48*(11), 1037-1038.

American Occupational Therapy Association, Inc. (1994c). Standards of practice for occupational therapy. *American Journal of Occupational Therapy, 48*(11), 1039-1043.

American Occupational Therapy Association, Inc. (1994d). Guide for supervision of occupational therapy personnel. *American Journal of Occupational Therapy, 48*(11), 1045-1046.

American Occupational Therapy Certification Board, Inc. (1994). *Certification examination for occupational therapist, registered and certified occupational therapy assistant: Program directors reference manual.* Gaithersburg, MD: Author.

INTERVIEWING SKILLS

The role of interviews in occupational therapy is discussed, and examples of interviewing techniques are given.

LEARNING OBJECTIVES

At the end of this chapter, you should be able to:

1. Explain what is meant by communication.
2. Explain the difference between a conversation and an interview.
3. Describe movements of the eyes, jaw, hands, and legs to observe during an interview, and give an example of how movements of each can give information that conflicts with or confirms simultaneous verbal comments.
4. Explain what is meant by active listening.
5. List four specific interviewer behaviors that can indicate active listening.
6. Give two examples each of open-ended and closed questions, and explain why they are open ended or closed.
7. State appropriate interviewer behaviors when the person being interviewed verbally abuses or threatens the interviewer.

Occupational therapy practitioners communicate with many people every day. Communication may occur in writing, by telephone, by electronic mail and other technology, or face to face by verbal and nonverbal means. An interview is usually a verbal, face-to-face form of communication. In most occupational therapy settings, the interview is a private meeting between the practitioner and the patient. In some instances, a relative or a person who can add information may accompany the patient.

A successful interview requires effective communication between the interviewer and the person interviewed. Interviewing differs from conversation by its goal. Conversations may or may not have a goal of acquiring information. Conversations may or may not have a time limitation. An interview has both a goal of obtaining information and a time limitation.

THE ASSISTANT'S ROLE

The certified occupational therapy assistant (COTA) may need to interview the patient to obtain background information not found in the patient's chart. Specific information may be needed on the patient's self-care, home management, and work skills, as well as on the patient's leisure interests. The COTA may interview the patient to obtain information on how the patient feels about his or her disabling condition and how the feelings relate to the occupational therapy program. The COTA also may need to interview the patient's family or the facility's staff to obtain information in order to help plan or carry out an effective occupational therapy program.

Skillful interviewing techniques are essential to effective occupational therapy. The time limitation naturally imposed on interviews requires the efficient use of time. Interviewing techniques should be used within the framework of the COTA's personality.

INTERVIEWING TECHNIQUES

Genuine interest and sincere concern are basic to effective communication, whether in an informal conversation or in a formal interview. Interest and concern are expressed verbally and nonverbally by a skillful interviewer.

The purpose of the interview should be stated early and clearly understood by the patient. The professional attitude of confidentiality and the value of the interviewer's objectives are frequently sensed from the interviewer's nonverbal behavior; however, the patient should be verbally reassured anyway. Normally, when a COTA conducts an interview, a form with a checklist and space for additional comments is used. The following are suggestions for observing, listening, and speaking to the patient during an interview:

1. *Observing*

Keep in mind that a certain amount of anxiety can be expected during the initial interview. A cluster of behaviors can give clues to the patient's feelings and cognitive functioning.

The interviewer should observe the patient's general body movements. Does the patient appear alert, interested, angry, or distracted?

Is there a comfortable amount of eye contact, avoidance of eye contact, or constant, piercing eye contact? Are the jaws tightly clenched or in excessive motion? Does the mouth seem unusually dry? Is there excessive saliva during verbalization? Are the hands held in a relaxed manner or in a clenched fist, or are they in constant motion? Are the legs on the floor in a natural, relaxed way? Are the individual's legs or feet in constant motion, or is one leg entwined around the other?

Observe what is said and how it is said. Are questions answered with just one word? Are appropriate comments made upon request? Are the answers and comments rambling and irrelevant? Does the voice sound natural, barely audible, or unusually loud? Is there frequent sighing during sentences and throughout the interview? Do the patient's statements sound resentful or angry?

In general, it is not possible to interpret exactly the meaning of observed behaviors, but any behaviors observed during an interview, especially those that seem out of the ordinary, should be noted, since they may be important to the overall evaluation of the patient.

2. *Listening*

Listen actively. Active listening means that you are attempting to receive all of the information and messages the person being interviewed is giving. It is a way of encouraging a person to talk freely and with genuine feeling. By looking at the person, by turning your body toward him or her, and by showing appropriate facial expressions, you can demonstrate that you are paying attention in an undemanding, nonjudgmental way. Nonverbal movements or utterances can be used to let the patient know that you have heard his or her comments. A summary statement or other verbal comment can acknowledge your having heard the essence of the patient's message. Whenever possible, avoid writing while listening; notations can be made after the interview (Bernstein & Bernstein, 1985). If it is necessary to write comments on a form or complete a checklist, it is better to let the patient know that such notations must be made, make the notation, and then give full attention to the patient after making each notation (Benjamin, 1969).

Active listening means that you are watching, hearing, and physically reacting to what the patient is saying. Active listening is not possible if you are trying to compose the next words you are going to say while the patient is speaking.

Silences may feel uncomfortable to the novice interviewer, but are often valuable moments of the interview. Silent moments may indicate to the person being interviewed that you are genuinely interested in and actively listening to what he or she is saying. Silences may even let the patient know that there is time to express other concerns which affect the current situation. It is not necessary to fill every second of the interview with spoken words.

3. *Questioning*

If a checklist is to be completed, certain questions need to be asked in specific ways. If the objective is to obtain general background information and the patient's feelings about certain matters, it is better to use questions that cannot be answered by "yes," "no," or short answers. Open-ended questions are preferred (Bernstein & Bernstein, 1985). An open-ended question gives the patient an opportunity to answer as fully and honestly as desired. Following are some examples of open-ended questions (or statements, or even phrases), together with explanatory comments:

How do you feel about it? This can be answered with "Okay," but the words *how* and *feel*, in addition to appropriate interviewer behaviors, are likely to elicit a longer answer about the patient's feelings.

Will you fill me in on the background? This question is likely to give the patient the perception that you are interested in and need to know parts of the patient's background that are missing from current recorded information.

Will you please explain what you mean by that? This question lets the patient know that, rather than assume that you understand them, you prefer to have the patient clarify previous statements.

Please tell me about it. This request can be interpreted to mean that you are seeking any information about *it* that the patient wishes to relate. Such a request can be a way of learning what the patient feels is most significant about the topic being discussed.

Describe it in your own words. This statement gives the patient freedom to express thoughts in his or her own language. The expressions the patient uses in response, and the enthusiasm or lack of enthusiasm the patient shows, may demonstrate what is meaningful to the patient about what is being described.

For instance.... Occasionally a word, phrase, or utterance will encourage the patient to continue to express his or her thoughts and feelings.

Give me an example. This request can be used to allow the patient to clarify comments or descriptions.

Anything else? This question, together with a time for silence, allows the patient to express any additional thoughts and feelings he or she might have.

An interview is not a time for mutual exchange of information. Nor is it a time to ask questions to satisfy your curiosity. The person being interviewed may attempt to learn more about the interviewer. When this happens, the interviewer may answer briefly and refocus on the interview. Frequently, the interviewer will not want to answer a personal question. Such questions should be handled tactfully, so that the one being interviewed is not offended or embarrassed. A comment such as "This is your time, we can't take time now to talk about me" may suffice. Humor also may be helpful, but it needs to be used cautiously and thoughtfully. It is wise to reflect on the possible reasons that personal information is being requested.

4 *Language*

Use language that the person being interviewed will easily understand. A patient who has had prolonged or frequent treatment may have a good understanding of the professional jargon used at the particular setting. It is appropriate to speak to such a person using terminology employed by the staff. Another patient, however, may not be familiar with the meanings of the words common to practitioners. For example, instead of requesting a patient to "Flex your right shoulder," the interviewer could say, "Raise your right arm as if to touch the ceiling with your fingertips." Or the interviewer might demonstrate what is being requested. The purpose of each request for information must be kept in mind during an interview.

If it is important to obtain precise information, be clear about the patient's response. The patient may use relative terms such as "a little" or "sometimes." A better understanding can be obtained by requesting that the patient state a particular amount, of time, distance, or whatever. For example, the interviewer may ask, "When you say that you read a little, how many hours do you spend reading each day?" or "In the last five times when you have wanted to call your friend, how many times did you actually dial your friend's phone number?"

5. *The Patient's Behavior*

A patient may verbally express anxiety or show nonverbal signs of anxiety. Do not deny the anxiety or the need for it. Comments such as "You aren't afraid, are you?" or "There's nothing to be anxious about" devalue the patient's real feelings (Bernstein & Bernstein, 1985). It is usually helpful to recognize the patient's feelings with a comment such as "I can see that you are a bit uneasy. I hope you will feel more comfortable as we continue." Letting the patient know of any anxieties that you as an interviewer have are of little value, and, in general, the interviewer should avoid commenting on his or her own personal problems and feelings.

A patient may begin to cry during the interview. It is usually better to allow the patient to cry than to try to prevent him or her from crying. Make the patient as comfortable as possible, and remain silent and available. A condescending manner, such as patting the patient, or saying, "Oh, you don't have to cry," should be avoided. Such comments deny the value of the patient's feelings.

Patients may ask for advice during the interview. No matter how harmless the question seems, it is wise not to give advice. Rephrasing, such as "You are wondering whether to have the surgery?" may help clarify the intent of the patient. "I am sorry that I am not qualified to advise you on that," or "I cannot advise you, but I can tell the doctor of your concerns," may be helpful comments.

Patients sometimes become angry at the interviewer (Bernstein & Bernstein, 1985). Unless there is danger of direct physical attack, it is usually helpful to allow the verbal expression of anger. Keep in mind that the anger in most instances is not due to the interviewer. Challenging the angry patient with hostility and making threatening comments will usually make matters worse.

The interviewer should always be alert to potential physical harm. If the patient has a history of aggressive behavior, it should not be ignored. If there is such a history and an interview is scheduled, the interview should be conducted in a safe place, with escape routes planned and assistance available. Signs of aggression or running away (such as rapid breathing, darting looks, tense body movements, and perspiration) are indications that the interview should be terminated and assistance sought.

If a patient expresses values, biases, and behaviors that are intolerable, and your feelings are interfering with the goals of the interview, it is advisable to terminate the interview. If you cannot resolve your feelings, it may be wise to ask that the patient be referred to another staff person.

Patients sometimes make derogatory remarks about another staff person. Any such remark can be acknowledged without signifying agreement with it, and the patient can be redirected toward the interview. A matter-of-fact comment that may help to continue the interview is "It sounds as though you are annoyed with Mr. Smith right now. Would you like to talk to him now about what is bothering you, or may we complete our business first?"

A depressed patient usually has difficulty talking. He or she may sigh frequently. Do not pressure the patient for answers; the particular information can be obtained later. Any pressuring you put on the patient may increase his or her negative feelings. Any comments the patient makes about wishing to die or harm him- or herself should be accurately recorded and reported to the supervisor. When interviewing a mentally ill patient, the specific techniques advocated by the facility should be used. These techniques vary from allowing the patient to speak freely to refusing to listen to any comments the interviewer considers irrational. Appropriate information on the matter should be obtained from the supervisor prior to the interview.

SUMMARY

An interview is a planned meeting with a goal of obtaining specific information from a person or group of people. Many factors will influence the interview, from the patient's condition to the ages, life-styles, and values of both the patient and the interviewer. A comfortable and positive interview depends upon mutual understanding, trust, and respect.

REVIEW QUESTIONS

1. Define communication.
2. How does interviewing differ from conversing with a person.
3. a) Describe a person's body movement(s) and a simultaneous comment that would probably be incongruous. b) Describe a person's body movement(s) and a simultaneous comment that would probably be congruous.
4. What is active listening?
5. Describe nonverbal signs that often accompany active listening.
6. Give an example of a) an open-ended and b) a closed question.
7. Give appropriate actions for the interviewer to take when he or she is asked a personal question?
8. What actions should the interviewer take when the person being interviewed makes verbal threats of physical harm and begins clenching his or her fist, hyperventilating, and pacing?

ANSWERS

1. Giving and receiving information, signals, and messages.
2. Interviewing has a goal, usually has a time limit, and is a search for information. Conversations may or may not have any of these elements.
3. a) Avoidance of eye contact, eyes darting about the room, and a somber face while saying, "I like this place and really trust everyone here." b) A flushed face and tearful eyes while saying, "I am so upset with what I was told, that I don't know what to do or whom I can talk to."
4. Attending to a person's verbal and nonverbal messages, encouraging the person to communicate, and helping the person feel that the listener has been attentive by summarizing the message.
5. Eye contact, the body turned toward the speaker, arms relaxed, a facial expression showing interest without judgment or objection, and movements and utterances designed to encourage comments.
6. a) How did you feel about the lunch? This is an open-ended question that encourages the respondent to talk about any feelings he or she

had about the setting, food, or people, or indeed, any aspect of the lunch.

　　b) Did you enjoy your lunch? This can be answered with "yes" or "no" and is considered a closed question.

7. Answer the question if desired, and redirect questions toward the person being interviewed. The interviewer should tell the person that the question cannot be answered if the interviewer does not wish to answer a personal question.

8. Terminate the interview as calmly as possible. If the behavior has been anticipated, another person should be alerted to assist in the event of an emergency. If an attack cannot be prevented, the interviewer should do whatever is necessary for self-protection.

ADDITIONAL LEARNING ACTIVITIES

1. Interview a willing person about a specific topic—for example, his or her leisure interests, educational experiences, and special talents. After the interview, write down the smiles, frowns, signs of uneasiness, anger, or other nonverbal expressions you noted. When did these occur? Did you achieve your the goal of your interview?

2. Be interviewed. After the interview, write down the feelings you had during the interview. Did you have any feelings such as pride, pleasure, a desire for secrecy, anger, or distrust? What statements, questions, or nonverbal expressions caused these feelings?

3. Volunteer to role play an interview for your class when this topic is scheduled to be discussed. Discuss with your course instructor possible points to emphasize.

REFERENCES

　　Benjamin, A. (1969). *The helping interview.* Boston: Houghton Mifflin Company.

　　Bernstein, L., & Bernstein, R. S. (1985). *Interviewing: A guide for health professionals* (4th ed.). Norwalk, CT: Appleton-Century-Crofts.

8

REPORTS AND RECORDS

This chapter describes the purpose of patients' records and provides suggestions for recording data and writing reports. The problem-oriented reporting system is introduced.

LEARNING OBJECTIVES

At the end of this chapter, you should be able to:

1. Define the words *report, record,* and *document* in the context of occupational therapy.
2. State four main reasons for having records and reports in treating patients.
3. State five categories of information usually included in a patient's chart.
4. State four ways to make patients' reports more objective and clear.
5. St Explain the meaning of each letter of the acronym for problem-oriented report writing.
7. Given a descriptive paragraph, and identify words and phrases that describe facts.

A patient's complete medical treatment is generally recorded in the patient's chart. After the patient is discharged, the chart is usually retained in its original form in the medical records file for a given period of time. After the established period, determined by the administrators, the information is usually preserved on microfilm, on disk, or in some other form that conserves space and is easily retrievable.

CONTENTS OF PATIENTS' RECORDS

A patient's record will generally contain the following kinds of information:

1. *Identification.* At the time of admission, current information identifying the patient will be obtained from the patient or his or her family. The patient's name, age, sex, religious preference, marital status, address, educational background, and employment, as well as additional information, are recorded.
2. *Present Condition.* The patient's physical condition on admission will be recorded. This usually includes weight; height; physical appearance; orientation to time, place, and person; capabilities and disabilities in mobility; self-care capabilities; ability to communicate; and other functional skills.
3. *History.* If the patient has had prior medical care, related information usually is included in the patient's record. In some cases, however, such information cannot be obtained for a variety of reasons. The staff at the present facility would then question the patient and family to obtain as much information as possible. The social worker is usually the staff person who gathers the family, education, and work history.
4. *Medical Treatment.* The physician's evaluation, diagnosis, and treatment plan are recorded. Physicians' orders and nursing observations are usually found in this section of the patient's chart. Consultation reports and laboratory findings may be included in this section or placed on the back of the chart.
5. *Other Therapy.* The type of facility may determine the additional treatment provided the patient. Occupational, physical, recreational, respiratory, and speech therapy may be included in a patient's treatment plan in a rehabilitation hospital. In a general hospital, special cases may need those therapeutic methods. If the patient receives therapy, reports documenting it are in the patient's chart. Each therapeutic service record includes information identifying the patient, an evaluation of the patient's condition, a treatment plan with goals and methods if therapy is given, progress reports, and a discharge summary when therapy is discontinued.
6. *Legal and Financial Information.* The patient's record includes consent forms of various kinds—forms consenting to surgery or other special treatment, consenting to the occasion to be photographed or videotaped, and consenting to the occasion to be presented before an audience for educational purposes. The record also may include information on the patient's private possessions at the hospital, insurance, or financial status. Special legal forms and information may be included as well.

PURPOSE OF PATIENTS' RECORDS

The purpose of having patients' records is to preserve information, in as accurate a fashion as possible. Records serve four main purposes:

1. They assist in the efficient and effective treatment of a patient.
2. They assist in efficient management and control of the facility and various departments within it.
3. They provide data for research and information for the hospital.
4. They comply with legal regulations and substantiate or refute claims.

Patients' records provide a means for large numbers of people to give and obtain accurate information in a short amount of time. Whether large or small, facilities usually provide 24-hour care for patients. It is crucial for staff on all shifts to have access to information about patients in order to provide the communication that is essential for efficient and effective health care.

Records enable physicians to write orders for medication or other treatment, even though the person who will carry out the order is not present. The person who has carried out the order can record the completion and results of carrying it out. Staff can gather significant information quickly from the records. Recorded information enables the physician to review the effects of treatment, current treatment, and future plans with the patient and patient's family.

Research provides a means of determining the effects of treatment. Surveying patients' records for the results of a specific treatment may provide valuable information to improve medical care. Statistical information from records offers an insight into the causes of various problems and may aid in planning treatment. Trends, such as the lengths of stay for certain conditions, can be predicted by analyzing data from records.

Records serve as legal documents. They may be subpoenaed to evaluate a claim of wrongdoing or malpractice, or they may be used as evidence in claims for compensation or insurance coverage. Records may serve as evidence that the physician was ethical in his or her practice and that the best treatment possible was provided.

Records are considered the property of the facility. All information contained in them is privileged and is not to be circulated outside of the facility without permission.

REPORTS

A report is an abstract of a record. In a report, significant information is presented briefly, in written or oral form. *To report* means to give information about something observed or investigated. The purpose of a medical report is to disseminate information to a group of people who are concerned with the particular patient and his or her treatment.

Occupational therapy personnel report and record information about a patient's evaluation, treatment plan, treatment, progress, and discontinuation from treatment. It is important to present the information accurately, concisely, and in a readable and understandable manner.

RECORDING OBSERVATIONS

It may be difficult to determine the most important events in a treatment session because of the holistic nature of occupational therapy. The difficulty is compounded when patients are treated in a group. Then, the effect of their interactions, the accuracy of the observations concerning their treatment, and the practitioner's memory can all pose problems.

Observing patients as they are being treated in an occupational therapy session and then discussing the session with the therapist will help focus on important information to record. In general, the significant information will be related to treatment goals and objectives.

A good command of language and good writing ability are prerequisites to effective recording and reporting. Translating visual, auditory, and cognitive perceptions into written language on a few lines in a patient's chart for another person's understanding requires great skill.

Observations of an event should be recorded as soon as possible after the event has happened. Reports are generally written 1) after an evaluation or treatment, 2) for conferences with patients, or 3) when requested by professionals of other disciplines.

HOW TO WRITE RECORDS AND REPORTS

To write clear, cogent records and reports, one must do all of the following:

Learn the established procedures for the specific setting. If only black ink is to be used, use black ink. If reports are generated by computer, learn the particular program that is used. If errors are to be crossed out with a line through them and identified by the word *error* and the *writer's name* and *professional designation,* follow the procedure exactly. If the occupational therapy student or assistant needs to have a report countersigned by the occupational therapist, see that the required signature is on the report.

Sign and date all reports and records. The date and time are required whenever one signs a document. The term *signature* means a person's first and last name, followed by his or her professional designation.

Use commonly understood language and accepted professional terminology. Use the abbreviations, words, and phrases that are prevalent within the facility. Some facilities may not use terminology that is specific to occupational therapy. Some words that are used within a specific professional group may have little or no meaning to others. Use words that communicate your ideas clearly.

Organize information logically. The information in a report or record should be easily read and understood by the reader. Write the information in chronological order, order of importance, categories, or any other order that is logical. The facility may have an established format to follow.

Be concise. Limited staff time for reviewing written reports and limited writing space on the patient's chart require clear, concise statements. Of course, meaning should not be sacrificed for brevity, but most facilities use common abbreviations and shortened professional phrases and language for efficiency.

Categorize information. Relate the patient's performance to the stated goals. Any activities used can be categorized rather than named. Describe activities as structured when the objective of treatment is for a patient to organize items—say, to prepare a meal. Describe activities as expressive when the objective of treatment is for the patient to express his or her feelings verbally.

Write reports and records on a systematic schedule. In rehabilitation centers and hospitals, treatments are usually recorded on the patient's chart immediately following a session. In long-term care programs, treatment and progress are summarized after a given number of days, weeks, or months. In such situations, it is important to record information in a separate file until summarizing it in the patient's record. Relying on memory is more likely to result in inaccuracy and the omission of importan

Be factual and objective. Phrases such as "seems to be" and "for some time" should be avoided because they reflect the writer's perception without providing factual information. Documenting information objectively and quantitatively is essential (Dunn, 1973).

RECORDING OBSERVATIONS OBJECTIVELY

To record observations in an objective manner, one must adhere to the following guidelines:

Describe behaviors in observable terms. Descriptions are frequently stated in terms of the observer's interpretation, rather than in terms of what was actually observed. Interpretations depend upon the observer's past experiences, expectations, and value system. If there is need to include the observer's interpretation, the reason should be stated. Words such as "lacked interest" and "was frustrated" describe the observer's interpretation of events. Words such as "He sat with head down and did not speak" and "After making an error, she threw her project across the table" describe the observed behavior without judgment or interpretation.

Describe the situation in which the behavior occurred. Behavior is the patient's response to environmental stimuli. Analyzing a given behavior is aided by having as complete as possible a description of the events and environment associated with that behavior.

Describe what happened, rather than what did not happen. Never report behavior in terms of what the patient did not do. A statement such as "Pat did not eat most of his lunch" is probably trying to describe a mealtime problem. "Pat ate two bites of mashed potatoes for lunch" gives a clearer picture of the patient's food intake. Additional specific information would aid in analyzing the problem and perhaps suggest the need for changes in the food, consistency of the food, setting, or other factors associated with the meal.

Describe behavior in terms of frequency, rate, or duration. Most behaviors can be described in numbers, which are less likely to be misinterpreted than are qualitative descriptions. For example, how frequently does the behavior occur? We might respond with "Tom voluntarily lifted his head three times during the 15-minute period." At what rate does the behavior occur? "Jim placed 10 pegs in the peg board in a 15-minute period." How long did the behavior last? "Jan voluntarily remained in her chair for the first 10 minutes of a 30-minute session."

Begin each statement with an action verb. Eliminate unnecessary words to save time. As long as the patient's name appears on the report form, the name need not be repeated in each recorded observation. For example, the statements in the previous paragraph can be condensed by using an action verb and omitting certain words: "Lifted head voluntarily three times in 15 minutes"; "Placed 10 pegs in peg board in 15 minutes"; "Remained in chair voluntarily for first 10 minutes of a 30-minute session." These statements give a clear picture of the observed behavior, although they are not complete sentences. They can be condensed further by using abbreviations and commonly used symbols, such as *min* in place of *minutes* and *3x's* in place of *three times.*

Use a direct style of writing. All words used in an observational report should have meaning. Provide factual information as clearly and thoroughly as possible. Omit unnecessary words. The aim of recording observations is to give the reader a clear picture of the patient's behavior during the observation period and to preserve the information obtained. The aim is not to guess why the behavior occurred or predict what will occur.

Record as soon as possible after observing. Generally, forms for recording observations will be available. When a number of tasks are requested of a patient or a number of patients are evaluated, memory is unreliable.

PROBLEM-ORIENTED RECORDS

Facilities differ in recording style and method. The Problem-Oriented Medical Record system, developed by Weed (1971) for use in psychiatric hospitals, has been effective in other treatment settings. This logical and sequential system of recording patient care documents problems identified by the patient and the care givers, plans to resolve problems, and the results of treatment. The system focuses on the actual needs of patients and develops logical patterns of thinking (Kuntavanish, 1987).

The key elements of the problem-oriented record are:

1. The data base
2. The problem list
3. The plans
4. The progress notes

The data base includes all of the background information known about the patient upon his or her entering the facility. The information is gathered from interviews with the patient and family and from evaluations and examinations by physicians, nurses, and others.

The problem list, which is developed from the data base, contains anything of concern to the patient and to the staff from whom the patient seeks help. Problems may be medical, psychological, socioeconomic, or demographic, as well as active or inactive. Each problem is assigned a number, not necessarily in order of importance. The list of problems with assigned numbers is kept at the front of the patient's chart. Any problem can then be cited or recorded by referring to its number, rather than writing it out, thus shortening the time for making entries in the patient's chart. After certain problems are successfully treated, any remaining ones retain their original numbers, thereby maintaining efficient and effective communication and documentation.

A plan of intervention is formulated for each problem identified. The plan includes means of gathering more information, details the treatment of problems, and indicates how the patient will be taught to deal with the problems. All plans are charted on the same sheet, regardless of the specific discipline. All are dated, titled, numbered, and signed. Plans are periodically reviewed and updated.

Various staff members record their progress notes chronologically on the same sheet. The progress notes are dated, numbered, and titled to correspond with the problem list and then are signed.

Progress notes contain subjective impressions, objective measures, assessments, and plans (SOAP). The acronym helps to remember essential parts of a progress report. Subjective impressions include the patient's view of himself or herself relative to the patient's feelings, abilities and disabilities, past and current goals, relationship to others, place in the community and at work, and socioeconomic status. Objective measures include the diagnosis, the results of the evaluation, what the patient does in treatment, and what is done to the patient in treatment. Assessments are the professional judgments made about the subjective and objective data collected. The patient's strengths, deficits, motivation, priorities, primary and secondary concerns, and short- and long-term goals are included. The plan is a plan of action to achieve the patient's goals based on the assessment. It can include the need for further evaluation or the need to contact the family for more information. The plan should give an estimate as to when the goals will be achieved and should be documented for the record and the third-party payer.

When the patient's goals have been achieved, a reassessment, discharge summary, and follow-up plan of care are included in the progress notes.

Among the advantages of the problem-oriented record are the following:

1. *Improved communication.* All disciplines have access to plans and treatment results of other disciplines. Significant information is recorded immediately and chronologically.
2. *Documentation.* A document is anything written or printed to record or prove something. Documentation of services is required for insurance coverage, reimbursement by agencies, licensure requirements, and other legal and financial reasons. The problem-oriented record is a thorough, concise system of documenting service provided.
3. *Identification and measurement of goals.* The problem-oriented record system helps staff identify treatment goals and logically plan treatment methods. The sequential reporting system enables staff members to review and evaluate the effectiveness of treatment methods as frequently as they need to.
4. *Establishing treatment priorities.* Establishing a problem list enables the team of care givers to analyze the patient's problems logically, develop priorities, and plan a holistic treatment program.

The problem-oriented system of recording patients' treatment regimens provides a review of any treatment that is in progress. Problems can be noted and corrected quickly. The patient's performance is communicated objectively by the staff and subjectively by the patient. The system meets professional standards of practice, provides objective data to measure a facility's quality of care, and assists in obtaining proper reimbursement for services. The documentation system provides users with an effective means of communication, makes them accountable for their performance, and educates them through continued feedback on the patient's response to the intervention they are using.

SUMMARY

Records are maintained to preserve events in a permanent form. Patients' records assist in efficient treatment and efficient management of the facility. They also provide information for research, hospital reports, and legal use. Records should be written in a clear and concise manner. The Problem-Oriented Medical Record system is a frequently used method of recording observations in many treatment settings.

REVIEW QUESTIONS

1. Explain the difference between a record, a report, and a document.
2. List four reasons why patient treatment records are needed.
3. Name the categories of information usually included in a patient's chart.
4. What are four ways to write objectively?
5. State six basic guidelines for recording observations.
6. What do the letters SOAP mean in problem-oriented records?
7. In each of the following student observation reports, underline the words and phrases that give objective information in terms of frequency, rate, or duration:
   1) Felt sick but felt better later. Worked on necklace for wife. Very good worker. Worried about others watching. Talked to another patient 10 minutes.
   2) Eager to work on project, but at first, when she got stuck, she didn't call until a couple of times. Then she started calling for help. Worked until project was completed. Very quiet and cheerful for the half-hour session.
   3) Fooling around at first. Then got project done with three stitches in 20 minutes and quit. Got depressed talking about marriage because of her husband's death.
   4) Didn't settle down, paced, came in and took some pretzels. Kept coming in and out. Didn't say very much.
8. For an extra exercise in report writing, rewrite the following notes to state what was probably meant. The notes are said to have been actual notes written by nurses, therapists, and physicians.
   1) The left leg became numb at times, and she walked it off.
   2) On the third day the knee was better, and on the fourth day it had completely disappeared.
   3) By the time she was admitted to the hospital, her rapid heart had stopped and she was feeling much better.
   4) Coming from Detroit, Michigan, this man has no children.

ANSWERS

1. A record is a factual statement of events, usually written or maintained in some permanent manner. A report is an abstract or summary of events or occurrences for the purpose of communicating the infor-

mation to others. A document is anything written, printed, or preserved in a permanent manner that is used for future viewing or to prove something. Records and reports can be used as documents.

2. Patient treatment records are needed:
   1) To assist in efficient and effective treatment of patients.
   2) To provide data for research or special projects.
   3) To assist in efficient management of the facility.
   4) To comply with the law or substantiate claims.
   5) To measure the quality of services provided.

3. Charts include information that identifies the patient and his or her present condition, history, and medical treatment, lists other therapies the patient has had, and present legal and financial information about the patient.

4. Observations will be written more objectively if:
   1) They are described in observational rather than interpretive terms.
   2) The situation in which the observation was made is described.
   3) What happened, instead of what did not happen, is described.
   4) They are described in terms of frequency, rate, or duration.

5. Guidelines for recording observations are:
   1) Always sign and date reports and records.
   2) Use commonly understood language.
   3) Organize information in a logical manner.
   4) Write concisely.
   5) Categorize information.
   6) Write reports and record observations on a systematic schedule.

6. The letters SOAP mean:
   S = subjective—the patient's views and information on symptoms.
   O = objective—includes data from tests and examinations.
   A = assessment—includes evaluations and interpretations of objective and subjective information.
   P = plan—includes plans and methods for treating the patient, plus an estimated date for achieving the stated goals.

7. The objective words and phrases are:
   1) 10 minutes (duration).
   2) half-hour (duration).
   3) three stitches in 20 minutes (frequency).
   4) No objective information is given.

8. The notes probably are more accurately written as follows:
   1) The occasional numbness in her left leg disappears when she walks.
   2) The problem with the knee was not evident on the fourth day following the complaint.
   3) After the patient was admitted to the hospital, her heartbeat was normal, and she reported feeling better.
   4) The patient resides in Detroit, MI. He has no children.

REFERENCES

Dunn, D. J. (1973). Recording observations. *Consumer Brief, 1*(1), 4-6.

Kuntavanish, A. A. (1987). *Occupational therapy documentation: A system to capture outcome data for quality assurance and program promotion.* Bethesda, MD: American Occupational Therapy Association, Inc.

Weed, L. L. (1971). *Medical records, medical educations, and patient care.* Chicago: Year Book Medical Publishers.

SUGGESTED READINGS

Gilandas, A. J. (1972). The problem-oriented record in a psychiatric hospital. *Hospital and Community Psychiatry, 23*(11), 336-339.

Llorens, L. A. (1982). *Occupational therapy sequential client care record manual.* Laurel, MD: RAMSCO.

Potts, L. R. (1972). The problem-oriented record: Implications for occupational therapy. *American Journal of Occupational Therapy, 26*(6), 288-291.

9

EVALUATION

This chapter explains and diagrams the sequence of events beginning with referring a patient for occupational therapy and ending with discharging the patient after treatment. Areas of occupational therapy evaluation and types of evaluations used are introduced.

LEARNING OBJECTIVES

At the end of this chapter, you should be able to:

1. Give a general explanation of evaluation, screening, assessment, and reassessment.
2. Explain, with words or a diagram, the actions taken by occupational therapy personnel when a patient is referred for therapy.
3. State at least one basic difference between a standardized and nonstandardized test.
4. Explain what is meant by clinical assessments and discuss their value in occupational therapy.
5. State the names of the following assessments, and give the general purpose of each: DDST, SIPT, MMT, JROMT, and TVMS.

In occupational therapy, *evaluation* refers to the process of determining whether or not a patient needs occupational therapy intervention. If a decision is made that intervention is needed, evaluation includes estimating the amount of time the patient will be treated, as well as estimating the level of personnel and coordination of the intervention process. Evaluation includes gathering information through skilled observation, interviews, reviews of records, and tests (both standardized and criterion referenced) and, subsequently, documenting all evaluation activities and findings. Undergoing evaluation is a prerequisite to treatment (AOTA, 1994b).

Figure 9.1 shows the steps a therapist takes after a patient is referred for occupational therapy. Evaluations accompany these steps throughout the entire process. A brief explanation of each step follows the figure.

FIGURE 9.1

FLOW CHART FOR OCCUPATIONAL THERAPY REFERRAL TO DISCHARGE

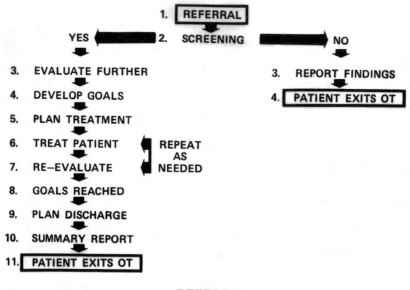

REFERRAL

When the patient's primary reason for treatment with occupational therapy is medical or psychiatric, referrals are usually made by the patient's medical doctor or psychiatrist. When an individual is under 22 years of age and the primary need is special education, the student's teacher is usually the person making the referral. In some situations, a treatment team or the patient him- or herself may make the decision to be referred for occupational therapy.

To *make a referral* means to direct a request for service to someone or something, or to direct a request for a change in a service already being provided by someone or something. A referral is usually, but not always, made in writing. Most hospitals and agencies have their own referral forms with appropriate identification. An oral, person-to-person or telephone referral is sometimes made to expedite the process. Oral referrals are followed by a written referral. Occasionally, a certified occupational therapy assistant (COTA) may receive an oral referral. In some settings, the COTA may have the responsibility for acknowledging a referral and conducting a screening, whether the referral is written or oral. The COTA should follow the procedure used in the specific setting. The supervising occupational therapist (OTR) should be informed of all referrals. Occupational therapy practitioners must follow the requirements of the federal, state, and local governmental agencies, third-party payors, and all regulatory agencies affecting referrals for health care (AOTA, 1994a).

All referrals must be acknowledged and processed, and a response returned to the originator of the referral. The response is usually a report that includes the results of a screening and the OTR's recommendations.

SCREENING

Screening includes the various activities used to gather general information about the patient's current physical and psychosocial status and needs. The aim is to make an early decision about the potential value of occupational therapy for the patient. Information may be gathered from a screening test, interviews with and observations of the patient, a staff conference at which new patients are discussed, a review of the patient's record, or a combination of these.

If screening indicates that occupational therapy will not be of value to the patient, a report is written setting forth the findings and stating why occupational therapy is not recommended. If screening indicates that occupational therapy may be of value to the patient, a report is written setting forth the findings and stating recommendations for further assessment and the expectations of treatment.

ASSESSMENT

Assessment includes the tests and procedures used to gather information to identify the specific performance components and contexts that create dysfunction in the patient. The information is essential in planning a treatment program that is individualized for each patient. The specific tests and procedures selected will depend upon the patient's existing sensorimotor, cognitive, psychosocial, and psychological condition, his or her chronological and developmental age, and the environmental factors, including the physical, social, and cultural aspects of the environment, that influence the individual's performance. Assessment may include additional or detailed discussions with the patient, significant staff, and family members, a review of the patient's history, and the administration of specific tests. The findings garnered from the assessment are documented and, usually, discussed formally and informally with the members of the treatment team.

TREATMENT GOALS

Treatment goals are formulated following assessment. The patient's subjective view of his or her problems and needs, in addition to the objective test results, are considered when developing treatment goals. The treatment goals will be affected by the patient's age, mental status, cognitive ability, language ability, work environment if the patient is employed, family situation, life-style, and other environmental factors affecting the patient's daily living routine.

Treatment goals are planned specifically for each patient. They will generally be similar for patients with the same injury or condition, but rarely will they be exactly the same.

Treatment goals may be referred to as either long term or short term. Long-term goals are the final goals desired. Short-term goals are the more immediate goals needed to reach the final, long-term goals.

Short-term goals are also referred to as treatment objectives. In most treatment plans, the objectives or short-term goals are the abilities, achieved sequentially, needed to reach the long-term goals.

TREATMENT PLAN

The treatment program is planned in such manner as to establish guidelines for achieving the goals formulated. The treatment plan is subject to change. Treatment plans should outline methods and target dates for achieving specific goals. If the goals are not achieved at the expected times, a review of the plan may indicate a need to alter its methods, target dates, or even goals.

The following considerations are taken into account in planning the treatment program (the student is referred to sample treatment plans in other texts (Linder, 1993; Pedretti & Zoltan, 1990)):

1. *Priority of goals.* What are the patient's goals? Which goals need to be achieved first? Will the achievement of goals in occupational therapy depend upon the patient's progress in other therapies?
2. *Target dates.* Are the target dates for achieving the goals realistic?
3. *Methods.* What techniques and methods will be used? Will these methods be compatible with those used by other disciplines? If a special technique or method is to be used, have all the team members been informed of it? Do all the team members agree with or understand the reason for the technique?
4. *Schedule.* What is the patient's current schedule? When is the patient available to be scheduled for occupational therapy? When is the therapist free to treat the patient? Will schedules need to be adjusted? If so, is it possible to adjust them? Which professionals in other disciplines need to be consulted?
5. *Staff.* Who has the special skills needed to treat the patient? Is the person available at the time the patient is scheduled for treatment? If

the primary therapist or assistant is unavailable, will another staff member provide treatment, or will the treatment be canceled?

6. *Supplies, equipment, and space.* Where will the patient be treated? Will space be available at the time it is needed? Will necessary equipment and supplies be available at the time of the scheduled treatment? Is it possible to obtain additional or new equipment if needed?

TREATMENT

Treatment (i.e., intervention) usually results in changes in the patient. In some treatment procedures, formal assessments are part of each session. For example, when a patient has a limited range of motion in a joint, the range of motion of that joint may be measured at the beginning of the treatment session and again at the end of the session. In that way, both the effects of the treatment in a given session and the effects over the entire series of treatments can be measured.

In another situation, informal observation of changes in the patient's condition may indicate a need for a formal reassessment. The latter may then reveal a need to begin a new phase of the treatment, to begin a different kind of treatment, or even to discontinue treatment.

In some cases, unexpected changes occur. In other cases, changes do not occur as expected. Both situations indicate a need for reassessment. The reassessment may then reveal a need to add, delete, or alter the goals and methods of treatment. In some cases, target dates may need to be changed. The reassessment and treatment continue alternately as many times as needed until some formal set of goals is achieved.

ACHIEVEMENT OF GOALS

Ideally, all goals will be achieved before the patient is discharged, enabling the patient to function optimally upon leaving the setting. In practice, however, the ideal is rarely attained. Instead, the patient is discharged from the hospital as soon as possible.

Discharge may be to a subacute facility, to the patient's home with home care service, or to some other setting, even though the final desired goal has not been reached. In some cases, a reassessment may result in a change from the original final goal, so that a new final set of goals is actually achieved.

DISCHARGE PLAN

The patient's discharge from the treatment facility is under consideration from the time of admission. The patient's ability to function as independently as possible after discharge is a prime consideration in occupational therapy.

Formal discharge planning begins as progress toward the final goals is observed. The discharge plan may be to return the patient to the former home situation or to return the patient to another treatment facility. The plan considers those aspects of the patient's daily life that were affected by the problem and that required treatment.

The following factors are considered, whether the problem is physical or psychosocial:

1. *Living arrangement.* If the patient has physical limitations, can he or she compensate for them and manage independently? Do architectural barriers need to be removed? Are family members or others available for assistance? If the patient has psychosocial limitations, is there a need for supervision? Is supervision available? Can the patient function safely without harm to him- or herself or others?
2. *Mobility.* Is the patient independently mobile? Is the patient able to manage the equipment he or she needs? Does the patient know where to get help in the community?
3. *Self-care.* Can the patient dress, eat, bathe, and perform other self-care activities independently? If not, can arrangements be made for assistance?
4. *Work.* Does the patient have adequate work skills to return to his or her previous job? Does the patient need retraining? If so, has the patient been referred to the proper agency?
5. *Treatment.* Is additional treatment necessary? If so, can the patient get to the treatment facility? If exercise or special activities need to be done at home, does the patient have instructions and know how to do the activities? If special equipment is needed, does the patient know how to care for and use the equipment?

EXIT FROM OCCUPATIONAL THERAPY

In some cases, the patient is discharged from occupational therapy before being discharged from the facility. In other cases, occupational therapy plays a major role in determining the patient's discharge plan from the facility. For example, occupational therapy personnel may evaluate the patient's home and recommend changes to make it safe, such as removing scatter rugs and thresholds in doorways or installing grab bars in the bathroom. Or the patient and therapist together may decide that architectural remodeling should be done. Whatever the future occupational therapy needs may be, when the goals that were established at the setting are reached, the patient is discharged from the occupational therapy provided by that setting.

OCCUPATIONAL THERAPY EVALUATION

Occupational therapy evaluation is an attempt to judge the patient's ability to function as he or she needs or desires in activities of daily living, work and productive activities, and leisure or play activities.

Activities of daily living include basic activities such as grooming, oral hygiene, bathing, eating, dressing, managing medication, and managing devices needed to maintain health, as well as activities that require interaction with the larger society and environment. Socialization, functional mobility, and communication are included in activities of daily living.

Work and productive activities include those tasks done to care for the place of residence or to care for other persons, in the place of employment, in school, or in the community.

Leisure and play activities include recognizing the need for leisure and recreation, finding personnel and community resources to meet one's leisure needs, and selecting and performing appropriate activities to meet leisure-time needs.

The ability to function in activities of daily living, work and productive activities, and leisure or play activities requires an integration of the sensorimotor, cognitive, psychosocial, and psychological components of the specific activities within the temporal and environmental context in which the activities are performed.

Dysfunction in sensorimotor skills may require testing the patient's ability in many areas, such as the processing of tactile, vestibular, and other sensory input, as well as perceptual processing, including stereognosis, response to pain, and right-left discrimination. Physical dysfunction may require testing the patient's neuromusculoskeletal orientation, such as the range of motion of the joints, muscle strength, and reflexes, as well as the motor abilities of gross- and fine-motor coordination, bilateral integration, and other abilities. The patient's cognitive status, including his or her orientation to time, place, and person, ability to comprehend and communicate information, and other relevant cognitive skills, is evaluated. Among the patient's psychosocial skills and psychological components that are considered in evaluation are the patient's values, interests, self-concept, role performance, social conduct, interpersonal skills, self-expression, and self-management skills of coping, managing time, and self-control. The "Uniform terminology for occupational therapy—third edition" (AOTA, 1994c) provides complete information on the performance areas, components, and contexts that are evaluated before planning occupational therapy intervention.

METHODS OF OCCUPATIONAL THERAPY EVALUATION

Evaluation is the process of gathering data or significant information related to the patient's condition and determining the patient's abilities to perform necessary activities. Information may be gathered from the following sources:

1. *Medical record.* The medical record provides information about the patient's diagnosis, medical and other previous treatments, current condition, social and employment background, and educational history, as well as the patient's age, address, and other kinds of information. It is helpful to have information from the medical record before seeing the patient, but the information may not be available before the scheduled evaluation.
2. *Patient interview.* The interview with the patient provides an opportunity to establish rapport and a feeling of mutual trust. The therapist or assistant should explain the purpose of the interview and the need for recording information. The initial interview may provide information on how the patient views his or her present condition, problems, and future goals. However, the patient may not be ready to reveal any feelings or answer questions completely during the initial interview and should not be pressured to do so.
3. *Clinical observation.* Skilled observations provide valuable information. Many formal evaluations do not reveal the patient's response in a low-anxiety, normal setting. The patient may respond as he or she believes a patient should respond. Anxieties, attitudes, and other feelings may be revealed by facial expressions, hand gestures, and other nonverbal expressions. An experienced observer can gather valuable information on the patient's neuromuscular status and other physical and psychosocial conditions. Many of the performance skills of concern to occupational therapy personnel can be evaluated only by clinical observation. These performance skills include, but are not limited to, the ability to dress, eat, bathe, brush one's teeth, shave, and manipulate objects. The patient's equilibrium reactions and ability to move about with or without a wheelchair, walker, or cane also need to be evaluated by clinical observation. Information about all these skills and abilities that is obtained from close family members may be accurate in many cases, but more often, information that an occupational therapy practitioner gains from clinical observation is missing from secondhand reports.

Formal assessments of muscle strength, motion of the joints, response to sensations, and other physical attributes make use of instruments that give quantified measures. Examples of such instruments are the goniometer, for measuring the range of motion of joints; the dynamometer, for

measuring the strength of the grip; the Purdue pegboard test, for measuring dexterity; and the work simulator by Baltimore Therapeutic Equipment, which tests a person's upper extremity functioning using simulated work motions. Although these instruments give quantified measures, clinical observation of how the patient is using the body, how the
patient is feeling, and other factors are an important part of the assessment. Clinical observation in evaluations of physical dysfunction are
described in detail in other texts (Hislop & Montgomery, 1995; Pedretti &
Zoltan, 1990). Research suggests that some standardized occupational
therapy assessments fail to provide sufficient information to plan appropriate intervention programs and that clinical assessments may provide
the information needed (Settle & Holm, 1993).

Standardized tests

Standardized tests are tests that have been given to large numbers of
individuals to establish responses that are said to occur within a normal
range. To standardize tests, the same test is given to large numbers of
people. The same predetermined test items are administered to the sample
population in the same way. Giving the tests in the same way to large
numbers of people within a particular age range provides information
from which expectations can be established. For example, the test may
be to draw a triangle. After thousands of children between 3 and 10 years
old have been observed drawing a triangle under the exact same conditions, it can be established that the ability to draw a triangle generally
has developed by age 5 years. It can then be said that the normal age at
which the ability to draw a triangle should be present has been established for a given group of children. Standardized tests are those that
have established normative data.

Standardized tests require a period of training and testing for proficiency. Some standardized tests, such as the Sensory Integration and Praxis
Test (SIPT), are administered only by individuals certified to do so. The
SIPT requires the evaluator to have a background in tests and measurements in order to reliably evaluate and analyze the information obtained.
Ayres (1989) included a clinical evaluation procedure in combination with
the SIPT (Fisher, Murray, & Bundy, 1991).

One must exercise caution with standardized tests. For example, one
should realize that the normative data have been established only for
that group on which the test was standardized. As a case in point, the
Denver Developmental Screening Test (DDST; Frankenburg, Goldstein,
& Camp, 1971) was first standardized on children aged 2 weeks to 6.4
years and born to middle-class parents in Denver, Colorado. The aim of
the test was to establish normative data on development in areas of personal, social, fine-motor adaptive, language, and gross-motor skills. Ad-

ditional information was obtained later, and the test was revised and standardized for children of other regions and cultural backgrounds.

In a second case, the Southern California Sensory Integration Test (SCSIT) battery (Ayres, 1980) was first standardized on children in specific schools and care centers in Southern California in order to establish normative data on perceptual motor skills, later described as the ability to integrate and make appropriate use of sensory input and make an appropriate motor response. Ayres's intent in standardizing the test was to evaluate and correct sensorimotor and learning dysfunctions. Researchers administered two of the subtests to 98 children who were born in Japan and lived in Japan at least 1 year and to 82 children who were of Japanese descent and were born in America. The scores were compared with those of American children. The scores of the children born in Japan were highest, followed by the scores of the children of Japanese descent, and the American children's scores were the lowest (Saeki, Clark, & Azen, 1985). This research is cited here to point out that even standardized tests do not necessarily provide exact normative measures. Scores that place an individual outside the normal range on a given test may not be significant, even though the test is standardized. Knowing the population upon which the test was standardized may help the examiner decide whether or not the test is appropriate for the person being evaluated.

A second caution to observe is that the value of standardized test results depends upon the administrator of the test. Thus, the person using the test should be adequately trained to administer it and to evaluate the results.

The SCSIT, later revised and called the Sensory Integration and Praxis Test (SIPT), the Wechsler Intelligence Scale for Children (WISC), and the Gesell Developmental Examination are examples of standardized tests that require administration by skilled, certified examiners. Standardized tests can be used by COTAs who have been trained to administer them. The supervising OTR is responsible for verifying the proficiency of the COTA to administer any tests and procedures used to assess patients.

Nonstandardized tests

Nonstandardized tests used by occupational therapy personnel are formal evaluations with specific procedures for their administration. The manual muscle test, abbreviated MMT, is a traditional nonstandardized test generally used by therapists to measure muscle strength (Pedretti & Zoltan, 1990).

The results of the MMT are reported as zero, trace, poor, fair, good, and normal. Except for zero, which means that there is no muscle contraction at all, the results are reported in relative measures. Two people may be judged to have normal muscle grade, yet their muscle strengths, as measured by the MMT, may or may not be equal.

The MMT gives valuable information that may be used in planning treatment and in intervention. Other nonstandardized evaluations used in occupational therapy are the joint range-of-motion test (JROMT), eye-hand coordination tests, sensory tests, function tests, tests of feelings, and tests of leisure-time interest. The value of these evaluations is dependent upon the knowledge and observation skills of the examiner.

As computerized instruments that accurately record muscle strength and range of motion of the joints become affordable for most practice settings, tests such as the MMT will become obsolete, even for screening.

As with standardized tests, the supervising OTR is responsible for verifying the proficiency of the COTA to administer any nonstandardized procedures used to assess patients.

THE ASSISTANT'S ROLE

Both state licensure regulations and the supervising OTR determine how the COTA will assist in evaluation. The experienced COTA's responsibilities in evaluation vary from setting to setting and within settings. The COTA may be responsible for gathering data from medical records, interviewing the patient and significant family and staff members, and independently assessing the interests, activities of daily living, work and productive skills, and leisure and play skills of the patient. The experienced COTA may be trained to administer some clinical and standardized assessments, such as dressing and grooming skills and the JROMT, sensory test, DDST, and other tests. In some settings, the OTR administers all the assessments. A COTA who administers tests is considered competent to do so by the supervising OTR, since the OTR is responsible for the results of all assessments.

The variations in the COTA's responsibilities depend upon the knowledge, attitudes, and experiential background of the COTA and the OTR, the prevailing rules and regulations of the setting, the agency, and the state, and, finally, the sources of funding of the agency.

SUMMARY

The COTA assists in assessment and reassessment of the patient from the first referral to discharge. There are a number of commonly used assessment methods, and the COTA must exercise caution in using them. The background and attitude of the COTA and the supervising OTR, as well as current state regulations affecting funding and health care greatly influence the COTA's role in the evaluation process.

REVIEW QUESTIONS

1. Explain the words *evaluation, screening, assessment,* and *reassessment.*

2. Number each item so that they will be in proper sequence.

_____ Screen   _____ Treat

_____ Referral   _____ Plan Treatment

_____ Evaluate   _____ Patient Exits OT

_____ Develop Goals   _____ Discharge Summary

Circle the correct answer to complete the next two statements.

3. (1) A standardized test is a test
   a. used only by psychologists and OTRs.
   b. using standard, normal test items.
   c. having normative data.
   d. giving accurate information.
   e. to measure normal intelligence.
   (2) A nonstandardized test
   a. can be given by anyone.
   b. is the manual muscle test.
   c. does not require any use of language.
   d. uses normal test items.
   e. is the DDST.
4. What are clinical assessments, and why are they of value? Give some examples of results of clinical assessments.
5. Spell out the following abbreviations in full: DDST, SIPT, MMT, JROMT.

ANSWERS

1. *Evaluation* is the entire process of gathering information about a patient to determine whether or not the patient will benefit from occupational therapy. If intervention is to be provided, the process includes further evaluations and procedures beyond the initial screening to plan a treatment program. *Screening* is usually the initial step following a referral of a patient for occupational therapy. It is used to gather general information to determine whether or not occupational therapy is warranted for that patient. *Assessment* is the process of gathering detailed information about the patient and his or her problem. *Reasessment* measures a patient's progress or lack of progress, in order to determine whether treatment should continue, whether it should change direction, or whether the goals of therapy should be modified.

2.

2	6
1	5
3	7
4	8

3. (1) c; (2) b.
4. Clinical assessments are observations of a patient's abilities and dis-abilities made by practitioners. Information such as the patient's feelings, quality of movements, behavior, and motivation that is at present impossible or difficult to measure by specific tests are important for planning treatment. Among the results that may be found upon administering a clinical assessment are the substitution of one set of muscles for another when making a requested movement; visible difficulty or pain (which may or may not be verbally expressed) upon attempting to make a requested movement; observable problems with dressing, eating, and performing other activities of daily living; and other behaviors and attitudes that cannot be measured except by observation. Clinical assessments are of value because substitution of one set of muscles for another in order to perform movements, unsatisfactory quality of movements, inappropriate behavior, or lack of motivation have a bearing on treatment goals and whether a patient will return to his or her former role in society. Yet these observations, made clinically, may not be reflected in test results that objectively measure performance.
5. Denver Developmental Screening Test, Sensory Integration and Praxis Test, Manual Muscle Test, joint range-of-motion test.

ADDITIONAL LEARNING ACTIVITIES

1. Check the campus library, and review available assessments.
2. Visit some occupational therapy programs, and find out what kinds of evaluations are used in specific settings. Ask why those particular assessments are preferred.
3. Ask practicing COTAs what their responsibilities are in evaluating patients. Do they assist OTRs during evaluations? Do they perform any evaluation procedures independently? Do they analyze and record any of the results independently? At what stage of the patient's treatment does the COTA have a greater role in the evaluation?

REFERENCES

American Occupational Therapy Association, Inc. (1994a). Statement of occupational therapy referral. *American Journal of Occupational Therapy, 48*(11), 1034.

American Occupational Therapy Association, Inc. (1994b). Standards of practice in occupational therapy. *American Journal of Occupational Therapy, 48*(11), 1039-1043.

American Occupational Therapy Association. (1994c). Uniform terminology for occupational therapy—third edition. *American Journal of Occupational Therapy, 48*(11, 1047-1054.

Ayres, A. J. (1980). *Sensory integration test manual* (rev. ed.). Los Angeles, CA: Western Psychological Service.

Ayres, A. J. (1989). *Sensory integration and praxis tests.* Los Angeles: Western Psychological Services.

Fisher, A. G., Murray, E. A., & Bundy, A. C. (1991). *Sensory integration: Theory and practice.* Philadelphia: F. A. Davis Company.

Frankenburg, W. K., Goldstein, A. D., & Camp, B. W. (1971). The revised Denver Developmental Screening Test: Its accuracy as a screening instrument. *Journal of Pediatrics, 79,* 988-995.

Hislop, H. J., & Montgomery, J. (1995). *Daniels and Worthingham's Muscle Testing: Techniques of manual examination* (6th ed.). Philadelphia: W. B. Saunders Company.

Linder, T. W. (1993). *Transdisciplinary play-based intervention: Guidelines for developing a meaningful curriculum for young children.* Baltimore: Paul H. Brookes Publishing Co.

Pedretti, L.W., & Zoltan, B. (1990). *Occupational therapy: Practice skills for physical dysfunction* (3rd ed.). St. Louis: The C.V. Mosby Co.

Saeki, K., Clark, F. A., & Azen, S. P. (1985). Performance of Japanese and Japanese-American children on the Motor Accuracy-revised and Design Copying tests of the Southern California Sensory Integration Tests. *American Journal of Occupational Therapy, 39*(2), 103-108, 1985.

Settle, C., & Holm, M. B. (1993). Program planning: The clinical utility of three activities of daily living assessment tools. *American Journal of Occupational Therapy, 47*(10), 911-918.

10

PLANNING TREATMENT

The purpose of planning treatment and some general procedures for planning treatment are described. Sample formats of treatment plans are included.

LEARNING OBJECTIVES

At the end of this chapter, you should be able to:

1. Explain what is meant by a treatment plan.
2. State the basic reason for writing a treatment plan.
3. Name the performance areas and components that can be included in occupational therapy plans.
4. Discuss what information is needed before a treatment plan is formulated.
5. List the team members usually involved in formulating a total treatment plan for a patient.
6. Diagram headings of a sample treatment plan.
7. Discuss steps to take when the treatment plan is not effective.
8. State the assistant's role in planning treatment.

Planning a treatment program for a patient is a way of organizing data and strategies to eliminate or reduce problems interfering with the patient's performance of daily living tasks. It is a systematic way to formulate intervention methods and activities to achieve the patient's treatment objectives and goals.

The major problems that interfere with the patient's performance of daily living activities are typically identified during the initial assessment. The patient's capabilities, interests, and usual daily activities are also identified at that time.

The patient's long-term goals and more immediate goals are identified following the initial assessment. These goals are determined after considering the patient's present physical and mental condition, age, employment or other productive occupation, family status, social and economic status, and perceived goals and desires. The treatment goals should be compatible with the patient's life goals. If the present problems alter these, the patient should be helped to develop satisfactory modified life goals.

TREATMENT-PLANNING CONFERENCE

In most facilities, treatment-planning conferences are held at regularly scheduled times. All disciplines concerned with the patient are usually represented at these conferences. The physician, social worker, psychologist, nurse, and occupational, physical, and speech therapist are typically present. In psychiatric settings, the physician is usually a psychiatrist. In a physical rehabilitation setting, the physician is usually a physiatrist. In a school setting, the parents of the student, the teacher, and an educational supervisor are usually present. A physician or nurse is rarely in attendance at planning conferences in school settings. Specialists such as rehabilitation engineers may be present at some conferences.

The format of the conference is usually determined by the information that needs to be presented within a set time limit. The order in which the information is presented by the people present may be determined by the chairperson. If the primary treatment concerns a medical problem, the chairperson is usually a physician, but that is not always the case. If the intervention is to treat a rehabilitation problem, the chairperson's professional background can be any discipline in the health care field. If the intervention is educationally based, the chairperson is usually a supervisor in the educational setting. A common format is to request from each discipline an oral summary of formal, documented, evaluative findings and recommendations for treatment. The patient may or may not be present during the reports. If not present during the general presentations, the patient may be called in following formal reports. The chairperson interviews the patient, who, together with staff members, is given an opportunity to ask questions or comment on any area of concern. The patient is then usually excused.

The chairperson concludes the conference by summarizing the reports and discussions presented, as well as treatment to be initiated. Following the conference, each discipline develops specific treatment plans within its purview.

Treatment-planning conferences are usually held in a conference room, but brief, ongoing planning may take place at the patient's bedside during ward rounds. Rounds are more common in acute-care general hospitals than in long-term care facilities. During rounds, the physician in charge reviews the patient's chart, examines the patient, and sometimes asks pertinent questions of specific staff members. Whether treatment is to be continued or changed is noted.

OCCUPATIONAL THERAPY PLAN

Occupational therapy is concerned with the patient's ability to function in activities of daily living, work, and play or leisure. The ability to function in these three performance areas is specific to each individual. Each skill and task in these areas is made up of numerous sensorimotor, psychological, and cognitive components. To function in the desired or required performance areas requires the integration of many components of the skills and tasks.

Independent dressing, a task in the performance area of activities of daily living, for example, requires many complex skills. Basic motor abilities for dressing include postural balance in standing and sitting; trunk control to stabilize, rotate, flex, and extend the trunk; and head and neck control to stabilize, extend, and flex the head and neck forward and to either side. Coordination of the upper extremities requires extension and flexion of the shoulders, elbows, wrists, and fingers; abduction and adduction of the shoulders, wrists, and fingers; rotation of the shoulders externally and internally; supination and pronation of the forearm; and possession of the prehension patterns.

Visual and tactile perceptual skills are normally used in dressing. An individual who dresses independently has an understanding of directions, such as inside, outside, up, down, top, bottom, left side, and right side. Texture, weight, size, temperature, and color are other cognitive and perceptual components of dressing. Body image, self-concept, and interpersonal relationships also influence independent dressing.

A dysfunction or inability in any of the basic skill areas may indicate a need for specific training provided through occupational therapy.

Treatment plans in occupational therapy are usually developed by making a list of problems that interfere with the patient's general long-range goal. Short-term objectives needed to reach the goal are identified and listed. Methods and specific activities that can reduce or eliminate the problems and attain the objectives are then listed as well (Pedretti & Zoltan, 1990).

Should the patient not attain the objectives in the prescribed time, the treatment plan needs to be reviewed to determine whether the objectives, methods of intervention, or time schedule needs to be altered. Treatment plans are not static; they need to be monitored and altered in accordance with the changing progress and needs of the patient.

Treatment plans are set out in certain formats. Although these formats may vary slightly, all treatment forms identify the patient's problems, goals, and objectives, the expected date for achieving the goals and objectives, and the treatment methods.

SAMPLE TREATMENT PLANS

The following three examples, using a single goal for the patient, illustrate the variations in format of treatment plans:

EXAMPLE I

E.S., a 26-year-old woman, is being treated for psychiatric problems related to substance abuse and depression. Her goal is to interview for a job. She is careless in her hygiene and dress. She lacks judgment in how to spend her time and has been irresponsible in keeping appointments. She has adequate sensorimotor abilities, average intelligence, and appropriate social interaction skills when motivated. She lacks self-esteem.

Treatment Plan for ES		Date: 4/11/95
Goal: To be interviewed for a job		
Problem	Objective	Activities
1. Lacks proper hygiene. To brush teeth. To apply lotion and deodorant.	1. To bathe or shower each morning. of each task each morning. Give a predetermined reward upon fulfillment of criteria.)	1. Make a chart to check completion
2. Inappropriate clothing selection. Careless in appearance.	2. To select and wear clothes appropriate for each occasion. To button, zip, tie clothing as needed. To apply makeup (optional). To comb hair. appearance.	2. Collage of clothes appropriate for interview, work, movie, etc. Group discussions on clothing. Trips to clothing store to simulate Check appearance in a mirror.
3. Not dependable in keeping appointments. To report for meals at scheduled times.	3. To report to therapist at designated times. Chart in dining room to check when on time (reward as in #1).	3. Chart in OT to check when on time (reward as in #1).
4. Low self-esteem.	4. To identify and verbalize positive self-attributes. To identify and demonstrate work skills. To avoid making self-deprecating remarks. To acknowledge compliments.	4. Group activities. Supervised assignment in OT, ward, or other areas in the facility. Provide suggestions for improvement and positive comments on achievements. Record positive feelings, accomplishments, compliments received at end of each OT session.

EXAMPLE 2

In school settings, occupational therapy plans are included in the Individualized Educational Program (IEP) developed by a multidisciplinary team (Chandler, Dunn, & Rourk, 1989). Student goals are reviewed each school year. The plan includes the following information: the annual goal or goals of therapy, the objectives of the therapy, the dates treatment began for each objective, the dates of any revisions in treatment, the dates the status of the goals and objectives were reviewed, the dates the goals and objectives were reached, and the signatures of the members of the multidisciplinary team.

A number of annual goals may be identified. This abbreviated example will show one goal of an 8-year-old with mild cerebral palsy who shows problems in postural stability and reflex activity.

Student: Richard Dow		Date: 9/4/95
Annual goal #1: Stabilize sitting balance		
Short-Term Objectives	*Methods*	*Activities*
1. Maintain sitting position on a tilted board 5 of 5 times. variety of positions	Methods require body adjustments to maintain sitting in a rocker seat.	1. Beanbag toss and other throwing games while on a while engaged in activities.
2. Maintain sitting position on a T-stool while engaged in ball play for 10 min.		2. Rolling, tossing, kicking ball while on T-stool.
3. Maintain sitting position on a large ball moved by therapist for 10 min.		3. Therapist manipulates large beach ball, requiring child to make body adjustments of trunk rotation, shoulder abduction /adduction, and other postural movements needed to remain seated on the ball.
4. Maintain sitting position while engaged in play, classroom, and ADL activities.		4. Seated on a bench or stool; activities require bending forward, bending to the sides, and reaching up.

EXAMPLE 3

The Problem-Oriented Medical Record (POMR) makes information about a given patient and treatment more accessible to all persons involved in treating and caring for that patient (Llorens, 1982). The four elements of the POMR are the data base, the problem list, the plan, and progress notes.

The data base contains all the initial data on the patient collected through the history, examinations, and test reports. The problem list is a numbered listing of all problems found in the data base. The initial plan consists of all plans for the management of all numbered problems.

The physician or team orders the implementation of the plan. As the treatment plan is carried out, progress reports are written. The progress notes report the results of treatment, new information, any new problems, and the resolution of problems.

In the POMR, progress reports are written in what is commonly referred to as the *SOAP note*. The progress report is divided into four areas and is recorded accordingly. The first letter of the four areas is written on the chart and circled, followed by one or two short statements that report the patient's progress. The information for each area relates to the following:

Subjective data — the patient's view of his or her condition.
Objective data — significant findings from the initial assessment.
Assessment   — the interpretation of the findings from the assessment and a summary of what appears to be the patient's major problems.
Plan   — the goals, frequency, and length of treatment and the plans for achieving the goals.

The following condensed report illustrates an occupational therapy SOAP report.

Mrs. E. White	Date of Evaluation: 6/10/95

65-year-old Caucasian female, admitted 6/7/95.
Diagnosis: right cerebrovascular disease with left upper paralysis, left lower paresis.

S   I had a stroke. My left arm is paralyzed.
O   1. Speech was slow, deliberate, and slurred. Gave correct name, age, and address, but incorrect date and time. Hearing adequate. Loss of vision in left visual field.
　　2. AROM (active range of motion)—RUE (right upper extremity): WNL (within normal limits); LUE (left upper extremity): none.

PROM (passive range of motion)—RUE: WNL; LUE: full.
3. Strength—RUE: good; LUE: zero.
4. Sensation—RUE: WNL; LUE: diminished.
5. Coordination—RUE: good; LUE: none.
6. ADL (activities of daily living)—feeding independently, diminished oral motor control, further ADL tests to be done.

A   Paralysis in LUE, possible disorientation to time, diminished sensation in LUE, diminished ADL skills.

P   OT daily.
1. LUE: ROM (range of motion) and strengthening, muscle reeducation.
2. Maintain ROM and strength in RUE.
3. Reality orientation activities and cognitive activities.
4. Improve ADL skills.

Activities:
1, 2, 4: ADL activities emphasizing use of bilateral Ues.
3: Conversations directed toward recent events.
1, 2, 3, 4: Visual motor activities.

ALTERNATIVE PLANS

The aim of most treatment plans is to eliminate the problem interfering with the patient's normal performance. If the problem cannot be eliminated, the patient should be helped to develop alternative plans to resolve any remaining problems and to function maximally to his or her satisfaction. Alternative plans can include substitution of muscles or body parts, using therapeutic equipment or devices, or coping techniques.

Substitution of one normally used muscle or body part for another may be the most acceptable solution for the patient who wants to be independent. For example, if a patient is right dominant and cannot develop normal strength and coordination in the right upper extremity to enable the patient to write, the patient may learn to use the left extremity. Substitution may involve helping the patient who has a special pride in his or her handwritten letters to accept the notion that letters processed on computer are socially unobjectionable.

Another possible plan is to use a writing aid that attaches to the right hand and provides enough support to allow writing. If some movement and strength remain in the right hand, the patient may prefer this alternative.

If substitution or therapeutic devices do not enable the patient to perform the task, helping the patient to cope with the permanent disability may be part of the treatment plan. Occupational therapy plans include psychological as well as physical daily living skills.

THE ASSISTANT'S ROLE

The certified occupational therapy assistant (COTA) usually assists the occupational therapist (OTR) in planning treatment. The extent that the COTA is involved in such planning depends on the setting, the COTA's experience, and the predilections of the OTR. In some situations, the OTR may be responsible for developing the treatment plan independently of the COTA because of limited time or because of a policy at the particular setting.

The COTA needs to be familiar with the treatment plan in order to treat the patient. The COTA is responsible for understanding the plan in order to carry out duties related to the intervention. Progress or lack of progress should be reported to the supervising OTR so that changes can be made in the treatment plan. Effective communication about the plan is essential to providing the most efficacious occupational therapy intervention.

SUMMARY

The purpose of a written treatment plan is to systematically record the decisions made about the patient's problems, treatment objectives, goals, methods, and activities, as well as the expected time for achieving the objectives and goals. An overall treatment plan is developed collaboratively by all disciplines, with each discipline being responsible for specific areas of treatment. The format for occupational therapy plans may vary, depending upon the facility and the OTR. The OTR determines how the COTA assists in developing the treatment plan.

REVIEW QUESTIONS

1. What is a treatment plan?
2. Why should a treatment plan be written and available to the team involved in a patient's occupational therapy?
3. What components might be included in an occupational therapy treatment plan?
4. What information is needed before formulating a treatment plan?
5. Complete the following sentence: The total treatment plan is usually a cooperative effort by the treatment team, which is composed of

_____ .

6. State the section headings that are usually on treatment plan forms.
7. What needs to be done when objectives of a treatment plan are not being attained before or by the target date?
8. What is the COTA's role in developing a treatment plan?

Answer the following extra questions.
Circle the letter preceding the best answer.

9. Treatment plans are formulated and written in order to:
    a. meet state regulations for reimbursement.
    b. let the patient and family know what is planned.
    c. let each discipline know what the others are doing.
    d. systematically achieve the objectives and goals of the patient.

10. Specific occupational therapy plans are developed by the:
    a. treatment team chairperson.
    b. treatment team.
    c. OTR, COTA, and patient.
    d. director of occupational therapy.

11. The basic information in all occupational therapy plans consists of:
    a. goals, problems, and activities.
    b. problems, goals, objectives, target dates, and methods.
    c. problems, objectives, target dates, and results.
    d. assessments, objectives, methods, and results.

ANSWERS

1. A treatment plan is a way of organizing ideas about how to eliminate or reduce problems that interfere with a patient's performance of daily living tasks. It is a systematic way to formulate intervention methods and activities that will be used to achieve the patient's treatment objectives and goals.
2. A written treatment plan that is available to all members of the treatment team enables the team to know what is being planned.
3. One or all of the components (sensorimotor, cognitive, and psychosocial) of any of the occupational performance areas (activities of daily living, work, and play or leisure) might be included in an occupational therapy treatment plan.
4. The following information is needed to formulate a treatment plan: the patient's present problems, as perceived by the patient; the information from all evaluations related to the patient's problem, which would include the physical and mental status of the patient, any desires and interests on the part of the patient that will help to formulate the goal of treatment; and any other related information, including the patient's age, employment or other productive occupation, family status, and social and economic status.
5. The physician, social worker, psychologist, nurse, physical/occupational/speech therapist, patient, and patient's family. In school sys-

tems, teachers and educational supervisors are on the treatment team, and only rarely are physicians or nurses members. Specialists such as rehabilitation engineers may sometimes be included on the team.

6. Most treatment plan forms use as headings the patient's problems, goals, and objectives, the expected date for achieving the goals and objectives, and the treatment methods.

7. If the patient does not attain objectives in the time frame within which they are expected to be attained, the treatment plan needs to be reviewed to determine whether the objectives, methods of intervention, or time schedule needs to be altered. In general, treatment plans need to be monitored and altered in accordance with the changing progress and needs of the patient. If the patient does not reach his or her goal, alternative plans may have to be implemented. Among these alternatives may be the substitution of one set of muscles or body part for another, the use of therapeutic equipment or devices, and teaching the patient coping skills.

8. The COTA usually assists the OTR in planning treatment. The extent to which the COTA is involved in the planning depends on the setting, the COTA's experience, and the preferences of occupational therapist.

9. d.
10. c.
11. b.

ADDITIONAL LEARNING ACTIVITIES

1. Visit an occupational therapy department, and ask whether you may look at a treatment plan.
2. Ask an occupational therapy practitioner how decisions are made as to which of the patient's problems will be treated first.
3. Ask an occupational therapy practitioner how decisions are made as to which activity to use for specific problems the patient has.
4. Ask an occupational therapy practitioner how it is decided that a certain activity will be best for the patient.

REFERENCES

Chandler, B., Dunn, W., & Rourk, J. (1989). *Guidelines for occupational therapy services in school systems* (2nd ed.). Bethesda, MD: American Occupational Therapy Association, Inc.

Llorens, L. A. (1982). *Occupational therapy sequential client care record manual.* Laurel, MD: RAMSCO, 1982.

Pedretti, L. W., & Zoltan, B. (1990). *Occupational therapy: Practice skills for physical dysfunction* (3rd ed.). St. Louis: The C. V. Mosby Company.

11

THE SUPERVISORY FUNCTION

Experienced certified occupational therapy assistants (COTAs) have supervisory responsibilities. The role of the supervisor is briefly described.

LEARNING OBJECTIVES

At the end of this chapter, you should be able to:

1. Define supervision and state how the supervisory and managerial roles differ.
2. List at least five employee actions the supervisor can theoretically take.
3. State the primary function of a supervisor.
4. State four basic functions of a supervisor, and explain the supervisor's actions in a hypothetical activities department.
5. State at least 10 attitudes desired of an effective supervisor.
6. List at least 10 specific skills desired of an effective supervisor. Explain why the skills are needed.
7. Explain why effective supervisors understand and agree with the organization's philosophy.

The experienced certified occupational therapy assistant (COTA) has supervisory responsibilities as a staff member in an occupational therapy department or as the head of an activities department in a long-term care facility. These responsibilities may include supervision of another COTA, an aide, a volunteer, or a student. A COTA who becomes director of an activities department is usually a full-time supervisor. This chapter describes and examines the supervisor's role.

DEFINITION

To *supervise* means to oversee or direct a project or people. A *supervisor* is a person who supervises. The words *supervisor* and *manager* are sometimes used synonymously. Imundo (1980) states that supervisors are managers. Certainly, supervisors use managerial methods, and managers who primarily oversee people are often called supervisors. The managerial role includes supervision of people, but overseeing other aspects of the organization is the primary role of the manager.

Supervision has been defined as a process of planning and controlling the activities of subordinates on a direct face-to-face basis (Sartain & Baker, 1978). Van Dersal (1968) defines supervision as the art of working with a group of people under one's authority to achieve the greatest amount of work most efficiently.

THE SUPERVISORY POSITION

A supervisor is the link between management and labor or between administrators and staff. A hospital organization or long-term care facility has many supervisors. A supervisor in a given profession usually oversees people who are in the same profession. For example, in an occupational therapy department with 30 or more therapists and assistants, several occupational therapy practitioners may be designated as clinical supervisors. The supervisor's title usually identifies the category of workers. Director of nursing, coordinator of activities, and office head are examples of titles given supervisors.

In theory, the supervisor has the authority to hire, fire, transfer, suspend, lay off, recall, reward, or discipline a subordinate. Such authority requires the supervisor to be knowledgeable and able to justify the action taken. A supervisor must have the technical and professional knowledge of the specific field. A supervisor must also have a broad, general knowledge of employment practices and of people (Imundo, 1980).

In reality, most supervisors have the authority to recommend any of the aforementioned actions, but usually do not act independently in taking them. The final decision on any action is generally determined by management. Unions, people's rights, and laws related to employment and working conditions influence the actions taken by a supervisor, manager, or organization.

A supervisory position is both challenging and demanding. The functions of supervision are described next.

FUNCTIONS OF SUPERVISION

The primary function of a supervisor is to create an environment in which employees are willing to work together to achieve common goals (Imundo, 1980). In the case of a COTA who is the director of an activities program in a long-term care facility, creating such an environment means working with many people from various disciplines. The director of activities generates enthusiasm and cooperation among the staff of the facility so that they not only work together to provide the activities, but enjoy carrying out their responsibilities as well. The director of activities also works with management and other supervisors to create the desired working environment in the entire facility.

The primary goal of activities personnel is to provide activities to each patient in the facility. Attaining this goal is dependent upon the cooperative effort of those employees below or on the same level as the supervisor. The working relationship among all the parties, which is ideally characterized by open, two-way communication, is shown in the following diagram:

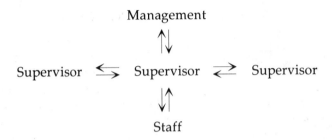

Supervisors exert influence over a variety of people, both formally and informally. The effective supervisor aims to influence people in positive ways for the mutual benefit of employees, patients, and the organization (Imundo, 1980).

The supervisor must have adequate conceptual skills. The supervisor decides *what* needs to be done to achieve the desired goals, *when* to do what needs to be done, and *who* is to do what needs to be done.

Following the planning stage, the supervisor organizes people, space, equipment, and whatever else is needed to achieve the desired goals. The supervisor then exerts his or her influence to control the achievement of the goals.

To accomplish the primary goals, the supervisor must have interpersonal relationship skills. These skills include knowing how to approach people, how to talk to people, and how to listen to them. The supervisor should have an understanding of people and their basic needs in order to help employees want to do their best.

Since supervisors usually have more responsibility than authority, the effective supervisor attempts to influence people to do the required tasks voluntarily, rather than ordering them to carry out the tasks. The work environment is more pleasant when employees feel responsible for doing their share of the required tasks to achieve the departmental and organizational goals.

The staff may surpass the supervisor in technical ability, since supervisors are not as frequently required to practice technical skills. However, the effective supervisor needs to maintain his or her technical knowledge and competence in order to be able to evaluate the competence of the staff and to assist in teaching them when necessary. The need to maintain technical knowledge places a demand on the supervisor to keep current through continuing education by attending workshops and reading current professional literature.

The evaluation of the competence of the staff is part of the supervisor's primary function. The evaluation should be fair and objective, which means that the supervisor must think and act like a supervisor to each staff member.

In sum, the supervisor creates an environment in which employees are motivated to work together to achieve the desired goals. The supervisor's basic functions are to plan, organize, control, and motivate. The supervisor's attitude influences the effectiveness of his or her efforts in fulfilling these functions.

SUPERVISOR ATTITUDES

Two supervisors may perform their functions adequately, yet there may be noticeable differences between the two groups of employees under them. These differences might be that one group may achieve its goals in a shorter time, have fewer employee absences, less employee turnover, or be superior in some other characteristic. The supervisor's attitude may be a factor in these differences.

Imundo (1980) identified the following desirable supervisory attitudes. The supervisor should:

1. be able to accept the final decisions made by higher management;
2. earn the respect, trust, and confidence of employees;
3. base decisions about controversial issues on facts and specific circumstances;
4. give credit, recognition, and praise to deserving employees;
5. accept responsibility for failures as well as successes;
6. be objective and fair in judging employees' actions;
7. consider corrective actions as rehabilitative measures;
8. allow employees to have as much control over their work as possible;
9. respect employee rights;
10. facilitate employee growth, both professionally and personally;
11. support employees when they are right;
12. maintain a work climate in which employees feel that they can openly express their feelings and concerns;
13. be honest and sincere;
14. keep personal feelings private; and
15. set an example as a leader.

The supervisor's attitude should communicate a feeling of respect and concern for the employee. In addition to having the proper attitude, the supervisor needs specific skills in order to gain respect from employees and carry out his or her functions.

SPECIFIC SUPERVISORY SKILLS

The COTA can expect to study supervisory skills in more detail in other courses. An effective supervisor continues to learn and practice appropriate supervisory techniques for his or her entire career as a supervisor. A supervisor's having knowledge of a variety of supervisory techniques is analogous to an occupational therapy practitioner's having knowledge of variety of occupational therapy techniques.

The following skills, among others, are required of an effective supervisor:

1. *Effective writing skills.* With such skills, the supervisor can compose letters, reports, and memorandums to all levels of personnel within the facility and to people outside the facility. Messages will then be clearly understood.
2. *Effective speaking skills.* With these, the supervisor can address all levels of personnel within the facility. People need to understand what is being said in order to achieve the desired goals. Most supervisors represent the profession and the facility when they speak before the general public. Effective speaking skills enhance public respect, which can influence the achievement of goals.
3. *Effective listening skills.* Then, messages from employees, management, and other supervisors can be communicated clearly. The ability to hear what is actually being said by individuals is essential to clear communication.
4. *Objectivity.* Biased and preconceived opinions can cloud a person's thinking. A supervisor must be as objective as possible. Objective criteria are needed when evaluating an employee, as well as when assigning a task.
5. *The ability to motivate workers.* Motivation is a major factor in achieving goals. A supervisor needs to understand the basic principles of motivation in order to motivate employees and then keep them motivated.
6. *The ability to solve problems.* Most supervisory positions are unique. This is because the problems that develop and that the supervisors are expected to solve often have unique elements, even when they fall into a category of similar problems. A supervisor needs to be creative and analytical in solving the problems that arise.
7. *The ability to set priorities.* A supervisor is frequently faced with deadlines. Setting priorities can be difficult because of differences of

opinion between employee and supervisor. A supervisor needs to hear the opinions of employees and be able to provide a rationale for rejecting such opinions if they are not relevant to the accomplishment of the stated goal. The supervisor must be able to make decisions and determine priorities, and then plan, organize, and control the accomplishment of the tasks by motivating employees to work on them.

8. *The ability to delegate responsibility.* Some supervisors find it difficult to delegate responsibility. The difficulty may be due to an employee not wanting to assume the responsibility. Often, a supervisor lacks faith in the employee's ability. A supervisor who does not delegate responsibility is soon overburdened with it and becomes ineffective on the job.

9. *Interviewing skills.* A supervisor needs to become a skillful interviewer. Selecting an inappropriate employee wastes time, energy, and money. Also, an inappropriate employee creates additional problems in the workplace through his or her lack of productivity and propensity to generate tension among the other employees.

10. *Counseling skills.* Most supervisors encounter situations in which an employee can be helped if the supervisor has some knowledge of counseling skills. The supervisor should know when to refer the employee to other professionals.

11. *Teaching skills.* Every supervisor should have teaching skills to help employees improve their own skills, to increase the employees' knowledge, and to motivate the employees to learn.

12. *Ability to laugh.* Every supervisor needs to appreciate the value of laughter and humor in a work situation. A supervisor should be able to recognize signs of stress, both in oneself and in employees. An effective supervisor attempts to counteract the detrimental effects of stress through humor, laughter, or other methods of relaxation.

13. *Ability to manage oneself.* Supervisors who understand themselves can lead others more effectively. Supervisors who manage their lives effectively can elicit maximum energy, creativity, competence, teamwork, and productivity from their employees (Johnson, 1983; Stout, 1984).

PHILOSOPHY AND SUPERVISION

A basic element in effective supervision is the philosophy of the organization and the supervisor's understanding of and feelings about that philosophy.

According to Ouchi (1981), a philosophy is needed to give staff a sense of values and objectives by which to work. The departmental philosophy suggests ways for staff to behave in the department and ways the department behaves in response to the patients, the facility, and the community. The departmental philosophy should include the objectives of the department, the means of achieving the objectives, and the limitations placed on the department by the facility, the community, and the larger society.

The departmental philosophy should be consistent with the facility's philosophy. To determine whether this is so, the supervisor needs to know the facility's true objective. Occasionally, a facility's true objective is disguised, or it is not possible to learn the true objective. In such cases, the supervisor works with the stated objective.

The departmental and facility philosophies should be discussed with staff members. An effective supervisor and effective employees understand and agree with the objectives of the department and the facility.

SUMMARY

To *supervise* means to oversee or direct another person, other persons, or projects. COTAs may supervise COTAs with less experience, occupational therapy aides, students, or volunteers. The supervisory skills and the attitude of the COTA influence the effectiveness of those under them.

REVIEW QUESTIONS

Circle the letter preceding the most correct answer.

1. A supervisor is defined as a person:
    a. who gives orders to subordinates.
    b. whose primary function is to oversee a group of people.
    c. whose primary function to is oversee an organization.
    d. can be a friend to subordinates.
2. A supervisor has the authority to:
    a. reprimand and suspend a worker for cause.
    b. recommend a promotion and an increase in salary for a worker.
    c. give departmental promotions, bonuses, and raises.
    d. transfer a person out of a department.
3. The basic supervisory functions are to:
    a. plan, organize, control, and motivate.
    b. interview, hire, train, and terminate.
    c. plan, delegate, influence, and motivate.
    d. direct, delegate, demand, and discipline.
4. An effective supervisor achieves goals:
    a. regardless of methods needed to achieve them.
    b. by creating the desired environment and motivating people.
    c. in the shortest time possible, since time means money.
    d. using reward and punishment techniques.

5. An effective supervisor:
   a. is able to ignore higher level decisions in order to show support for his or her staff.
   b. realizes that the opinions of his or her staff have little worth in the total situation.
   c. attributes good work to the department as a whole, and not an individual.
   d. helps staff understand and accept final management decisions.
6. An effective supervisor:
   a. does every task him- or herself.
   b. assigns tasks based on each person's avocational interests.
   c. writes and speaks effectively and listens to staff and others.
   d. has skills that are more technically advanced than those of any staff member.
7. A departmental philosophy:
   a. is most important for gaining accreditation for the department.
   b. includes objectives, methods, constraints, and a budget.
   c. is not needed if the parent organization has a philosophy.
   d. gives staff a sense of values and objectives by which to work.

ANSWERS

1. b.
2. b.
3. a.
4. b.
5. d.
6. c.
7. d.

ADDITIONAL LEARNING ACTIVITIES

1. Make an appointment to visit a director of an activities department in a long-term care facility. How many persons does the director supervise? What is the departmental philosophy? Does the director interview and hire staff? Does the director evaluate staff and recommend promotions or pay increases? How does the director feel about being a supervisor? Where did the director learn his or her supervisory skills?
2. Make an appointment to visit a COTA to learn the COTA's supervisory responsibilities. What are those responsibilities? Who assigns them? Where did the COTA learn supervisory skills? Would the COTA like to supervise a department, rather than provide direct treatment to patients? If yes, why?

3. Interview an occupational therapist who heads a department to learn his or her views about supervision. Where did the therapist learn to be a supervisor? What is the most difficult part of supervising people? What is the most rewarding part of supervision? What is the most important supervisory skill to possess?

REFERENCES

Imundo, L. V. (1980). *The effective supervisor's handbook*. New York: AMACOM, a division of American Management Associations.

Johnson, R. W. (1983). What you need to know to be a supervisor. *Supervisory Management, 28*(3), 35-42.

Ouchi, W. G. (1981). *Theory Z: How American business can meet the Japanese challenges*. Reading, MA: Addison-Wesley.

Sartain, A. Q., & Baker, A. W. (1978). *The supervisor and the job*. New York: McGraw-Hill.

Stout, J. K. (1984). The role of self-concept in interpersonal communications. *Supervisory Management, 29*(2), 12-16.

Van Dersal, W. R. (1968). *The successful supervisor in government and business*. New York: Harper and Row.

SUGGESTED READINGS

Blanchard, K., & Johnson, S. (1982). *The one minute manager*. New York: William Morrow and Company.

Blanchard, K., & Lorber, R. (1984). *Putting the one minute manager to work*. New York: William Morrow and Company.

Pollock, T. (1979). *Moving on up*. New York: Hawthorn Books.

Winston, S. (1983). *The organized executive*. New York: W. W. Norton and Company.

Section III

SPECIFIC OCCUPATIONAL THERAPY ASSISTANT SKILLS

The major role of the certified occupational therapy assistant (COTA) is to treat patients directly. The role requires knowledge of a variety of therapeutic activities relevant to occupational performance areas, components, and contexts. The knowledge base includes how to analyze a variety of activities, how to teach activities, and how to relate to the patient in such a way that the patient becomes an active participant in the treatment process. The COTA assists the occupational therapist (OTR) in evaluating patients, planning treatment, performing interventions, and planning the patient's discharge from the facility. This section covers some of the basic skills needed by the COTA.

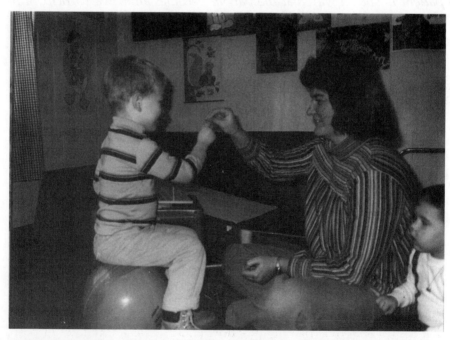

Deborah Kulich, COTA/L, helps Johnathon enhance sitting balance and visual-motor coordination.

12

THERAPEUTIC
USE OF SELF

The occupational therapist (OTR) and the certified occupational therapy assistant (COTA) are as important in the therapeutic process as are the methods or techniques used. The OTR or the COTA is the primary person who elicits responses from the patient that will lead to the achievement of the preestablished goals. Because the relationship between the patient and the COTA is so important, ways to create a therapeutic situation are discussed, with the emphasis on the COTA as a therapeutic agent.

LEARNING OBJECTIVES

At the end of this chapter, you should be able to:

1. Explain in one or two sentences what *therapeutic use of self* means in occupational therapy.
2. Name the three selves identified by Dr. Jerome Frank, and give a short explanatory statement of each.
3. Describe a therapeutic behavior observed at a treatment center that you feel is consistent with your behavior.
4. Give an example of behavior consistent with that of your ideal self.
5. Give an example of facilitating a person's self-confidence.

D r. Jerome Frank stated that *the self* refers to almost all aspects of the development and functioning of an individual's personality (Frank, 1958). In rehabilitation, the adjective *therapeutic* connotes all personal influences that facilitate positive change in the individual. In occupational therapy, the phrase *therapeutic use of self* is used to suggest that the occupational therapy practitioner, serves as a facilitator of positive changes in behavior in psychiatric patients as a result of his or her unique attributes, actions, and reactions. The practitioner is a therapeutic agent in any occupational therapy intervention, regardless of the diagnosis. Note that, although Dr. Frank's concepts were initially proposed for the psychiatric hospital treatment setting, they are important in any treatment setting.

THE GOALS

When using yourself as a therapeutic agent, you have two general goals. The first goal is to get the patient emotionally involved in the therapeutic situation. Unless the patient has some intrinsic investment in what is happening in treatment, there will be little lasting effect from the treatment. The second goal is to increase the patient's self-confidence in order to engage him or her in new interpersonal relationships. The practitioner can aid the patient in achieving the latter goal by reducing the patient's anxieties so that he or she becomes able to take risks and attempt new experiences (Early, 1993).

There are two prerequisites to reaching the two goals. The first prerequisite is self-understanding, which is a dynamic, ongoing process. Some people have the capacity to understand the behavior of others, but have difficulty understanding their own behavior. By contrast, some individuals are "tuned into" their own feelings and actions, but not those of others. Despite their being unable to understand the behavior of others, it is the latter individuals who have self-understanding. The second prerequisite is to have an understanding of the patient beyond the primary condition that created the need for treatment.

Both the COTA and the patient bring to the treatment situation unique backgrounds of cultural, societal, educational, and sensorimotor experiences. Each person comes with separate and distinct values, biases, and aspirations.

Regardless of the differences or similarities of the two individuals, communication between them is essential. The responsibility for creating a climate of trust and facilitating honest communication rests upon the staff person (Barris, Kielhofner, & Watts, 1983; Brill, 1990; Early, 1993).

THE SELF

Often, communication occurs freely between people, but substance and honesty are lacking. The absence of honesty and substance in communication may be due to the uncertainty each of us has about the genuineness, as well as the value, of our feelings and perceptions. We may also have questions about the genuineness of the person with whom we are communicating. If we have an understanding of our feelings and behavior, and if we try to communicate as honestly as possible in order to get across the feelings and behavior, there is a greater possibility of eliciting more meaningful and honest comments from another person. Communication may lack honesty and clarity because we, as well as the individual with whom we are communicating, are unaware of the incongruity in our own behavior and comments. The "mixed messages" we send make it difficult to have meaningful communication.

Frank (1958) identified three basic selves within each person: the *acting self,* the *perceived self,* and the *ideal self.* Normally, the individual is able to describe these three distinct selves, and normally, the three selves are congruent.

The *acting self* is the self that is revealed to others. This is the self that actively responds in certain ways or roles, depending on the responses of others. The core of the acting self remains consistent, despite the various roles it assumes.

The *perceived self* is the self the individual believes he or she is. The perceived self develops in childhood and is based on the parent's perception of the child. The child develops a basic sense of goodness and worth, or badness and unworthiness, depending on how he or she was treated in infancy and early childhood. When the child finally perceives him- or herself as a separate, physical entity, the realization leads to a sense of vulnerability. The individual attempts to preserve the constancy of the perceived self.

The *ideal self* is the self the individual would like to be. The ideal self is the caretaker of the values and standards that were developed by the perceived self. The perceived self is evaluated with the ideal self as a model. Normally, the individual likes the perceived self, but sees areas where improvement would make the perceived self more like the ideal self.

NIdeally, the acting self, the perceived self, and the ideal self are clearly defined in the individual's view. The individual can assume certain roles required by different situations, but each role assumed is consistent with the other roles. The acting self is also consistent with the perceived self. The individual can predict basically how he or she will respond in different situations and how he or she will be viewed by others. The perceived self and the ideal self are fairly similar. In this ideal process of the development of the self, the individual is self-respectful, is self-confident, and foresees a reasonable amount of success in the future (Frank, 1958).

THE USE OF SELF IN THERAPY

An understanding of the three distinct selves should help you communicate with honesty, clarity, and consistency. The realization that the patient also has these three selves will help you accept the patient's responses with greater understanding. For example, the person's behavior as a new patient may be quite different from her usual behavior known to her family and friends prior to her hospitalization. Or, the realization that the patient's acting self may have changed because a permanent injury has changed both his perceived self and his ideal self may help you accept the patient's comments with greater understanding. Such an understanding may then aid in eliciting responses from the patient that are honest and consistent with his other selves.

Occupational therapy involves engaging the patient in activity. The activity may be a self-help skill such as dressing, a creative craft such as a ceramics technique that assures success, or an exercise such as sanding wood to increase the range of movement in the joints and muscle strength.

The patient needs to engage consciously in the activity in order to benefit from it. The activity will have a greater benefit for the patient if he or she is enthusiastic about it. The activity will also be of greater benefit if the patient is enthusiastic about the environment in which it takes place, including persons in the environment. By contrast, the patient may emphatically refuse to engage in occupational therapy and may communicate this refusal with verbally abusive language. In that case, you might assume a certain role (the acting self) in response to the patient's behavior (the patient's new acting self responding to your acting self). Quite likely, the patient's new acting self in that particular instance is not consistent with his or her perceived self (well and capable) or ideal self (well, capable, productive, and independent). The realization that the refusal to participate in therapy and the verbal attack are not consistent with the patient's previous acting self or his or her other selves may enable you to respond therapeutically, rather than take the refusal as a personal affront.

In occupational therapy, you may assume many roles— supervisor, teacher, craftsperson, listener, motivator, evaluator, reinforcer, and more— while engaging the patient in productive and purposeful occupations (Early, 1993). In assuming these roles, you should maintain consistency in your acting self, because the therapeutic intervention is then more likely to be effective.

Patients may have difficulty keeping their three selves consistent following an acute injury, a disease, or a permanent state of dysfunction. The therapeutic climate should convey a sense of stability and predictability, to help the patient maintain consistency among the three selves. Since spontaneity, variety, and changes occur in an occupational therapy setting, you can convey a sense of stability and predictability by demonstrating consistency in your own behavior. As an experienced, confident COTA, you should be able to analyze the therapeutic situation objectively and determine the best response, based upon the patient's therapeutic needs and goals. In this regard, it is possible for your acting self to be spontaneous and flexible in the therapeutic intervention and still be consistent with your perceived and ideal selves.

SUMMARY

The COTA assumes many roles in the course of a workday. Using *the self* as a therapeutic agent is as important as using the proper technique or modality. Dr. Jerome Frank's analysis of self is used as a way to view a person's behavior in various situations. An understanding of the self is primary to creating a therapeutic climate.

REVIEW QUESTIONS

1. Is the self you reveal to patients and others *the acting self?* Justify your answer.
2. Match the following statements to the *acting self, perceived self,* and *ideal self.* A 14-year-old male patient who may have permanent paralysis of his lower extremities from an auto accident is (1) sullen and uncooperative during his first sessions in occupational therapy. His mother described him as previously (2) relating well to family members, peers, and others. (3) He was considerate and helpful to his neighbors. (4) He studied to achieve his academic goals and was pleased and proud to be on his school's honor roll. (5) He wanted to attend college and expressed a desire to teach because he liked to learn, study, and share information with people.
3. Give an example of your behavior which is consistent with that of an occupational therapy practitioner you have observed.
4. Give an example that describes your *ideal self.*
5. Give an example of facilitating the patient's self-confidence, and identify in your example the three selves described by Dr. Frank.

ANSWERS

1. Yes. With patients, I reveal myself as a therapist and respond to the response given by the patient. Depending on the setting and other persons present, I may be acting as an occupational therapist or as a faculty member responding to other persons' reactions and responses to me.
2. Perceived self: Statements 2, 3, 4.
   Acting self: Statement 1.
   Ideal self: Statement 2, 3, 4, 5.
3. The COTA waited patiently and appeared encouraging while waiting for a patient to express himself verbally. I believe that I have patience and can be attentive and encouraging both verbally and nonverbally.

4. I would like to be an excellent therapist in a school setting and to be an occupational therapy educator. I believe that I have an interest in education because my parents valued education and educators so highly.
5. When a patient is engaged in an activity and is expressing dissatisfaction because he cannot perform the activity as well as another patient can, I am able to find something that the patient is doing well and give positive reinforcement. *Acting self.* The patient is performing the activity in response to the therapy and therapists and is reacting with frustration because he believes that he is as capable as anyone else, but he sees that someone is performing the activity better than he is. I am responding to the patient's feeling of frustration and giving the patient reassurance and reinforcement, which is the therapeutic and expected response. *Perceived self.* The patient perceived himself as being able to do as well as the other patient. I perceive myself in the therapeutic setting to be a therapist with the appropriate response to give a patient. *Ideal self.* The patient would like to be the one performing the activity as perfectly as possible. I value helping a patient achieve therapeutic goals and providing encouragement and motivation for the patient to be independent as possible.

REFERENCES

Barris, R., Kielhofner, G., & Watts, J. H. (1983). *Psychosocial occupational therapy practice in a pluralistic arena.* Laurel, MD: RAMSCO Publishing Company.

Brill, N. I. (1990). *Working with people: The helping process* (4th ed.). New York: Longman Incorporated.

Early, M. B. (1993). *Mental health concepts and techniques for the occupational therapy assistant* (2nd ed.). New York: Raven Press.

Frank, J. D. (1958). The therapeutic use of self. *American Journal of Occupational Therapy, 12*(4), 215-224.

ANALYSIS OF THERAPEUTIC OCCUPATIONS

The purpose of occupational therapy is to help people be as independent as possible as they perform the daily life tasks and activities they need or want to do. Occupational therapy practitioners use occupations (activities) as part of the intervention process. Beliefs guiding the selection of occupations for intervention are discussed.

LEARNING OBJECTIVES

At the end of this chapter, you should be able to:

1. State the profession's belief about the value of occupations.
2. State five ways that engaging in purposeful activities affects an individual.
3. State two basic principles for selecting therapeutic occupations.
4. Discuss the certified occupational therapy assistant's role in the use of therapeutic occupations in the intervention process.
5. Name an activity and at least five of its performance components.

The words *occupation* and *activity* are used interchangeably in this chapter. Historically, the profession began when the general meaning of the word *occupation* was any activity in which a person was engaged. Currently, there is an effort to incorporate the word back into the professional language and literature; however, the terms *activity analysis* and *purposeful activity* are general in the profession and will be used here.

Occupational therapy was founded on the belief that participation in familiar, meaningful occupations aid a patient in recovering from an illness or injury. Active, rather than passive, participation in occupations is

believed to be more beneficial to the patient. Active participation in occupations elicits more responses from an individual. Responses from the
sensory, neuromusculoskeletal, motor, and cognitive systems are likely
to be elicited, as well as psychological responses such as motivation, enthusiasm, pleasure, and suspense. Psychosocial interests, beliefs, and values, and patterns of interpersonal behaviors, are also more likely to be
expressed when a patient is actively participating in purposeful activities.

Belief in the value of occupations was held not only by founders and
supporters of the occupational therapy profession, but also by educators,
such as John Dewey, who believed that engaging children in occupations
was essential for their development and education (Ratner, 1939). Professionals in the fields of rehabilitation and education held the view that
engagement in occupations had humanistic values, fostered the development of self-confidence, self-respect, and a sense of usefulness, and aided
the basic aim of their professions (Schwartz, 1992).

Some illnesses and injuries leave residual effects. Engaging in purposeful occupations enhances the patient's ability to cope with these effects. Occupations have therapeutic value when they have meaning to
the patient. Occupations permit patients to focus their mental and physical energy toward a goal and to receive stimulation from and interact
with the social, physical, and nonphysical elements of their environment.

DYSFUNCTION

A central belief of the occupational therapy profession is that human
beings are intrinsically motivated to interact with their environment.
Individuals have a curiosity about their environment and adapt to living
beings and nonliving things in the environment in order to find satisfaction and live in harmony with their surroundings (AOTA, 1979).

Conditions such as injury, illness, cognitive impairment, psychosocial
dysfunction, mental illness, developmental or learning disability, physical disability, sensory or emotional deprivation, and stress may interfere
with the individual's usual responses. Such conditions can cause abnormal responses to any environmental stimuli. Pain, fear, anxiety, embarrassment, or other sensations perceived by the individual can result in
overresponses or underresponses to relatively normal stimuli. When a
person's mental or physical response is abnormal, all body systems are
affected. It is likely that systems that seem peripheral to the affected
body part or system also respond abnormally.

Occupational therapy practitioners provide intervention to help patients regain normal responses. When the condition results in a permanent state of dysfunction, the patient is helped to learn to accept the
abnormal state and function by using new patterns of response. These

new patterns may include substituting another part of the body to perform the activity, using adaptive equipment and devices, employing someone to perform the necessary activities, or learning techniques to help cope with the situation.

THERAPEUTIC EFFECTS OF OCCUPATIONS

The therapeutic effects of occupations are determined by the outcomes of the interventions, as viewed by the patient. If the patient feels that treatment goals have been met, the intervention can be considered successful. This does not, of course, mean that a therapeutic activity used successfully with a particular patient will be similarly successful with another patient with the same condition. The occupational therapy profession does not have sufficient scientifically based findings to be able to predict outcomes for each activity used in therapy. The profession does have almost 80 years of empirical findings, in addition to formal research on which to base its intervention methods. However, even with such findings and research, as well as increasing scientific knowledge, as in most outcomes involving human relationships, much of occupational therapy is still an art. Because the occupational therapy practitioner plays a major role in intervention, practitioners use their own particular personality and style in different ways to meet the needs of each patient. Practitioners analyze the patient's behavior, language, gestures, and nuances of all kinds and act accordingly in providing intervention.

There are two principles to consider when selecting therapeutic activities. First, the treatment goals are established by the patient's needs. The patient is unique, has functioned in a given way, and will need to and wants to function in a particular way in a particular environment. Thus, what the patient considers important needs to be taken into account in establishing goals. Second, the activities selected for intervention should be compatible with the patient's goals. The activities must have meaning to the patient in order to be purposeful. An activity that is purposeful for one patient may not be purposeful for another patient with the same diagnosis.

Only when activities are purposeful for the patient will they be therapeutic. Inappropriate occupations can have a detrimental effect on the patient. Just as a purposeful activity can motivate the patient to participate actively and with a positive attitude during treatment, an inappropriate activity can destroy motivation, create frustration or anger, and result in premature termination of the intervention.

THE ASSISTANT'S ROLE

The certified occupational therapy assistant (COTA) assists the occupational therapist (OTR) in selecting purposeful activities and engaging the patient in them. Depending upon the patient, the diagnosis, the setting, the intervention plan, and the COTA's knowledge and skills, supervision may be close, routine, general, or minimal. The COTA may be given responsibility for selecting additional or alternative activities that have characteristics which will meet the needs of the intervention goals as the patient makes progress in his or her treatment and as the patient's needs change from session to session. The COTA is generally the occupational therapy practitioner with whom the patient spends the most time during intervention.

When you are assigned to a particular patient (or a group of patients), you are responsible for preparing the area where intervention is to take place with all needed equipment and supplies. You will motivate the patient in ways that are suitable for him or her. You will teach the activity, make any needed alterations or substitutions in the activity, and terminate the activity and session. Following the intervention session, you may be responsible for clearing the area and transporting the patient to the next treatment program or, if the patient is an inpatient, to the patient's living area. In many settings, occupational therapy aides assist in preparing and clearing the intervention area and transporting patients. In some settings in which many patients need to go from one area to another to receive their treatments, employees or volunteers are specifically assigned to transport the patients to and from their treatments and living areas.

You must prepare for each intervention session by confirming that the treatment area is ready with all needed materials and equipment. You must be prepared to teach the selected activity in an organized, step-by-step fashion and, if necessary, to alter the activity to conform with the patient's intellectual, emotional, and physical capabilities and disabilities. Knowledge of a wide variety of activities and the components and characteristics of each is essential. Interest in a variety of activities and the ability to solve problems are assets in fulfilling your role as a COTA (Hirama, 1992).

The selection of appropriate activities for a patient is dependent upon many factors. To select a purposeful activity for a specific patient, communication with the supervising OTR who evaluated the patient is crucial. You must take responsibility for reviewing pertinent information and having knowledge of the goals of the occupational therapy intervention plan.

The focus of occupational therapy intervention is to help the individual function as independently as possible, in a manner in which he or she desires, in a particular physical, social, and cultural environment. Such an all-encompassing concept requires examination of the person, the activity, and the components that make up the person, the activity, and the environment.

SELECTION OF THERAPEUTIC ACTIVITY

Because any number of factors, in addition to the primary condition requiring intervention, can affect the patient, therapeutic activities need to be selected with care. Occupational therapy practitioners select purposeful activities after analyzing activities and matching particular ones to the needs of the patient and the goals of treatment (Allen, Earhart & Blue, 1992; Early, 1993; Pedretti & Zoltan, 1990).

The selection of an activity for its therapeutic value is based on many factors. The supervising OTR will provide the COTA with pertinent information from the assessment, and much of the information will be included when the COTA receives the assignment to treat the patient. The COTA is responsible for using the information appropriately during intervention sessions, for being knowledgeable about the rationale for the techniques and occupations used, and for being able to relate the information to appropriate persons.

The patient. You should have as much information as possible about the patient. The following basic information will be helpful: demographics, such as age, sex, family status, and place of residence; education and educational goals; vocation and vocational goals; avocational interests and significant leisure experiences; social, economic, and cultural background; mental and physical capabilities and disabilities; and attitude toward the present condition and situation.

The condition. Information about the patient's medical and psychosocial condition is essential for selecting appropriate activities and engaging the patient in them. In general, the following information is needed: the nature of the condition causing the disability or dysfunction; the precautions to be taken in dealing with the condition; whether the patient's medical treatment can affect the use of activities in occupational therapy; the patient's specific schedule with regard to any other treatment he or she is receiving; and the patient's attitude toward the current condition.

Additional information that can be helpful in selecting activities are whether the patient has any limitations or needs in areas unrelated to the present condition. There are six such areas: 1) *Medical.* Does the patient have a normal healing response? Are there residual effects from previous medical conditions? 2) *Activities of daily living.* Can the patient perform all daily self-care, administer medication to him- or herself, and engage in other activities of daily living in a normal manner? 3) *Sensorimotor responses.* Are there any dysfunctions? Is there sensory awareness, sensory processing, perceptual processing, and perceptual discrimination? 4) *Neuromusculoskeletal responses.* Are there any limitations in the range of motion of the joints, strength and endurance, postural control, or gross-motor and fine-motor coordination? Is the body properly aligned? Is the body symmetrical? Are there any unusual body postures or movements? 5) *Cognitive.* Are there any limitations in the patient's attention span, memory, sequencing ability, spatial operations, problem-solving ability, or ability to learn or generalize information? 6) *Psychosocial.* Has the patient expressed values, beliefs, or attitudes that would influence his or her engaging in given activities? Will the patient's self-concept, social conduct, interpersonal skills, self-expression, self-control, coping skills, or ability to manage time affect his or her engaging in certain activities?

Cause of the condition. Knowledge of the cause of the condition can help in selecting appropriate activities for the patient. Occasionally, when patients are hospitalized, the cause of the condition is undetermined at the time occupational therapy is begun. In some cases, the cause may be known, but is not revealed to the patient. It is important for you to be aware of any such information. Degenerative conditions or terminal conditions may be treated differently from those that will not show lasting effects. The activities selected need to be appropriate for each patient's treatment goals and psychological and emotional needs. The patient's involvement in selecting the purposeful activity will usually result in an appropriate selection.

Projected duration of the intervention. The projected hospitalization stay and the length of time for which occupational therapy has been prescribed will affect the selection of activities. Activities completed in a short time may be preferred for medical and psychiatric patients with short-term, acute-care conditions. Activities that can maintain the patient's interest over a relatively long period may be more appropriate for long-term residential patients.

The length of the hospitalization is only one factor that is operative in deciding whether a short-term or long-term activity is appropriate. Other considerations include the patient's attention span, memory, interests, therapeutic needs, and physical and mental abilities. For example, short-term activities that provide immediate gratification will be needed for a patient with a short attention span, even when the patient is in a long-term care facility. In contrast, a long-term activity may be desired when a person is in an acute-care setting, but will return home for a long convalescence.

Available activities. The cost of supplies and equipment, as well as the need for storage space and for space for engaging in therapeutic activities, places constraints on the availablity of a variety of activities. Therapeutic activities include, but are not limited to, artwork, use of the computer, taking community trips, cooking, crafts, games, gardening, horticulture, music, needlework, verbal or nonverbal group interactions, writing, and any other mental or physical activities.

It is seldom possible to have available all supplies and equipment needed for the numerous activities in even one of the categories just listed. Most occupational therapy practitioners are familiar with a number of activities in each of the categories and have available a variety of activities for use in intervention. Fortunately, several activities have similar characteristics and can be equally effective in meeting the patient's needs. Occupational therapy practitioners are able to analyze and select activities that can be adapted and graded to make them suitable for the patient, regardless of age, sex, intellectual ability, social, economic, and cultural background, or the condition being treated.

Equipment and materials. The physical requirements of the activity are considered in selecting it. Physical requirements include the kinds and amounts of equipment, tools, and materials needed for the activity, the need for space, and the mobility of the equipment, tools, materials, and activity. Among the questions to consider are the following: 1) *Tools and equipment.* Is the equipment stationary or movable? How much space is needed? Are the size and weight of tools appropriate for the patients? How much noise will the tools make when being used? Are there potential dangers involved in using the tools? What are the safety features of the tools? 2) *Materials.* How much material will be needed? Will materials need to be stored? Is there sufficient storage space for the materials needed? Will the size, weight, shape, texture, color, and odor of the materials be appropriate for the setting? Can the patient injure him- or herself or otherwise irritate some part of the body when using the material? 3) *Space.* How much space is needed for the equipment, for the materials, and for engaging in the activity? Is appropriate space available? 4) *Time.* How much time is needed to prepare the materials and equipment for the activity? How much time is needed for the patient to engage in the activity? Can the activity be divided into segments of time so that it can be resumed at the next session? Does the activity meet the patient's psychosocial temporal needs? That is, can the patient attend to the activity for as long as he or she is expected to do so, or can the activity sustain the patient's interest for as long as it is expected to do so? How much time is needed to clear the area after completion of the activity? 5) Can the activity, equipment, materials, and tools be adapted to meet the needs of many patients, or are they designed for only a small number of patients?

Other space and time considerations. The space that is available and the time it will be available need to be considered in selecting an activity for therapy. In most treatment settings, including the private home, space is not available for such activities as art, ceramics, or gross-motor skills and games. How family members use space in the home and at what times they use it will affect the selection of activities. Occupational therapy practitioners frequently rely on their problem-solving skills and creative thinking to alter therapeutic activities to fit the space available. For example, activities have been modified to fit the space available in vans and mobile homes. Among the temporal aspects that are involved in selecting an activity are the length of time needed to engage in the activity, how the activity can be adapted to meet the time requirements of the treatment goal, and the patient's temporal needs.

The staff. Practitioners have their own skill levels and preferences for using activities in occupational therapy. Some prefer therapeutic exercises and electronically and mechanically controlled activities, some prefer group activities, and others prefer individualized craft activities. Although similarities exist among physical rehabilitation settings, long-term psychiatric settings, school settings, and other settings, there are differences among settings serving similar types of patients.

The differences in the types of activities in occupational therapy settings, the analysis of activities, and the therapeutic use of activities usually reflect the skills, interests, and frame of reference of the occupational therapy practitioner, even though activities have been used therapeutically for years. Grading and adapting the activity for a particular patient will also reflect the creative thinking and problem-solving abilities of the occupational therapy practitioner. Research may eventually result in more uniformity in the use of therapeutic activities for evaluation and intervention in given settings; however, the effectiveness of activities will be largely influenced by the skills and knowledge of the occupational therapy practitioner.

In the rest of this chapter, a few activities will be described and analyzed in terms of some of their performance components. The performance components are described fully in the *Uniform Terminology* document prepared by AOTA. Instructors in other occupational therapy courses or supervisors in actual settings may require more extensive analyses and may also request an activity analysis based on a particular frame of reference or treatment model that is being studied or used at the setting.

FINE-MOTOR ACTIVITIES

Ceramic products made of clay require many gross-motor and fine-motor activities before completion. In many treatment settings, partially prepared clay is used to avoid spending time mixing dry clay and water. Partially prepared clay is obtained in slightly moist blocks or in thick liquid form.

If the clay is in block form, a portion of the block is first wedged (i.e., manipulated by hand and repeatedly thrown against a canvas-covered board) to remove air bubbles and to create the desired consistency. The properly prepared clay can then be formed into objects by a variety of methods (Headquarters Department of the Army, 1980; Pedretti & Zoltan, 1990; Wankelman & Wigg, 1982). The wedged clay can be formed on a potter's wheel or sculptured with tools. The clay can be hand rolled into coils or into flat pieces with a rolling pin. The coils and flat pieces are then made into objects by adding additional coils or flat pieces. A handful of wedged clay can be pinched into any desired shape.

Liquid clay can be poured into prepared plaster-of-paris molds of the desired object. The clay is shaped by the mold as the mold absorbs the liquid from the clay. When the clay reaches a given consistency, it is removed from the mold.

The formed clay is allowed to dry until the object can be handled for sanding and smoothing. The dry, smoothed object is then placed in a kiln for bisque firing, after which it can be decorated by glazing and firing again as many times as desired.

Each procedure or method used in ceramics can be analyzed to determine its therapeutic value. For example, wedging the clay requires squeezing it, throwing it against a plaster bat, picking up the clay and slicing it against a taut wire, and repeating the process until the desired consistency is achieved. The wedging process may be therapeutic for a person who needs to strengthen the upper extremities and the range of motion of the joints or for someone for whom the texture of clay and the physical acts of slicing the lump of clay and throwing it may be relaxing and reduce tension.

To illustrate the process of analyzing an activity, let us next consider the making of a ceramic pinch pot.

Pinch Pot

Small pots, figurines, costume jewelry, and ornaments can be made by pinching or manipulating the properly wedged clay between the fingers. For a pot, the clay is shaped into a 3-inch or smaller ball and is then gradually formed into a pot by pushing in the center with the thumb, maintaining the desired outer shape with the fingers and palms. Evidence of fingerprints and other hand-molded effects may be left on the surface of the pot or may be sanded smooth. The edge is smoothed, the bottom flattened, and the pot is allowed to dry. The pot is glazed by dipping it into glaze or by painting the glaze on with a brush. Small designs can be painted with underglaze and finished with a clear glaze, or the surface can be finished as desired after bisque firing.

Special clay that does not need kiln firing is commercially available. Such clay is convenient for making a pinch pot in clinics, classrooms, and wherever a kiln is not available.

The following are some of the performance components involved in making a pinch pot:

Sensory: Vision is normally used, but a pinch pot still can be made by a person who is visually impaired or blind. Proprioception should be adequate to maintain the trunk and body parts in positions needed to manipulate the clay to form the pot. The hands receive tactile stimulation. Clay has a distinctive odor, but the olfactory sense is not crucial to this activity. Hearing is needed for verbal instructions and conversations with the supervisor of the activity, but an intact auditory sense is not essential for this solitary activity.

Neuromusculoskeletal and motor: Wedging a 6-inch or larger clump of clay is usually performed while standing or sitting erect in front of the wedging board. This activity requires normal postural control and alignment, integrated reflexes, strength, endurance, normal range of motion of the joints, and soft tissue integrity. Significant demand is placed on the dominant upper extremity. Both upper extremities are used during wedging when squeezing, slicing, and lifting the clay. If a small piece of clay is wedged for an individual pinch pot, the clay can be prepared by squeezing, twisting, and pushing it in the hands. Forming, sanding, sponging, and glazing the pinch pot all require bilateral use of the upper extremities, muscle control, bilateral integration, gross-motor and fine-motor coordination, visual-motor integration, laterality, and praxis.

Cognitive: Making a pinch pot requires a certain level of arousal, an orientation to and a recognition of the materials and objects to be used, and an attention span sufficient to engage in parts of the activity for a given period of time. The clay can be kept moist and can be worked on at a later time. The activity requires cognitive abilities such as initiating the activity, remembering and ordering the sequence of procedures involved, and categorizing various aspects of the activity. It also requires motor planning, in handling various tools and the clay to form the desired object and in terminating the activity and generalizing the information learned to similar activities. Concepts of size, shape, mass, wetness, dryness, space, and design can be learned. Problem-solving abilities and judgment are required as well.

Psychosocial: Forming the clay into an object requires an interest in doing so and self-expression from the individual and reveals some of the person's feelings and values. Because the clay can easily be manipulated and formed into an acceptable end product, a sense of achievement can arise, and the person's self-concept can be elevated. Self-control is exercised, since the clay and tools need to be handled in designated ways to yield satisfactory results. Interpersonal and social skills are used in relation to the supervisor of the activity and to other persons in the area. Time management is exercised because the clay changes its consistency over time. Coping skills are used when learning a new activity, when following instructions that sometimes do not yield expected results, and when waiting for materials to change their characteristics or for time to pass before being able to proceed to the next step. Immediate gratification can occur during each step and upon completion of each step of the process. Delaying gratification can be experienced if the kiln cannot be fired for a period of days or if repeated firings are required.

Making a pinch pot is an individual activity requiring no social interaction after the initial teacher-learner encounter. Group interaction may be facilitated by having individuals work on their projects in close proximity.

Temporal aspects:

Age and sex: Pinch pots can be made by individuals of either sex age 7 years or older.

Time required: Making ceramic products by the method just outlined is usually a short-term process. The completion time for the pinch pot can be as little as 15 minutes if the clay is already prepared and provided to each person in small balls. If the person prepares the clay and forms the pot, the activity can take as long as 45 minutes. Ceramic activities can be stopped and then started whenever supplies and areas in which to work are available. The completion of the project is measured in days or weeks, depending on the drying and firing schedule.

Precautions: Making a pinch pot is a relatively safe activity. Potential hazards exist for very young children and for disoriented individuals, who may attempt to ingest clay and glazes. The ceramist should be alerted to look for possible allergic reactions to the clay and the effect of abrasive clay on tender skin. Some individuals may object to handling clay.

Additional Learning Activities

1. Make an appointment to visit a local senior citizens' center or retirement village where ceramics classes are held. Observe the individuals as they handle the ceramic objects. Learn which type of method is most popular.
2. Practice analyzing other activities that are performed primarily with the upper extremities, such as a card game, discussed next.

Card Games

Card games using commercial or handmade cards can be used alone, by two people, or a group of people. Card games may involve concepts of matching (concentration), sequencing (rummy), categorizing (fish), or mathematics (gin rummy), or any combination of such concepts. The games can range from simple to complex. Card games may end after one set or may continue for hours or even days. Most card games may be interrupted and resumed at a later time, depending upon the player's decision. In your analysis of a card game, use the following performance components to answer questions about the activity:

Sensory: Are sensory awareness and sensory processing needed to perform the activity? What sensory systems are used to maintain the body and body parts in the required positions? What sensory systems are used to participate in the activity? Is discrimination of various sensory responses necessary? That is, is it important to have olfactory discrimination, visual discrimination, or any other sensory discrimination? What perceptual processing is needed to engage in the activity?

Neuromusculoskeletal and motor: What is the position of the body and body parts during the game? What is required to maintain the body in that position and to move the body and body parts during the activity? Is it necessary for some parts of the body to remain stable while other parts are moving? Is a certain amount of coordination or dexterity required to engage in the activity? Is a given amount of strength, range of joint motion, or level of endurance needed?

Cognitive: What levels of recognition, attention, and orientation are required? What concepts are required? What level of memory is needed? Is the ability to solve problems, order things in sequence, or organize or classify information required? Should the individual be able to begin and end his or her participation in the game?

Psychosocial: How much will personal values, interest, and motivation affect one's participation in the game? Is a certain level of self-concept, self-control, social conduct, self-expression, or interpersonal skills needed to engage effectively in the activity?

Temporal Aspects.

Age and sex: What is the recommended age range for the activity? Can the activity be engaged in by either sex?

Time required: What is the recommended time span for the activity? Can the time span be adapted to any of the individual's characteristics—for example, a short attention span? Can the activity be stopped and resumed later in the day or any number of days later?

Precautions. What are precautions surrounding the activity? Is the activity safer in given physical areas? What conditions will make a safer environment? What are the psychosocial precautions to take? Are any precautions needed that relate to the diverse nature of the group members?

GROSS-MOTOR ACTIVITIES

Gross-motor activities refer to those sensorimotor activities requiring large muscle movements—for example, of the head, the trunk, or the extremities. The activities elicit adaptive body responses and integration of body systems. Body balance, coordination, motion of the joints, and muscle strengthening can be improved by gross-motor activities.

Gross-motor activities may or may not need equipment. Running, jumping, and similar gross-motor activities involving games, such as "May I?" and "Simon Says," do not require equipment.

The parachute is a popular item that can be used for physical, psychological, and social benefits in gross-motor activities (French & Horvat, 1983). Occupational therapists initially used regular military parachutes. In many settings, when it became popular to use parachutes, smaller sized as well as large parachutes became available commercially.

The entire body can be involved in parachute activities. Among the positions and movements that are possible are standing, moving in a side step, holding the parachute with one hand and moving forward or backward, and extending and flexing all joints of the upper and lower extremities by lifting the parachute as high as possible and lowering it to the ground. Psychosocially, a group is formed when individuals grasp the edge of the parachute and face each other. Individuals learn that each person affects what happens with the parachute. The entire group can work together on a particular activity, or individuals opposite each other can form teams and compete in activities. Individuals can be active participants, even without speaking. Depending upon the activities performed, the parachute can develop a person's sensorimotor, perceptual, cognitive, or psychosocial skills. Handling a large item that is affected by both the air in the environment and the participants usually elicits motivation, interest, and the desire to be a member of the group. The gross-motor movements of running, skipping, walking, and crawling, as well as the range of motion of the joints, muscle strength, and endurance can be developed, depending upon the activities selected and the time taken to complete them. Postural balance can be practiced with parachute activities.

Simon Says, "Use a Parachute"

The purposes of this activity are to increase one's general physical strength, endurance, and cooperation by moving the joints and to contribute to the group effort by using the parachute and identifying body parts. The individuals face the center of the parachute and grasp the edge of the parachute with the dorsum of the hand on top. The overhand grasp places the upper extremities in the proper anatomical position for shoulder flexion. The size of the parachute will determine the maximum number of participants. A space that allows each person to abduct the upper extremities about 45 degrees will be ample.

The participants are first introduced to the effect of lowering and raising the parachute. Each person can see and feel that individual actions have an effect on what happens to the parachute.

The staff person or a selected group member calls out the instructions.

For example, the instruction may be "Simon says, 'Drop the parachute to your knees,'" or "Simon says, 'Raise the parachute above your head.'" The performance components of the activity are as follows:

Sensory: To hold and manipulate the parachute while maintaining control over and moving the body and body parts requires sensory awareness and sensory processing of the tactile, proprioceptive, and vestibular systems. To see the objects and persons in the environment and hear the instructions requires adequate functioning of the visual and auditory senses. Adequate perceptual processing of kinesthesia, body scheme, and right-left discrimination will allow appropriate responses to instructions and movement. An adequate sense of pain is needed in any gross-motor activity with a group, in order to alert the individual and others when the individual experiences pain, since the potential for injury exists. Visual discriminations of figure versus ground, depth perception, and spatial relations will enable the individual to handle the parachute as instructed.

Neuromusculoskeletal and motor: To hold the parachute and follow instructions to make gross body movements in unison with other group members requires reflex integration, postural control and alignment, the full range of motion of the joints, and strength and endurance for the duration of the activity. Because movements will need to be made as soon as instructions are given, motor-planning ability, bilateral integration, motor control, and gross-motor and visual-motor coordination are needed. Midline crossing and laterality may be needed as well, depending on the instructions given.

Cognitive: To work as a group following instructions using a parachute requires the participants to have and maintain a level of arousal, to be oriented to time and place, to recognize objects and persons and be aware of environmental influences, to recognize and respond to the instructions, to know when to initiate and terminate segments of the activity, and to remember the instructions long enough to carry them out.

Psychosocial: Since cooperation is needed in performing the activity, the individual should value other persons. Interest in the activity will enhance the level of performance as each person assumes the role of a group member. Social conduct, self-control, and time management are also needed for effective participation. Self-expression and interpersonal skills are exercised as well. Self-expression is possible through joining or not joining the group, through performing physical actions, and through verbalizing feelings. Coping skills are developed as individuals work at group efforts to handle the parachute as instructed.

Temporal aspects:

Age: This activity is suitable for ages 7 and above, since it requires knowledge of body parts, responding to verbal instructions, and working together with others. A relatively homogeneous group in age and physical size is most appropriate.

Time required: The length of time required to carry out the activity will depend on the endurance of the group members. Parachute activities can be planned for about 30 minutes, with rest between short sessions.

Precautions: Watch for fatigue. Ask participants periodically how they are feeling, and give them an opportunity to rest as a group or individually. Watch for fear or dizziness when activities involve persons being under the parachute or being on top of the parachute and rocked or bounced. All parachute activities should be done only under supervision, with caution, and with the participants exercising responsibility for each other. The activities require a large room such as a gymnasium or should be performed outdoors in a relatively level area. If the activities are held outdoors, the temperature should be mild and there should be no strong breezes or other inclement weather. The group should be able to understand the language being used for the instructions. Allow time after the activities for individuals to discuss how they felt about their participation.

Additional Learning Activities

1. Make an appointment to visit an elementary school or a Head Start or special education program to observe the adaptive physical education or occupational therapy program used.
2. Ask occupational therapy practitioners if they use indoor or outdoor games for gross-motor therapeutic activities.

GROUP INTERACTION ACTIVITIES

Some therapeutic activities are aimed at helping patients develop group interaction skills. These activities can be nonverbal, verbal, gross motor, intellectual, educational, or musical, or they can have another focus, depending upon the patient's need and interests.

The soapbox debate will be analyzed next for its psychosocial therapeutic uses. Group members should meet the recommended criteria in order to form the foundation for a successful activity.

Soapbox Debate

The soapbox debate (Remocker & Storch, 1992) is a verbal group activity whose purposes are to help a person develop confidence in a group situation and to speak in a group. Participation in the activity aids decision making and logical reasoning. Group members should be fairly comfortable with each other and be able to read and verbalize in the same language.

The time available for the activity may determine the maximum number in the group. A maximum of 10 minutes is allowed for each person to read the statement to be debated, present a personal view, and hear responses to his or her presentation. Four or five people in a group is the recommended number.

The activity is essentially a modified debate. The staff person prepares a set of cards, on each of which is a different statement to be debated. One or two cards more than the number of people in the group are used. Each statement should be capable of being answered with the words "I agree" or "I disagree." For example, one card may state, "Hunting wild animals with bows and arrows should be outlawed." The cards are placed in a box on a table so that group members cannot see the written statements. The participants are invited to sit around the table. The first debater takes a card out of the box and reads the statement aloud. The debater then agrees or disagrees with the statement and justifies his or her opinion with three reasons. Other group members listen until the debater finishes speaking. At this point, the topic is open for debate by the other group members. Ten minutes are allowed for each statement to be debated. After that time, the next person selects a card, and the process is repeated. The activity should not exceed 1 hour; a shorter session of 30 to 40 minutes is recommended. A small group helps each group member feel more comfortable speaking.

The staff person sets the stage for the debate, explains the rules, maintains freedom of speech for the speaker, and, when necessary, clarifies comments. For example, if a speaker rambles or combines three reasons in one sentence, the staff person intervenes, clarifies what was said, and facilitates the continuation of the activity.

At the end of the session, the staff member acknowledges the end of the debate. Positive comments may be made about the group's or each individual's performance. If individual behaviors are to be reinforced, be sure to have a positive comment for each member of the group. Examples of such comments are "Everyone in the group followed the rules and stayed within the time allowed," "Jane, you spoke clearly and projected your voice, so we heard your statements," "Dan, you maintained eye contact with each person who responded to you. [To the group:] Did that make each of you feel better as you talked to Dan?" and "Bill, I liked the way you stated your response so concisely." The activity ends with the group members being thanked for participating.

The following are the performance components of the soapbox debate:

Sensory: Sensory awareness and sensory processing of tactile, proprioceptive, visual, and auditory systems, perceptual processing of stereognosis and kinesthesia, and discrimination of depth perception and spatial relations are needed to reach into the box without looking into it, select a card, read the statement written on the card, and hear statements read by others.

Neuromusculoskeletal and motor: Reflex integration and postural control and alignment are needed to sit in a normal position at the table. An adequate range of motion of the joints, motor control, fine-motor, gross-motor, and visual-motor coordination, and muscle strength and endurance are needed to reach into the box, select a card, hold and release the card, and participate in the activity for its duration. The motor skills are not prerequisites for the actual debate, since it is primarily a verbal activity. Any body position that allows verbal participation may be assumed. The desired positioning of the participants is to have members speak to each other face to face.

Cognitive: The activity requires a certain level of arousal, orientation, recognition, attention span, memory, and generalization of past learning. Participants must be able to read the words on the card, formulate concepts, use language effectively, reason logically, and speak coherently about the statement.

Psychosocial: The participants express their personal values and interests as they debate the various statements. The self-concept is enhanced as each person is given full attention when he or she debates the statement in a safe situation and when those who respond agree with the debater's position on the statement. Interpersonal skills, social conduct, and roles are exercised during the activity. Time management is exercised as the participants deal with the time limit set for them. Self-control and coping skills can also be expressed as each participant becomes the center of attention as the debater, following the rules of the debate and waiting for a turn to participate.

Precautions: The issues and statements to be debated should be appropriate for the group's cognitive level, psychosocial functioning, and cultural situation. Nonpersonal and nonthreatening issues are easiest for discussion.

Preparing more statements than the total number in the group may alleviate suspicious feelings. Group members may themselves submit statements for debate when appropriate. The debate can take place indoors or outdoors. The space should be relatively quiet and free from the possibility of intrusion.

Additional Learning Activities

1. Suggest other verbal activities that focus on developing or enhancing one's self-concept, speaking in front of a group, or expressing one's opinions.
2. Suggest nonverbal activities that aid in expressing one's feelings or opinions in a safe way.

3. Think of ways to adapt the activities you have suggested so that they can be used with a preschool group, school-age children, and other age groups.

SUMMARY

Therapeutic occupations (activities) are analyzed by OTRs and COTAs and are judiciously used in the intervention process. Analyzing activities and adapting them to meet the many needs of the patient are constant challenges for occupational therapy practitioners. The variety of occupations that can be used allows for highly individualized treatment, depending upon the occupational therapy practitioner's knowledge and skills, the patient's needs and treatment goals, the available activities, and the ability to grade the activities and adapt them to the patient's level of functioning. Each activity can have different performance components, depending on how it is presented and used.

REVIEW QUESTIONS

1. Give the basic belief about occupations upon which the profession of occupational therapy is founded by circling the best answer to complete the sentence:
   Occupations are considered therapeutic when:
   a. the patient selects and enjoys completing the activity.
   b. the patient's mind and body are engaged in the activity.
   c. they are purposeful and aid in achieving treatment goals.
   d. they are selected by the occupational therapy practitioner.
2. State five ways that engaging in purposeful activities affects an individual.
3. What two principles should be considered when selecting therapeutic occupations?
4. Discuss the COTA's role and possible tasks related to therapeutic occupations.
5. Select one of the following activities, and identify its performance components. Or name your own activity, and identify its performance components. State the precautions to take in implementing the activity you have selected.
   1) Make a mixed-leaf vegetable salad.
      a) Select the ingredients_____. b) Wash, cut, or tear the leaves_____. c) Mix the salad_____. d) Divide and put the salad into individual bowls_____. e) Select a dressing, and place it onto the salad_____.
   2) Play the card game concentration.
      a) Shuffle the cards_____. b) Place the cards on the

table face down, in equal rows and columns_____. c) Pick up two cards one at a time, look at them, and replace them face up on the table_____. d) Remove cards or replace them, depending on whether they match_____. e) Wait for your turn_____. f) Begin and complete play_____.

ANSWERS

1. c.
2. Engaging in purposeful activities can affect one's cognition, emotions, social relationships, motivation, sensorimotor abilities, muscle strength, range of motion of the joints, physical and mental endurance, and sensory integration.
3. 1) The patient's needs should be considered to determine whether the occupations will affect his or her problem that is to be treated, abilities and disabilities, mental and emotional state, and physical condition, as well as whether they will affect individuals in the patient's life and the physical, social, and cultural environment in which the patient has been living. 2) The activity should aid in achieving the patient's therapeutic goals.
4. The COTA assists the supervising OTR in the selection of therapeutic activities. This may include analyzing activities that will meet the needs of the patient and the goals of intervention, suggesting activities similar to those selected by the OTR, and adapting the activities that have been selected as the patient's intervention needs to be changed. The COTA educates the patient about the value of the occupation in meeting the treatment goals, motivates the patient to engage in the activity, teaches the procedures that make up the activity, provides reinforcement for the patient who has performed the activity well, corrects any misconceptions the patient has and any wrong motions the patient makes in carrying out the activity, and evaluates and reports on how the patient has been participating and progressing during the intervention. The COTA may arrange the therapeutic setting, assure the safety of the equipment and materials that will be used, and maintain the required supply levels.
5. 1) Make a mixed-leaf vegetable salad.
   a) Select the ingredients___*Sensory (visual), Cognitive (nutritive value, safe food), Psychosocial (values, interest)*___. b) Wash, cut, or tear the leaves___*Neuromusculoskeletal and motor (postural control, range of motion, gross-motor, fine-motor, and visual-motor coordination*___. c) Mix the salad___*Neuromusculoskeletal and motor (same as b)*___. d) Divide and put the salad into individual bowls___*Cognitive (spatial operations, problem solving), psychosocial (value, social conduct, time*

management, role performance, interpersonal skills___. e) Select a dressing, and place it onto the salad_*Sensory (visual, auditory), psychosocial (values, social conduct, role performance)___*.

Precautions: Teach the participants to wash the vegetables properly. If a knife or pair of scissors is used to cut the vegetables, remind the patient of its proper use. Caution the participants to keep the floor clear of liquids and vegetables to avoid falls. If any unprepared vegetables or utensils fall to the floor, they are to be washed again; however, vegetables that have been peeled and cut into pieces should be discarded rather than used for the salad.

2) Play the card game concentration.
a) Shuffle the cards___*Neuromusculoskeletal and motor (postural control, integration of reflexes, upper extremity range of motion, gross-motor, fine-motor, and visual-motor coordination, dexterity, strength___.* b) Place the cards on the table face down, in equal rows and columns___*Neuromusculoskeletal & motor (same as a), sensory (awareness, processing of tactile, proprioceptive, vestibular, visual, and auditory systems, visual discrimination of figure from ground, depth perception, spatial relations), cognitive (orientation, recognition, initiation and termination of activity, sequencing, spatial operations)___*.
c) Pick up two cards one at a time, look at them, and replace them face up on the table___*Neuromusculoskeletal and motor, sensory, cognitive (same as b), psychosocial (role performance, social conduct, interpersonal skills, self-expression)___.* d) Remove cards or replace them, depending on whether they match___*Neuromusculoskeletal and motor, sensory, cognitive (same as c), psychosocial (same as c, plus coping skills, time management, and self-control___.* e) Wait for your turn___*Psychosocial (role performance, social conduct, coping skills, self-control)___.* f) Begin and complete play___*Cognitive (recognition, attention span, spatial operations, initiate and terminate activity, memory, sequencing, categorization), psychosocial (role performance, social conduct, self-control, time management)___*.

Precautions: The potential for physical injury is minimal. The person supervising the game should be alert to psychosocial effects and should provide reinforcement to all players for their effort, involvement, social conduct, interpersonal skills, coping skills, and other positive behaviors.

ADDITIONAL LEARNING ACTIVITIES

1. Make appointments to visit occupational therapy programs in state and private psychiatric hospitals, school programs, retirement villages,

rehabilitation hospitals, and other settings to observe their use of therapeutic activities. Discuss with the occupational therapy practitioner how the particular activity meets the patient's therapeutic needs.

2. If you selected one of the activities listed for review question 5 and included more performance components than were given in the answer, your answer is likely to be correct and more complete. Congratulations for a great start in analyzing activities! You can also think about other aspects of the activity. For example, is it noisy or quiet? Is it clean or dirty? Is it messy or orderly? Is it active or sedentary? Is it relaxing or tension building? Is it an aggressive activity? Is it considered a masculine, feminine, or neuter activity? How much verbalization is required to perform the activity? Is it a group activity that allows a newcomer to feel welcome? And finally, what potential does the activity have for meeting the physical, emotional, intellectual, social, and cultural needs of a particular patient?

3. Can the activity you selected in review question 5 be adapted to a range of intellectual levels? Can it be adapted for a person in a wheelchair? For someone with the use of only one upper extremity?

4. Review videotapes and movies on different craft activities. Jot down ideas on how persons with physical disabilities can engage in these activities. Think of ways to adapt the use of the tools, the materials, and the positions in which the activity is done to patients with disabilities. Discuss your ideas with occupational therapy practitioners.

REFERENCES

Allen, C. K., Earhart, C. A., & Blue, T. (1992). *Occupational therapy treatment goals for the physically and cognitively disabled.* Bethesda, MD: American Occupational Therapy Association, Inc.

American Occupational Therapy Association, Inc. (1979). The philosophical base of occupational therapy. *American Journal of Occupational Therapy, 33*(11), 785.

American Occupational Therapy Association, Inc. (1994). Uniform terminology for occupational therapy—third edition. *American Journal of Occupational Therapy, 48*(11), 1049-1055.

Early, M. B. (1993). *Mental health concepts and techniques for the occupational therapy assistant* (2nd ed.). New York:

French, R., and Horvat, M. (1983). *Parachute movement activities.* Bryon, CA: Front Row Experience.

Headquarters Department of the Army (1980). *Craft techniques in occupational therapy.* Washington, DC: Superintendent of Documents, US Government Printing Office.

Hirama, H. (1992). *Activity analysis: A primer.* Baltimore: CHESS Publications, Inc.

Pedretti, L. W., & Zoltan, B. (1990). *Occupational therapy: Practice skills for physical dysfunction.* St. Louis: The C. V. Mosby Co.

Ratner, J. (1939). *Intelligence in the modern world: John Dewey's philosophy.* New York: Random House.

nRemocker, A. J., & Storch, E. T. (1992). *Action speaks louder* (5th ed.). London: Churchill, Livingstone, Inc.

Schwartz, K. B. (1992). Occupational therapy and education: A shared vision. *American Journal of Occupational Therapy, 46*(1), 12-18.

Wankelman, W. F., & Wigg, P. R. (1982). *A handbook of arts and crafts for elementary and junior high school teachers* (5th ed.). Dubuque, IA: William C. Brown Company, Publishers.

SUGGESTED READINGS

Allen, C. K. (1987) Activity: Occupational therapy's treatment method. *American Journal of Occupational Therapy, 41*(9), 563-575.

Blakeslee, M. E. (1981). *The wheelchair gourmet: A cookbook for the disabled.* Don Mills, Ontario: General Publishing Company Limited.

Cox, B. (1981). *I can do it! I can do it! Cookbook for people with special needs.* Newport Beach, CA: K & H Publishing Company.

Creighton, C. (1992). Origin and evolution of activity analysis. *American Journal of Occupational Therapy, 46*(1), 45-48.

Depew, A. M. (1960). *The Cokesbury game book.* New York: Abingdon Press.

Di Joseph, L. M. (1982). Independence through activity: Mind, body and environment interaction in therapy. *American Journal of Occupational Therapy, 36*(11), 740-744.

Drake, M. (1992). *Crafts in therapy and rehabilitation.* Thorofare, NJ: Slack, Inc.

Gibson, W. (1970). *Family games America plays.* Garden City, NY:

Lamport, N. K., Coffey, M. S., & Hersch, G. L. (1993). *Activity analysis handbook* (2nd ed.). Thorofare, NJ: Slack, Inc.

Lyons, B. G. (1983). The issue is: Purposeful versus human activity. *American Journal of Occupational Therapy, 37*(7), 493-495.

Manchester, R. B. (1980). *The 2nd mammoth book of fun and games.* New York: Hart Book Associates.

Mosey, A. C. (1973). *Activities therapy.* New York: Raven Press.

Olszowy, D. R. (1978). *Horticulture for the disabled and disadvantaged.* Springfield, IL: Charles C. Thomas.

SUGGESTED LISTENING/VIEWING

Allen, C. K. (1991). *Why occupational therapists use crafts.* Bethesda, MD: American Occupational Therapy Association, Inc. VHS (30 min).

Check your campus and community library for films on recreational and leisure activities.

Check your campus and community continuing education departments for courses on recreational and leisure activities.

14

THERAPEUTIC EXERCISE AND THERAPEUTIC ACTIVITIES

The definition and purpose of activities and exercise are given. The current use of activities and exercise in occupational therapy is discussed.

LEARNING OBJECTIVES

At the end of this chapter, you should be able to:

1. Define therapeutic exercise.
2. Define therapeutic activities.
3. State four purposes of therapeutic activities.
4. Explain the difference between therapeutic activities and therapeutic exercise.
5. Discuss the advantages of therapeutic activities and therapeutic exercise.

Although the human body is a mobile structure, it may be affected, temporarily or permanently, by disease or injury. When normal movement is limited, specific repeated movements of the affected joints may help to restore such movement. For example, when the hand is injured, therapeutic exercise helps restore mobility and maintain the gliding planes of motion. Therapeutic exercise also prevents scar tissue from becoming dense or restrictive and maintains the mobility of connective tissue. When contractures and tendon adhesions develop, therapeutic exercise is used to restore motion (Stanley & Tribuzi, 1992).

Therapeutic exercise refers to body movement or muscle contraction that is prescribed to correct an impairment, to improve or maintain musculoskeletal function, or to maintain a state of well-being (Kottke, Stillwell, & Lehmann, 1982). *Taber's Cyclopedic Medical Dictionary* defines therapeutic exercise as "Scientific supervision of exercise for the purpose of preventing muscular atrophy, restoring joint and muscle functions, increasing muscular strength, and improving efficiency of cardiovascular and pulmonary function" (Thomas, 1993, p. 1976).

Therapeutic exercise, which is specific to each patient, is prescribed by a physician. The physician will usually refer the patient to a physical therapist, an occupational therapist, or some other qualified professional, depending upon the particular needs of the patient. As the patient's condition changes, the prescribed exercise or the way it is to be performed changes. Therapeutic exercises must be carefully supervised by the therapist.

Physicians who prescribe and supervise therapeutic exercise and therapists who supervise patients in their performance of the exercise are knowledgeable in the biophysical and neurophysiological aspects of kinesiology and the basic principles of therapeutic exercise. The entry-level occupational therapy assistant who lacks such knowledge should receive supervision when engaging a patient in therapeutic exercise.

PURPOSE OF THERAPEUTIC EXERCISE

Therapeutic exercise is usually prescribed to achieve one or more of the following broad goals:

1. To increase or maintain mobility of joints.
2. To develop, improve, or maintain coordination.
3. To develop, improve, or maintain strength and endurance.
4. For relaxation (Kottke, Stillwell, & Lehmann, 1982).

Specific goals and exercises are established for individual patients (Pedretti & Zoltan, 1990).

Mobility

Most people without disabling conditions move their joints through their full range of motion many times in the normal course of their daily activities. If the range of motion of their joints is restricted for a period of time, tightness develops.

Tightness in a joint may develop into a limitation on the motion of the joint, which is disabling. Exercise may be prescribed to prevent tightness and maintain the joint's full range of motion.

Injury, pain, weakness, or treatment that immobilizes a joint also may reduce the joint's normal range of motion. Exercise may be prescribed to increase the range of motion if such potential exists.

Coordination

Coordination is the combination of many movements performed by many muscles in smooth patterns of motion. Coordination is dependent upon the integration of neuromuscular activity with cerebral activity, plus practice of precise movements through many repetitions.

Initially, attention is required to obtain the movements desired. Gradually, as extraneous movements are inhibited and the precise desired movements are performed many times, the movements are performed automatically. For example, rising from a chair and walking, as well as riding a bicycle, requires precise, coordinated movements. When initially being learned, both activities require mental concentration and repeated practice. When finally learned, walking and bicycling become automatic. Concentrated repetition of movements is needed to relearn coordinated patterns of movement following injury or disease.

Strength and Endurance

Strength is the maximum tension that can be exerted by a muscle during a contraction. *Endurance* is the ability of the muscle to contract and to exert tension for a period of time. *Power* is the rate of work done per unit of time (Kottke, Stillwell, & Lehmann, 1982).

Therapeutic exercise to develop or maintain strength, endurance, or power is classified as *assistive, active,* or *resistive.* Additional descriptors, such as active-assistive, are used for more definitive classifications at some settings.

Passive exercise does not develop or maintain strength, endurance, or power, but is still a therapeutic exercise. The purpose of passive exercise is to maintain the range of motion of a joint and prevent contractures, adhesions, and deformity. Passive exercise does not increase the range of motion of the joint because no force is applied to the joint. Similarly, muscles are not strengthened because no muscle contraction occurs (Pedretti & Zoltan, 1990).

In assistive exercise, equipment or a therapist assists the patient in performing the exercise. If muscles cannot lift the body part against gravity, the effect of the force of gravity is eliminated by the equipment or the therapist. This may be done by supporting the extremity on equipment such as a skateboard or a suspended sling. For example, to enable horizontal abduction and adduction of the upper extremity with assistive exercise, the patient's right forearm can be strapped to a skateboard. The patient, who is seated at a table, rolls the skateboard from the midline of the body to the right edge of the table and back to the midline 10 times. If the patient is unable to complete the full range of motion, the therapist or equipment assist in completing it.

Active exercise requires the patient to move the affected body part through the available range of motion independently. During the first stages of active exercise, the patient may need to have the effect of gravity eliminated. A powdered surface, skateboard, deltoid aid, or suspension sling used in assistive exercise may be needed by the patient initially.

Resistive exercises are movements of the body part through the full range of motion, against gravity and applied resistance. Elastic bands, weighted wrist and ankle cuffs, sandbags, springs, and weights are used to add resistance. Resistive exercises are used to increase muscle strength.

Endurance is increased by repeated exercise against low or moderate resistance. Endurance can be developed only if fatigue is experienced. Because of the prolonged repetition of exercise needed to develop endurance, the exercise should be of interest to the individual. Interest can be created by self-competition and competition against time, as well as by exercising with others, keeping records, and receiving tangible reinforcement.

Relaxation

Anxiety is not uncommon among patients. Anxiety creates tension, which adversely affects many body systems. Prolonged muscle contraction due to anxiety may cause headaches, neck aches, dental problems, and discomfort in joints and muscles. Any of these symptoms can create anxiety, and a circular process develops. Anxiety has a detrimental effect on the patient's treatment program.

In many rehabilitation hospitals, treatment often includes relaxation exercises to reduce anxiety. Most relaxation exercises are based upon Jacobson's classic progressive relaxation technique (Jacobson, 1938, 1957). A member of the occupational therapy staff who has learned the technique may be responsible for administering the exercise. Or, another discipline may have the responsibility for administering it, depending upon the regulations of the facility.

THERAPEUTIC ACTIVITY

herapeutic activity consists of purposeful occupations prescribed to improve or maintain neuromuscular or psychosocial functioning. The occupations can be any tasks or skills an individual engages in for self-care or during work or leisure time. The patient's willing and active participation in the activity is needed to derive the greatest therapeutic benefit.

The specific therapeutic characteristics of the occupations to be used in therapy are determined by the occupational therapist planning the patient's treatment program. The occupational therapist or assistant, who is responsible for the direct intervention, selects those occupations which are best suited for the patient.

In the treatment of a patient, therapeutic activities may have the same purpose as therapeutic exercises. The disadvantage of therapeutic activities is their lack of precision of movements and the number of repetitions of movements they require, which make measurements and documentation of results more complicated and often unacceptable. On the other hand, therapeutic activities have the distinct advantage of providing many sensorimotor, cognitive, and psychosocial components that are not present in repetitive therapeutic exercises.

PURPOSE OF THERAPEUTIC ACTIVITIES

Therapeutic activities may be used in occupational therapy to achieve one or more of the goals related to the patient's activities of daily living, work activities, and play or leisure activities. The broad goals are to:

1. develop, maintain, improve, or restore the performance of necessary functions;
2. compensate for dysfunction;
3. minimize or prevent debilitation; and
4. promote health and wellness (AOTA, 1994).

Specific goals and activities are established for individual patients (Pedretti & Zoltan, 1990).

OCCUPATIONAL THERAPY AND THERAPEUTIC EXERCISE

Traditionally, rehabilitation to restore physical functioning included exercise for patients in need of treatment for joint motion, muscle strength, and endurance. Therapeutic exercise was considered more within the domain of physical therapy than occupational therapy. For example, a patient with limited strength and range of motion of the right upper extremity might exercise by moving the extremity in a given way for a definite number of times, with resistance as part of the physical therapy intervention. In occupational therapy, the same patient might use the same extremity and perform similar movements against similar amounts of resistance, but would do so while engaged in a project or an activity of interest that used many body parts.

Occupational therapy normally combines purposeful activity with exercise. The purposeful activity provides psychosocial benefits through interest, motivation, gratification, and a sense of self-worth, by producing a completed item. Normally, individuals use muscles and body parts in an integrated fashion rather than in isolation. Individuals also use the body and mind in relation to the environment, time, and the values they hold. The purposeful activity provides an opportunity to use the affected body part together with the rest of the body. As part of occupational therapy, therapeutic exercise thus benefits the whole person—physically, cognitively, and psychosocially. When specific repetitive exercise is used in occupational therapy, it is usually used in preparation for engaging in a functional activity. The exercise is a segment of the treatment process during a treatment session. Exercise would not normally be the complete treatment the patient engages in during the session.

Activities such as weaving on table and floor looms, woodworking, metalwork, leather craft, ceramics, block printing, and making square knots can be therapeutic and help to develop gross-motor and fine-motor coordination, dexterity, strength, concentration, a sense of accomplishment, and many other desired characteristics; however, there are often disadvantages in using such activities in therapy for physical rehabilitation. Space required for equipment and storage, time required for preparing and teaching many different activities, and the cost of replacing materials are disadvantages, compared to equipment and supplies that do not need to be replaced or changed. Also, it is difficult to document that certain results seen after engaging in therapeutic activities are actually *caused* by the activities, because it is difficult to quantify the numerous unique actions of the individual during the process. The lack of time, the need to provide service for more patients, and the need to document specific measurable results of therapy are some reasons that therapeutic activities are used less now than they were in the past.

SUMMARY

Specific therapeutic exercise or activity is prescribed to improve, increase, or maintain mobility of the joints, muscle strength, and coordination. Exercise or activity may also be prescribed to achieve relaxation, since excessive tension and stress adversely affect the body systems. The entry-level occupational therapy assistant who lacks the knowledge of how to use therapeutic exercise should have training and close supervision while treating patients.

REVIEW QUESTIONS

1. Define therapeutic exercise.
2. Define therapeutic activity.
3. What are four purposes of therapeutic activities?
4. How do therapeutic exercise and therapeutic activities differ?
5. Discuss the advantages of therapeutic activities and therapeutic exercise.

ANSWERS

1. Therapeutic exercise consists of specific repetitive body movements and muscle contractions prescribed to correct an impairment or to improve or maintain musculoskeletal functioning and a state of well-being.

2. A therapeutic activity is a purposeful occupation selected to improve or maintain neuromuscular or psychosocial functioning. Therapeutic activities are tasks an individual engages in for self-care or during work or leisure time.
3. The purposes of therapeutic activities are to: 1) develop, maintain, improve, or restore the performance of necessary functions; 2) compensate for dysfunction; 3) minimize or prevent debilitation; and 4) promote health and well-being.
4. Therapeutic exercises are repetitive movements and muscle contractions performed in a prescribed way for a determined number of times or a given length of time during treatment. The exercises are usually for a specific part of the body. Therapeutic activities are usually selected to achieve a specific goal. They usually take into account the patient's interest in the activity. In therapeutic activity, movements are not exactly replicated each time, as they are in repetitive exercises, and the same movement is not made for the same number of times or the same length of time, as is the case in therapeutic exercises.
5. Appropriately selected therapeutic activities afford physical movement and strengthen the affected body parts, while motivating the patient to engage in the activities. Therapeutic activities also can provide cognitive and psychosocial benefits. Therapeutic exercises provide the precise movements and strengthening needed for treatment, and the patient's progress can be easily measured and documented.

ADDITIONAL LEARNING ACTIVITIES

1. Visit an occupational therapy department of a rehabilitation hospital. Identify the therapeutic exercises used in that facility to improve a) range of motion and b) muscle strength and endurance.
2. Ask occupational therapy practitioners in various settings to comment on their use of therapeutic activities and exercise. Do the diagnostic groups in the settings determine whether therapeutic exercises or therapeutic activities are used?
3. Visit a physical therapy department to observe the use of therapeutic exercise by physical therapists and physical therapy assistants.

REFERENCES

American Occupational Therapy Association. (1994). Uniform terminology for occupational therapy—third edition. *American Journal of Occupational Therapy, 48*(11), 1047-1054.

Jacobson, E. (1938). *Progressive relaxation.* Chicago: University of Chicago Press.

Jacobson, E. (1957). *You must relax* (4th ed.). New York: McGraw Hill Book Company.

Kottke, F. J., Stillwell, G. K., & Lehmann, J. F. (Eds.). (1982). *Krusen's handbook of physical medicine and rehabilitation* (3rd ed.). Philadelphia: W. B. Saunders Company.

Pedretti, L. W., & Zoltan, B. (1990). *Occupational therapy: Practice skills for physical dysfunction* (3rd ed.). St. Louis: The C. V. Mosby Co.

Stanley, B. G., & Tribuzi, S. M. (1992). *Concepts in hand rehabilitation.* Philadelphia: F. A. Davis Company.

Thomas, C. L. (1993). *Taber's cyclopedic medical dictionary* (17th ed.). Philadelphia: F. A. Davis Company.

SUGGESTED READINGS

Fazio, L. S. (1992). Tell me a story: The therapeutic metaphor in the practice of pediatric occupational therapy. *American Journal of Occupational Therapy, 46*(2), 112-119.

Fick, K. M. (1993). Influence of an animal on social interactions of nursing home residents in a group setting. *American Journal of Occupational Therapy, 47*(6), 529-534.

Huss, H. J. (1981). From kinesiology to adaptation. *American Journal of Occupational Therapy, 35*(9), 574-580.

Kielhofner, G. (1982). A heritage of activity: Development of theory. *American Journal of Occupational Therapy, 36,* 723-730.

Neistadt, M. E., McAuley, D., Zecha, D., & Shannon, R. (1993). Analysis of a board game as a treatment activity. *American Journal of Occupational Therapy, 47*(2), 154-160.

Stevens-Ratchford, R. G. (1993). Effect of life review reminiscence activities on depression and self-esteem in older adults. *American Journal of Occupational Therapy, 47*(5), 413-420.

Tse, S.-K., & Bailey, D. (1992). T'ai Chi and postural control in the well elderly. *American Journal of Occupational Therapy, 46*(4), 295-300.

15

THERAPEUTIC EQUIPMENT

Factors to consider before recommending therapeutic equipment for a patient are reviewed. Some commonly used therapeutic equipment is examined. Safety measures for constructing or adapting equipment are given.

LEARNING OBJECTIVES

At the end of this chapter, you should be able to:

1. Discuss factors to consider in deciding whether therapeutic equipment will be useful for a patient.
2. Name at least three adaptations to wheelchairs, and state the intended value of each.
3. Name at least one piece of therapeutic equipment that will aid the performance of the following activities: sitting, eating, dressing, and leisure.
4. State at least five safety features to include when building or adding metal or wood adaptations to equipment.

Ideally, upon completion of an occupational therapy program, the patient regains all of his or her previous abilities. Unfortunately, the ideal does not always occur. The patient may regain the ability to function independently, but not to the previous level. Or the patient may regain only enough function to perform independently if changes in the physical environment are made. Or the patient may be able to function independently only with special equipment. Since an aim of occupational therapy is to enable the patient to perform daily living activities as independently as possible, evaluating the environment and the possible use of an adaptive device to maximize the patient's independence is an occupational therapy service.

177

Equipment that enables an otherwise dependent person to perform daily living activities independently is as valuable as therapeutic techniques used to improve muscle strength, range of motion of the joints, and endurance. Such equipment is commonly referred to as *therapeutic equipment,* or *therapeutic devices.* Whether or not therapeutic equipment is recommended for a patient will depend on a variety of factors.

Therapeutic equipment generally needs to be fitted to the particular patient. The time required to evaluate the prospect of the equipment helping the patient, to fit the equipment to the patient, and to train the patient in the use of the equipment, as well as the cost of the equipment, need justification in terms of what the resulting benefit will be to the patient.

A general rule is to recommend therapeutic equipment only when the patient cannot function without it. The equipment should be prescribed only for the period needed. As the patient's condition improves, the use of the equipment should gradually lessen. In some cases, however, the therapeutic equipment will be needed permanently.

The following characteristics of the patient need to be considered before recommending special equipment:

1. *Physical condition.* Is the patient's physical condition permanent? If so, is the condition stabilized? Will deterioration occur? If so, how soon will it begin? Will it be possible to use or adapt the equipment when deterioration begins? Will the patient physically be able to manage the equipment? If the patient needs assistance to use the equipment, is such assistance available? Will the patient's height and weight change rapidly?

2. *Mental status.* Does the patient have the intelligence, judgment, memory, concentration, and motivation to use the equipment safely? If not, is someone available to assist the patient? Can the equipment be adapted so that the patient can use it despite his or her mental limitations?

3. *Psychological status.* Does the patient accept the disability? Does the patient accept the equipment? Does the patient have the desire to function in the way the equipment will allow? Will the patient in fact use the equipment?

4. *Work situation.* If the patient is employed, is the equipment needed in the workplace? If so, is it possible to transport the equipment? Is space available at the workplace for the equipment? Does the workplace or the home need to be remodeled or otherwise rearranged before the equipment can be used? If so, is remodeling or rearrangement possible?

5. *Social situation.* Is the equipment needed in a social situation? Is the equipment cosmetically appropriate for the person's life-style?

6. *Financial status.* Is the purchase of the equipment covered by insurance? If not, can the patient pay for the equipment? If not, can the equipment be made less expensively by the patient's family? What other resources are available?

COMMERCIAL SUPPLIERS

When a decision is made that therapeutic equipment is needed by the patient, the equipment is either purchased or made. Commercial suppliers have valuable information to give to occupational therapy personnel. Many suppliers work directly with therapists and assistants to provide the most appropriate equipment for the patient.

Many supply companies are owned and operated by occupational or physical therapists who have a special interest and expertise in particular items in their inventory. Some supply companies employ therapists as permanent staff members or as consultants. These professionals can be particularly helpful.

OTHER RESOURCES

Frequently, when commercial equipment is not available or is too costly, private resources are available. Community organizations often seek special projects. Some organizations annually help special categories of people as one of the organization's purposes.

Sheltered workshops, vocational training schools, volunteers, and family members may be resources for the construction or adaptation of therapeutic equipment. In many facilities, the maintenance department works with therapists to construct and adapt special equipment. Some occupational therapy departments include a staff member whose primary role is to construct and adapt such equipment.

Local chapters of special-interest groups, such as Access, the Association for Retarded Citizens, the Easter Seal Society, and the Society for the Blind, offer literature and speakers to provide information on special equipment. These groups are listed in the blue pages of the telephone directory.

Professional therapy groups usually have state and regional chapters of their national organization. Colleges, universities, and health care facilities are good sources for information on various therapies and their use of equipment.

Literature on therapeutic equipment is available at public libraries, educational institutions, and hospital libraries.

Excellent information on therapeutic equipment can be found in commercial catalogues. Each year, the American Occupational Therapy Association distributes a buyers' guide to its members. Catalogues may be requested from companies that manufacture therapeutic equipment. The catalogues include photos, descriptions, and prices of the equipment and specify its purpose, all to aid the prospective purchaser in making an appropriate selection. Professional journals and texts authored by therapists and former patients contain photographs and descriptions of custom-made therapeutic equipment (Cromwell, 1984; Taylor, Trefler, & Nwaobi, 1984).

The remainder of the chapter discusses a few of the many kinds of equipment that are used in occupational therapy.

WHEELCHAIR ADAPTATIONS

Many physically disabled, developmentally delayed, and elderly individuals need to be in wheelchairs for long periods. The wheelchair should fit the patient properly and provide adequate support.

The depth of the seat should be 7.62 cm (3 inches) less than the length between the posterior part of the buttocks and the back of the knee. The width of the seat should be 5.08 cm (2 inches) wider than the width of the patient's hips or thighs when the patient is seated. The wider of the hip and thigh measurements should be used. Braces or heavy clothes should be included in the measurement. This measurement allows 2.54 cm (1 inch) of clearance on either side. The distance from the seat to the footrest should allow 5.08 cm to 7.62 cm (2 inches to 3 inches) of clearance between the lower thigh and the seat. The footrest should clear the floor by 5.08 cm (2 inches). The wheelchair arm height should be 2.54 cm (1 inch) more than the measurement from the seat platform to just under the elbow (Everest & Jennings, 1979). Wheelchair measurements should take into consideration cushions or other additions to assure a proper fit.

Frequently, patients are placed in wheelchairs with collapsible seats and backs. These wheelchairs are not designed for patients who lack normal mobility and spend hours in the chair. If these wheelchairs are to be used for long-term sitting, the seats and backs should be made firm.

In some cases, due to reflex action or weakness, patients tend to slide forward in a wheelchair. Adjusting the angle of the seat to less than the normal 90° may be helpful. Seat belts and shoulder holsters similar to those in automobiles help to maintain the patient in a proper sitting position. A stable platform footrest will provide more support and aid the patient in maintaining the proper position. The height of the wheelchair back may need to be increased if the patient has poor head control. Wheelchair trays may help maintain the hips in proper position, as well as serve as a work area for cognitive and leisure activities or for eating. Trays can be secured to the armrests, as well as strapped around the back of the chair. A special armrest can be attached to the wheelchair to elevate the forearm and hand for proper positioning or to prevent edema.

Finally, a mobile arm support or a suspension sling may be added to a wheelchair to reduce the force of gravity on weak upper extremity muscles. The freely moving horizontal support may permit motion of the upper extremity joints. The patient may gain the ability to feed him- or herself or perform other hand activities, depending upon the nature of the condition (Pedretti & Zoltan, 1990).

MEALTIME ADAPTATIONS

Food is, of course, essential for life. Even before the first attempts at finger feeding, an individual has the desire to control his or her food intake. Problems with food intake can be due to physical, neurological, emotional, or developmental causes.

A person with a spinal cord injury may be able to feed him- or herself if the person is properly fitted in a wheelchair with a mobile arm support or suspension sling and has been trained to use special mealtime equipment. A person with cerebral palsy in a wheelchair that is adapted to control reflex movements also may be able to eat independently.

Dycem is a material that temporarily holds another surface to either of its flat surfaces. It can be purchased by given lengths or in place-mat size. Dycem is used between the plate, bowl, or cup and the surface of the table to keep the food container in place. It is useful for patients who lack coordination or who have the use of only one upper extremity. Dycem may add enough stability to deter a patient from aggressively pushing a plate off the table or picking up the plate and throwing it.

Plates with deeper bowls, such as a scoop dish (a plate with a raised rim against which a spoon can be pushed to keep food in place on the spoon) or a sectioned plate, enable patients to fill a spoon or fork with food when they lack coordination or have the use of only one upper extremity. Plate guards, made of 1-inch-thick stainless steel or Plexiglas, are made to clamp onto the side of the regular plate for the same purpose.

Handles of spoons, forks, and knives are adapted in a variety of ways to enable independent feeding when movement of the joints is limited or when muscle weakness and lack of coordination interfere with or prevent normal hand-to-mouth movement. The numerous variations are illustrated in most supply catalogues. A few of these variations are as follows:

A long-handled spoon or fork may be useful for a patient with limited joint movement. An increase in the diameter of a handle may enable a patient with limited grasp to hold a spoon or fork. A patient with the use of only one upper extremity may find a "spork," which is a combination spoon and fork, and a rocker knife helpful. A person with minimal joint movement or limited grasp may be able to eat independently with the use of a universal cuff into which a spoon or fork has been inserted.

Gravity helps to hold the food in swivel spoons as the spoon is taken to the mouth. Swivel spoons and forks are helpful for those who lack forearm supination and pronation. These and other adaptations enable otherwise dependent people to eat independently.

CLOTHING AND HYGIENE ADAPTATIONS

Clothing and hygiene are basic to keeping the body protected and healthy. A person's psychological well-being is influenced by clothes, grooming, and cleanliness. Most individuals prefer managing these personal tasks as independently as possible (Kernaleguen, 1978).

Limited movement in the joints, muscle weakness, and incoordination prevent patients from performing many self-care tasks. Equipment that is adapted to their condition may enable patients to perform these tasks independently.

Long handles on combs, brushes, bath sponges, and shoehorns may be helpful. Reachers allow objects to be grasped from shelves or the floor. Dressing sticks, sock donners, trouser pulls, button aids, toileting aids, and other items foster independence in self-care.

Clothes can be constructed in special ways to allow independent dressing. Front- or side-opening garments, fasteners adapted to the individual, loose sleeves, and other features can be found in ready-to-wear garments or can be custom tailored to meet individual needs.

LEISURE ACTIVITY

Leisure activity is important to maintain a balance in an individual's life. A change in the kind of leisure activity one performs may be necessary for a patient who becomes wheelchair bound or who has the use of only one upper extremity. Many activities are possible without adaptive equipment. On the other hand, such equipment may enable a patient to continue to engage in activities of special interest (Pedretti & Zoltan, 1990).

Card holders are available for one-handed card playing. Large-print cards and braille cards are available for the visually impaired and the blind. Puzzle pieces with attached knobs enable children who lack a pincerlike grasp to work with puzzles. A variety of book holders enable people to read in various positions without holding the book. Embroidery hoops that clamp to the table allow needlework using one upper extremity.

Clamps, Velcro®, magnets, and other materials can be used to adapt leisure time games and materials appropriately to enable patients to engage in their favorite activities. Frames, tilted boards and tables, and other means of adapting viewing and playing surfaces are ways of helping patients engage in activities.

CONSTRUCTION SAFETY

The following precautions should be observed when buying or constructing furniture, equipment, and toys for patients:

1. Furniture and equipment should have a sturdy base. Many patients do not have adequate balance or the ability to make postural adjustments to maintain their balance.
2. Edges should be rounded and smooth.
3. Wood should be finished to prevent splintering.
4. Paint and other finishes should be and free of lead and other toxic ingredients.
5. Nails and screws should be countersunk, puttied, and properly finished.
6. Toys should be of sturdy construction so that small parts cannot be removed.
7. Toys with sharp edges or points should be avoided. Be especially cautious of metal and plastic toys and parts that can cause injury.
8. Avoid toys with small parts that can be easily removed.
9. Be cautious of toys with lengths of string, rope, or elastic. If these are used, they should be checked periodically and used under supervision.
10. Surfaces on toys, furniture, and equipment should be washable or easy to clean.

SUMMARY

The patient should be evaluated prior to any recommendation of therapeutic equipment. Consideration should be given to the patient's physical, mental, psychological, work, and social situation. Therapeutic equipment should be recommended only when the patient cannot function without the equipment and only for as long as will be needed. Numerous varieties of therapeutic equipment are available from various sources.

REVIEW QUESTIONS

1. What factors need to be considered when deciding on therapeutic equipment for a patient?
2. List at least three adaptations to wheelchairs, and give the purpose of each.
3. What therapeutic equipment would you recommend to aid the following patients?
   a. A patient with an above-the-elbow amputation of the dominant extremity wants to participate in leisure group activities while waiting for a prosthetic device.

    b. A woman wants blouses and dresses with buttons, but no longer has the dexterity or coordination to button her clothing.

    c. A child with cerebral palsy has reflex action that results in extension of the spine and inability to maintain a sitting position in a wheelchair.

    d. A person with a spinal cord injury wants to feed himself, has no limitation in the joints, but has weak upper extremities.

4. List at least five safety features to look for in therapeutic equipment made of metal or wood.

ANSWERS

1. The factors to be considered before deciding on therapeutic equipment for a patient are the patient's physical condition, mental status, psychological status, work situation, social situation, and financial status.

2.

    1) Angle the seat about 70° instead of the usual 90° to inhibit reflexive extension of the spine and to help the patient maintain a sitting position.

    2) A lapboard stabilized by strapping it around the back of the wheelchair so that the child with reflexive extension of the upper extremities will not push the device off helps the child to maintain a sitting posture, provides support of the upper extremities, and offers a work area for the patient.

    3) Extending the back of the wheelchair to the height of the crown of the head helps maintain head control in a person who lacks such control.

    4) A solid seat and back gives proper support to a patient who spends long hours in a wheelchair.

3. Therapeutic equipment and devices that may be helpful for the people described are as follows:

    a) A card holder would permit the patient to play cards. Velcro or dycem can be used if the bottom of an object needs to be stabilized. Masking tape can be used to tape down paper for writing and artwork. One-handed leisure activities, such as playing board games, can be suggested.

    b) Sew the buttons onto the buttonholes, and use Velcro dots to fasten the buttons. Have the woman change to a zipper, larger buttons, or larger snaps if she can manage any of them.

    c) A chair with the seat approximately 70° rather than the usual 90° degrees, a seat belt, a stabilized wheelchair tray, a solid footrest, and, if needed, straps covering the toes of the shoes to prevent the feet from slipping off the footrest should help the child maintain a sitting position.

d) A suspension sling or mobile arm support would help with self-feeding.
4. Some items that should be checked on metal and wood items are the following:
   1) Furniture and equipment should have a solid, sturdy base to prevent tipping.
   2) Finishes should be lead free and nontoxic.
   3) Small removable parts should be avoided on furniture, equipment, and toys.
   4) Furniture, equipment and toys should not have sharp, potentially dangerous edges and corners.
   5) Long cords, elastic, and strings should be avoided, or the child should be carefully supervised during their use.
   6) Nails and screws should be countersunk and carefully embedded in the equipment.

ADDITIONAL LEARNING ACTIVITIES

1. Scan some supply house catalogues for information on therapeutic equipment. .
2. Visit the local Society for the Blind. Ask to see aids for the visually impaired and blind.
3. Visit a telephone company store. Ask to see various aids for the hearing impaired and deaf.
4. Visit rehabilitation hospitals for the physically disabled. Ask to observe the various therapeutic equipment in use.
5. Locate a hospital or other facility where engineers are working on developing special equipment for the physically disabled. Arrange a visit if possible.

REFERENCES

American Occupational Therapy Association. (yearly). *Buyer's guide.* Bethesda, MD: Author.

Cromwell, F. S. (Ed.). (1984). *Occupational therapy strategies and adaptations for independent daily living.* New York: The Haworth Press.

Everest and Jennings, Inc. (1979). *Measuring the patient.* Los Angeles: Author.

Kernaleguen, A. (1978). *Clothing designs for the handicapped.* Manitoba, Canada: The University of Alberta Press.

Pedretti, L. W., & Zoltan, B. (1990). *Occupational therapy: Practice skills for physical dysfunction.* St. Louis: The C.V. Mosby Company.

Taylor, S. J., Trefler, E., & Nwaobi, O. (1984). Occupational therapy and rehabilitation engineering: Delivering technology to the severely physically disabled. In F. Cromwell (Ed.), *Occupational therapy strategies and adaptations for independent daily living.* New York: The Haworth Press.

16

SPLINTING

This chapter examines hand function and splinting. Some purposes, limitations, and precautions of splinting are discussed.

LEARNING OBJECTIVES

At the end of this chapter, you should be able to:

1. Discuss the characteristics of the normal hand that contribute to its functioning.
2. List the four phases of the complete functional action of the hand.
3. Name and demonstrate, draw and label, or describe six prehension and grasping patterns.
4. Describe or illustrate and label the resting position of the hand.
5. Describe or illustrate and label the functional position of the hand.
6. Name three basic purposes of hand splinting, and give an example of each.
7. State the difference between a static and dynamic hand splint.
8. Name four signs of an improperly fitted splint.
9. State at least four precautions to observe in wearing and caring for splints.
10. Compare the role of the occupational therapist and the assistant in hand splinting.

A *splint* is a rigid or flexible device used to immobilize, support, or correct injured, displaced, or deformed body parts. *Melloni's Illustrated Medical Dictionary* (Dox, Melloni, & Eisner, 1993) shows airplane splints and cervical splints and describes other kinds of splints.

THE HAND

The basic function of the hand is to hold or stabilize objects in order to perform functional activities. However, merely holding or stabilizing objects would limit hand function. The complete functional action of the hand requires movement, strength, endurance, dexterity, coordination, sensation, emotions, and cognition.

Normally, the hand has movement at each joint. When required, the joints can be stabilized in certain positions. The hand is attached to the rest of the upper extremity, which allows additional movements. The upper extremity is attached to the trunk at the shoulder, which permits the hand to carry out an even wider range and variation of movements.

The hand has the ability to regulate the strength required to hold a sewing needle or a 5-pound hammer. The hand also has the ability to respond to visual, auditory, tactile, and proprioceptive stimuli and coordinate movements, depending upon the size, shape, weight, texture, and temperature of an object. The hand has the ability to express its owner's feelings. The hand can even relay information about the owner's age, interests, and life-style to a skilled observer.

The complete functional action of the normal hand can be divided into four phases: the reach, the grasp, the carry, and the release. Dysfunction in any of these phases hinders normal hand function; however, since hand splinting is concerned mostly with the second phase, we next examine grasp and prehension patterns.

GRASP AND PREHENSION PATTERNS

In *fingertip prehension,* the thumb pad is in contact with the pad of the index or middle finger. This prehension pattern is used to pick up, hold, or manipulate small objects such as pins, nails, and buttons.

Palmar prehension is commonly called the "three-jaw chuck." The thumb, index finger, and middle finger pads are in contact with the object. Palmar prehension is used to pick up or hold cylindrical or spherical objects such as pens, eating utensils, marbles, or small cubes. It is used most frequently when performing daily activities.

In *lateral prehension,* the thumb pad is in contact with the lateral distal portion of the index finger. This prehension pattern is used to turn a key in a lock or hold a small plate. Lateral prehension is generally stronger than, but lacks the coordination of, fingertip and palmar prehension.

The *cylindrical grasp* is commonly called the "palmar grasp." The object is in contact with the palm of the hand, with the four digits holding the object against the palm. The cylindrical grasp is used to hold a water glass, a broom, and the handle of a hammer.

The *spherical grasp* is commonly called the "ball grasp." The fingers flex around an object. This kind of grasp is used to hold a ball, orange, or doorknob.

The *hook grasp* is so called because the fingers seem to hook around the object grasped. The hook grasp is used to carry a pail or briefcase or to hang from a narrow ledge. (See Figure 16.1.)

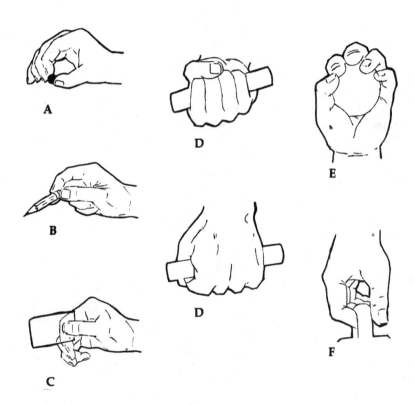

FIGURE 16.1
Basic types of prehension and grasp. A, fingertip prehension. B, palmar prehension. C, lateral prehension. D, cylindrical grasp. E, spherical grasp. F, hook grasp. (Reproduced with author's permission from Malick, M. H. *Manual on Static Hand Splinting*. Pittsburgh: Harmarville Rehabilitation Center.)

RESTING POSITION OF THE HAND

Normally, the hand assumes a relaxed position in which the muscles, joints, nerves, and vessels are in a state of rest. The wrist is extended or slightly dorsiflexed. All the finger joints are slightly flexed. The thumb is in partial opposition to the fingers and is abducted, so the thumb web space is maintained. The thumb pad faces the pad of the index finger. (See Figure 16.2.)

FUNCTIONAL POSITION OF THE HAND

Functional activities usually place the hand in some dorsiflexion at the wrist. All of the fingers are partially flexed, and the thumb is in opposition to the fingers. The hand, in a position of function, assumes a configuration resembling the spherical prehension pattern. The wrist is dorsiflexed about 30 degrees. The thumb is abducted and is in opposition to the four fingers. The middle joints of the fingers (the proximal interphalangeal joints) are flexed about 45 degrees. (See Figure 16.3.)

Generally, slight dorsiflexion of the wrist is necessary for adequate action of the fingers. When the wrist is dorsiflexed, the extensor muscles of the fingers relax. The fingers are then able to flex to the degree necessary for the action to occur. For functional activities, flexion of the fingers is more valuable than extension.

In describing the functional position of the hand, the importance of the thumb cannot be overemphasized. The thumb is the most important and the strongest digit of the hand. It is capable of all the movements of a ball-and-socket joint and has the ability to act as a stable pole against which objects can be held. Its range of movement, the myriad positions it can assume, and its strength and dexterity give the thumb the "most important digit" classification.

CLASSIFICATION OF SPLINTS

There are two basic types of hand splints: *static* and *dynamic.* Static splints have no moving parts. They keep the joint or joints and surrounding muscle parts fixed in one position. When treatment includes a period of exercise or mobile use of the splinted area, the splint is removed during that time.

An example of a static splint is a resting pan or resting hand splint. The splint keeps the wrist and hand in a normal resting position. The splint may be prescribed for a stroke patient to prevent the wrist from dropping, since the weakened or paralyzed muscles cannot maintain the hand and wrist in proper positions. When the stroke patient exercises the upper extremities, the splint is removed (Malick, 1979; Pedretti, 1990).

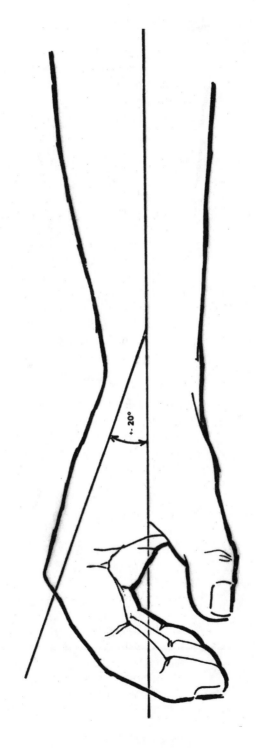

FIGURE 16.2
Position of rest, Lateral view, right hand. (Reproduced with author's permission. From Malick, M.H.: *Manual on Static Hand Splinting.* Pittsburgh, PA, Harmarville Rehabilitation Center.)

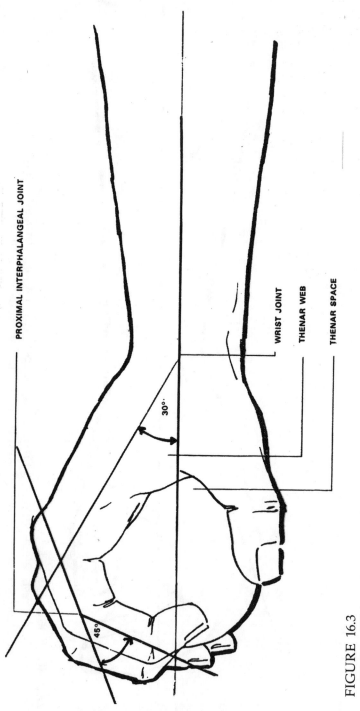

FIGURE 16.3
Position of function, Lateral view, right hand. (Reproduced with author's permission. From Malick, M.H.: *Manual on Static Hand Splinting.* Pittsburgh, PA, Harmarville Rehabilitation Center.)

A dynamic splint has an immobile part or parts, plus one or more parts that move. Movement is made possible by a hinge joint, springs, pulleys, rubber bands, or other additions. A dynamic splint stabilizes the proximal part of the extremity. It allows the patient to move the weakened part as far as possible and then completes the movement for the patient. An example of a dynamic splint is a splint that supports the forearm, wrist, thumb, and fingers in extension. A thin bar is attached to the splint and placed horizontally above the dorsum of the fingers. Rubber bands hang from the bar and are attached to the material supporting the fingers. The movable rubber bands assist the fingers in extension, and the immobile parts of the splint provide support to other areas of the extremity to make finger movement possible. The metacarpophalangeal extension-assist splint and other dynamic splints are illustrated and described in other texts (Malick, 1978, Pedretti, 1990).

A 1992 survey showed that therapists used both static and dynamic splints in their treatment procedures with patients with quadriplegia. Dynamic splints were used most for patients with spinal cord injuries at the cervical spinal levels 6 (C6) and 7 (C7). The most frequently stated purpose for using a splint was to prevent contractures of the wrist and hand and to prevent overstretching of wrist extensors. Other purposes were to protect and stabilize the joints and to maintain the arches and the thumb web space (Krainik & Bridle, 1992).

PURPOSE OF SPLINTING

Early splinting can prevent further problems with, and even permanent disability to, the hand. Lack of treatment for even 3 weeks can cause muscle atrophy, contractures, improper body alignment or, motor dysfunction.

Splints constructed by occupational therapy personnel are most frequently used in treating temporary conditions. Usually, splints are part of a total treatment plan, which may include therapeutic exercise and activities. Splints may be used in treatment plans for muscle weakness, limitation of movement in the joints, improper body alignment, or motor problems. Splints may be part of a treatment program for amputations, arthritis, burns, hand injuries, spinal cord injury, strokes, and other conditions.

Splints may be prescribed to achieve the following goals, among others:

1. Strengthening of weak muscles, by assisting movements (e.g., finger exercises following surgery for a hand injury);
2. Prevention of deformity, by maintaining body parts in correct positions (e.g., fingers in an arthritic hand);

3. Correction of deformity, by gradually placing body parts in the best possible positions (e.g., a drop foot following prolonged bed rest);
4. Protection of weak muscles from overstretching (e.g., weak wrist muscles following a stroke);
5. Temporary support for a painful body part (e.g., an arthritic wrist);
6. Substitution for a disabled or displaced part (e.g., an amputated thumb tip);
7. Maintenance of body parts in the best possible position (e.g., during healing or following surgery, skin grafts, burns, or injuries.

SPLINTING MATERIALS

The material most frequently used by occupational therapy personnel in constructing static hand splints is low-temperature plastic. The thermoplastic material becomes flexible and moldable at approximately 140°F to 160oF. The material can be heated in water with hot, dry air or a hot iron. It can be cut with scissors or a knife. Straps can be secured to the material with rivets, with plastic glue, or by imbedding the straps between two pieces of the plastic material so that the edges of the plastic bond together to secure the straps in place. There are various trade names for these materials, each of which has unique qualities.

Because many static splints are made of low-temperature materials, the patient needs to be instructed in the care of the splint. The splint should be kept away from temperatures that will change its shape. Splints should not be left on radiators, or on sunny window sills where the heat will affect the plastic material. Splints can be cleaned with soap and water below 140oF. If the splint has Velcro hook-and-pile straps, the patient should be informed of the abrasive effect the hook may have on other garments or the skin. Unheated splinting materials are quite sturdy, but should not be stepped on, left under heavy objects, or used to hit hard surfaces. The patient should be instructed to inform the physician or therapist if the splint loses its original shape or if any part of the splint creates a pressure point.

LIMITATIONS AND PRECAUTIONS

As mentioned earlier, the use of the hand is dependent upon muscle strength, endurance, mobility of the joints, body sensations, emotions, interests, and intellectual ability, as well as genetic, social, cultural, and economic factors.

A properly prescribed and fitted splint may protect, correct, support, or help strengthen a body part or prevent deformity; but a splint may also place limitations on the body. A splint prevents the normal movement of some part of the body. It also shields the skin surface from normal stimulation. The patient may feel that the splint is a grotesque addition to the body, may be unable to understand the purpose of the splint, or may be uninterested in activities that the splint enables the patient to do.

Following are some general precautions that may prevent further problems from being caused by splints:

1. When splints are necessary, they should be incorporated into the complete treatment program.
2. Cover only necessary parts of the body with splints.
3. Splint only those joints that it is necessary to splint.
4. Remove static splints at intervals, so that joints can be moved either passively or actively.
5. Gradually build up a tolerance for wearing splints.
6. Help the patient understand the purpose of the splint.
7. Help the patient accept the splint as part of the treatment program.
8. Help the patient accept responsibility for the care of the splint.
9. Watch for signs of improper fit of the splint and patient discomfort with it. Remember that not all patients will complain of discomfort. Watch for swelling, redness that does not disappear after the splint has been removed for 15 minutes, and whiteness beyond the pressure point, and ask the patient how the affected area feels.
10. Check the splint to see whether it is achieving its goal. If it is not, a reevaluation is needed.

THE ASSISTANT'S ROLE

The certified occupational therapy assistant (COTA) assists the occupational therapist (OTR) in constructing a splint. The OTR evaluates the patient and determines whether he or she needs a splint and, if so, what kind of splint. The experience and responsibilities of both the OTR and the COTA at the facility determine who will construct the splint or its parts. Generally, the COTA is qualified to make basic static splints and adjust them to the patient as needed. The physician and OTR reevaluate and determine whether the splint needs to be adjusted or removed.

The experienced COTA may become proficient in the construction of dynamic splints. Supervised experience and continuing education are the determining factors.

The COTA may be the person who teaches the patient how to care for the splint. An experienced COTA may carry out some aspects of the treatment under the direct or general supervision of the therapist.

SUMMARY

Normal hand function includes reaching for, grasping, carrying, and releasing objects. Coordinated and dexterous movements are required to execute the various grasp and prehension patterns needed to perform activities of daily living. When injury or disease prevents normal hand function, a splint may be used to protect or support muscles and joints or to prevent and correct deformity. The COTA has the basic knowledge and skills that are necessary to construct and apply static splints to maintain the patient's hand at rest or to support muscles and joints so as to permit use of the hand. The use of splints in treatment includes evaluating the splint in terms of how it fits and educating the patient in wearing and caring for the splint.

REVIEW QUESTIONS

1. Discuss the characteristics of the hand that allow controlled movements.
2. What are the four phases of complete hand function?
3. Circle the letter preceding the most appropriate ending to each numbered phrase.
   1) Fingertip prehension is used:
      a. by adults writing with a pen.
      b. to turn a key in a lock.
      c. to pick up a sewing needle.
      d. by infants learning to eat with a spoon.
   2) Lateral prehension is used:
      a. by adults writing with a pen.
      b. to turn a key in a lock.
      c. to pick up a sewing needle.
      d. by infants learning to eat with a spoon.
   3) Palmar prehension is used:
      a. by adults when writing with a pen.
      b. to hold the handle when carrying a pail of water.
      c. to pick up a 3-inch ball.
      d. by infants learning to eat with a spoon.
   4) The hook grasp is used:
      a. by adults writing with a pen.
      b. to hold the handle when carrying a pail of water.
      c. to pick up a 3-inch ball.
      d. by infants learning to eat with a spoon.
   5) The spherical grasp is used:
      a. by adults writing with a pen.
      b. to hold the handle when carrying a pail of water.
      c. to pick up a 3-inch ball.
      d. by infants learning to eat with a spoon.

6) The cylindrical grasp is used:
   a. by adults writing with a pen.
   b. to hold the handle when carrying a pail of water.
   c. to pick up a 3-inch ball.
   d. by infants learning to eat with a spoon.
4. When the hand is in a resting position:
   a. the wrist is slightly dorsiflexed.
   b. the finger joints are slightly flexed.
   c. the thumb web space is maintained.
   d. all of the above.
5. The functional position of the hand resembles the:
   a. palmar prehension pattern.
   b. spherical grasp pattern.
   c. cylindrical grasp pattern.
   d. hook grasp pattern.
6. Name at least three purposes of splinting.
7. Circle the letter preceding the most appropriate ending to each numbered phrase.
   1) A static hand splint:
      a. is stabilized to a treatment table.
      b. is made of metal so that the joints cannot be moved.
      c. has no movable parts.
      d. allows movement in only one joint.
   2) A dynamic hand splint:
      a. is removed during therapeutic exercise.
      b. has all movable parts.
      c. assists the patient in hand movements.
      d. corrects hand deformities.
8. Describe four signs of an improperly constructed or fitted splint.
9. What should you do to aid patients in accepting and learning to use a splint?
10. Discuss the COTA's primary role in splinting.

ANSWERS

1. The hand is a part of the upper extremity and shoulder girdle (and entire body) that enables a wide range of various movements. The hand has the ability to respond to sensory stimuli and initiate and coordinate movements, depending upon the individual's desire to do so and on his or her biophysiological and cognitive capacity.
   1) Reach, 2) Grasp, 3) Carry, 4) Release
3. 1) c 2) b 3) a 4) b 5) c 6) d
4. d
5. b

6. 1) maintain the body parts in a proper position to prevent deformity.
   2) protect weak muscles from overstretching.
   3) stabilize the affected area during healing.
   4) temporarily support a painful body part.
7. 1) c 2) c
8. 1) The splint material covers more skin surface than is necessary.
   2) The splint material covers joints unnecessarily.
   3) There are areas of pressure evidenced by redness after the splint has been removed for 15 minutes, there is whiteness beyond the splinted area, and swelling or bruises appear on or near the affected area.
   4) The patient does not wear the splint.
9. 1) Help the patient learn the purpose of the splint.
   2) Help the patient accept the splint as part of the treatment.
   3) Help the patient build up a tolerance to wearing the splint.
   4) Remind the patient to remove the splint when exercising the joints.
10. The COTA assists the therapist by constructing and adjusting splints and by participating in instructing the patient on how to wear and care for the splint, as specified and as the COTA's experience permits.

ADDITIONAL LEARNING ACTIVITIES

1. Look through catalogues that contain splinting supplies, and become familiar with some of the supplies and equipment used in constructing a splint.
2. Ask a COTA how much responsibility he or she has in splinting procedures.
3 Make an appointment to visit an occupational therapy department in a rehabilitation center, hand therapy center, or burn center in order to see some splints and learn about their purpose.
4. Read articles on splinting in the *American Journal of Occupational Therapy*. For what conditions were the splints described in the articles used? Were the splints static or dynamic splints?

REFERENCES

Dox, I., Melloni, B. J., & Eisner, G. M. (1993). *Melloni's illustrated medical dictionary*. Baltimore: The Williams and Wilkins Company.

Krainik, S. R., & Bridle, M. J. (1992). Hand splinting in quadriplegia: Current practice. *American Journal of Occupational Therapy, 46*(2), 149-156.

Malick, M. H. (1978). *Manual on dynamic hand splinting with thermoplastic materials* (2nd ed.). Pittsburgh: The Harmarville Rehabilitation Center.

Malick, M. H. (1979). *Manual on static hand splinting* (5th ed.). Pittsburgh: Harmarville Rehabilitation Center.

Pedretti, L. W., & Zoltan, B. (1990). *Occupational therapy: Practice skills for physical dysfunction* (3rd ed.). St. Louis: The C. V. Mosby Company.

SUGGESTED READINGS

DiPasquale-Lehnerz, P. (1994). Orthotic intervention for development of hand function with C-6 quadriplegia. *American Journal of Occupational Therapy, 48*(2), 138-144.

SUGGESTED LISTENING/VIEWING

Static splinting made easy. (1987). VHS (90 min.). Brookfield, IL: Fred Sammons, Inc.

Inhibitory casting of upper extremities for occupational therapists. (1986). VHS (three tapes, 60 min. each). Bethesda, MD: American Ocuupational Therapy Association, Inc.

Section IV

CONDITIONS REQUIRING OCCUPATIONAL THERAPY

The disabling conditions that create a need for occupational therapy are varied. A moderately mentally retarded individual may need special training in work skills, as well as socialization skills. A mother with weakness on one side of her body following a stroke may need training in personal care and home management, as well as in coping techniques and alternative methods for handling the responsibilities of a family. An acutely mentally ill person may need to be engaged in special activities to help her regain the sense of reality and to develop trust in preparation for returning to her employment. A worker with a hand injury may need special splinting and exercises to improve muscle strength, range of motion of the joints, and endurance in order to return to work.

The holistic nature of occupational therapy, with its emphasis on enabling individuals to be as functionally independent as possible in their daily lives, the general emphasis in society on preventative measures to maintain optimal health and a sense of wellness, and the rapid increase in scientific and technological information have resulted in a need for occupational therapy personnel in a variety of settings dealing with a variety of disabling conditions.

The next several chapters introduce a few of the conditions that benefit from occupational therapy.

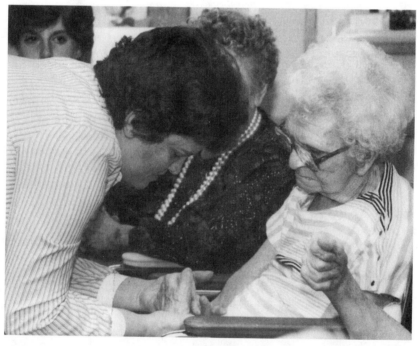

Dolores Blickley, COTA/L helps Lillian Swartz during a group exercise session. Photo courtesy of Phoebe-Devitt Homes.

17

DEVELOPMENTAL DISABILITIES

The definition of a developmental disability, including the major areas of disability and diagnostic categories, is given. Education for handicapped children is discussed.

LEARNING OBJECTIVES

At the end of this section, you should be able to:

1. Define a developmental disability, according to the public law.
2. Name seven areas of life activities that may prevent a person with developmental disabilities from becoming independent because of functional limitations.
3. Name three diagnostic categories that can result in developmental delays.
4. Name four major skills needed to perform most life activities.
5. State the original title and effective date of the law that provided for education for all handicapped children.
6. Explain the role of occupational therapy, as stated in the foregoing law.
7. State 10 of the 11 categories of handicapping conditions covered by the aforementioned law.
8. State the words that the letters IEP and IFSP abbreviate.
9. Name and discuss P.L. 102-119.

Former President John F. Kennedy felt strongly that national programs were needed for mental health and to combat mental retardation. In 1963, he presented Congress with a proposal, which they passed as the Mental Retardation Facilities and Community Mental Health Centers Construction Act (P.L.88-164). This act allowed states to improve facilities, establish community centers, train personnel, and try new programs relating to mental health and mental retardation. Although its impact was significant, the act limited what could be done. The individuals who could receive services were narrowly defined; it was apparent that individuals with other diagnoses needed intervention programs as well. A number of amendments and laws were subsequently passed to allow service to a larger population identified as having developmental disabilities (Hightower-Vandamm, 1979).

A *developmental disability* is defined as a severe, chronic disability of a person that "(a) [is] attributable to a mental or physical impairment or combination of mental and physical impairment; (b) is manifested before the person attains age 22; (c) is likely to continue indefinitely; (d) results in substantial functional limitations in three or more of the following areas of major life activity: 1. self-care; 2. receptive and expressive language; 3. learning; 4. mobility; 5. self-direction; 6. capacity for independent living; and, 7. economic self-sufficiency; and (e) reflects the person's need for a combination and sequence of special, interdisciplinary, or generic care, treatment, or other services which are of lifelong or extended duration and are individually planned and coordinated" (Rehabilitation Comprehensive Services and Developmental Disabilities Amendments of 1978, Public Law 95-602, Section 503 (b) (7) (E), p. 3005; cited in Hightower-Vandamm, 1979).

DIAGNOSTIC CATEGORIES

Developmental disabilities include a group of diagnostic categories, among which are mental retardation, cerebral palsy, autism, epilepsy, language delay, and specific learning disability. Current knowledge suggests that most individuals with developmental disabilities have a central nervous system that is not functioning in the normally expected manner (Johnston & Magrab, 1979).

The central nervous system, which includes the brain and spinal column, matures gradually during the first 21 years of life. Disease or injury to the central nervous system at any time during the developmental period can affect one or any number of developing skills. Major life activities are dependent upon the adequate integration of intelligence, language, and sensorimotor and adaptive skills.

PUBLIC LAWS

The Education for All Handicapped Children Act of 1975 (Public Law 94-142) became effective on October 1, 1977. Prior to that date, children could be excluded from education for various reasons. The criterion for being able to receive free public education was based on the child's ability to perform certain skills. Since September 1, 1978, all handicapped children aged 3 through 18 years were provided the opportunity to have a free, appropriate public education. Amendments to the original law provide opportunities for education and services to individuals from birth to 21 years of age if they have disabilities that hinder their educational progress.

Handicapped children were classified into 11 categories in P.L. 94-142: deaf, deaf-blind, hard of hearing, mentally retarded, multihandicapped, orthopedically impaired, other health impaired, seriously emotionally disturbed, specifically learning disabled, speech impaired, and visually handicapped. The number of categories and their titles may change.

Subsequent laws and amendments related to P.L. 94-142 had an impact on all education, not only special education. In 1986, P.L. 99-457 expanded and improved early intervention services for infants and toddlers with disabilities and at-risk infants and toddlers and their families. In 1991, the passage of P.L. 102-119, the Individuals with Disabilities Education Act (IDEA), incorporated P.L. 94-142 and P.L. 99-457 and expanded educational services to all qualified individuals. Part H of IDEA, the section dealing with infants and toddlers with disabilities, provided services to identify and track children at risk of having developmental delays, strengthened the participation of families in the services and supports, strengthened families' control over the services and supports, encouraged the provision of services in natural environments, included assistive technology services and devices, and made the transition between the Part H program and the preschool program more efficient (Gallagher, Harbin, Eckland, Clifford, & Fullagar, 1992; U.S. Department of Education, 1991).

The preceding laws provide opportunities for appropriate education in the most appropriate settings for children who were previously ineligible to be educated in public facilities. Thus, children who were ineligible to attend regular classes because of a handicap became eligible to attend such classes in elementary schools, high schools, and colleges when these were the most appropriate settings. Architectural barriers that prevented handicapped students from attending certain classrooms were modified to make those classrooms accessible. The effectiveness of the various educational programs is monitored by methods such as the individualized educational program (IEP) and each child's individualized family service plan (IFSP).

Occupational therapy was included in the original law as a service related to special education. The law stated that occupational therapy improves, develops, or restores functions that were impaired or lost. As a related, rather than a primary, service, occupational therapy must be associated with the academic focus of the child. This means that occupational therapy is believed to be necessary for the child to progress in his or her IEP.

Developmental disabilities are a chronic condition for the majority of individuals affected by them, and services are needed to help these people plan beyond the normal early education. New legislation can be expected as needs for this group are identified. The complete regulations and recent amendments on laws related to the education of handicapped children are available in the *Federal Register* and the *U. S. Statutes at Large* at many public libraries. Information also can be obtained from state and district representatives, as well as the U.S. Government Printing Office.

NUMBER OF STUDENTS SERVED

The U.S. Department of Education reported that 5,110,653 disabled students from ages birth to 21 years were provided educational programs in 50 states, the District of Columbia, and Puerto Rico in the academic year 1992-1993 (U.S. Bureau of the Census, 1995). The greatest percentage of students who received services described in the aforementioned public laws were those diagnosed as learning disabled (51.3%), followed by those diagnosed as speech impaired (21.7%) and those diagnosed as mentally retarded (11.3%). Eight percent were diagnosed as emotionally disturbed. The remainder of the disabled student population that received services were diagnosed as hearing impaired and deaf, orthopedically impaired, having other medical problems, visually impaired, multiply impaired, and deaf-blind (U.S. Bureau of the Census, 1995).

Education was provided to 44.8% of disabled students in regular classrooms, with the student receiving special education and related services less than 21% of the day. The resource room was used for 27.8% of disabled students, who received special services 21-60% of the education day, and 12.0% of disabled student were segregated in a separate classroom in which more than 60% of their day was receiving special education and related services. (U.S. Bureau of the Census, 1994). Other environments were public and private facilities, separate residential settings, correctional facilities, and the home and hospital (U.S. Bureau of the Census, 1995). These findings indicate that more disabled students are integrated into regular classrooms and receive less special education and related services than those disabled students who receive education in segregated classrooms.

OCCUPATIONAL THERAPY

The goal of occupational therapy is to assist the person with developmental delay in improving or becoming functional in the performance of various life activities. An occupational therapy evaluation is indicated when an individual presents problems in functioning in the occupational performance areas of activities of daily living, work, or play and leisure.

The evaluation may identify a delay in or lack of the sensorimotor, cognitive, or psychosocial components that are needed to perform skills in the occupational performance areas.

Occupational therapy that relates to activities of daily living, such as dressing, grooming, hygiene, mealtime behavior, functional mobility, functional communication, and managing medication, may be included in the IEP. The therapy may be related to sensorimotor components that are preparatory to learning skills such as printing and cursive writing, cutting with scissors, and manipulating objects. Such classroom skills require gross- and fine-motor coordination, muscle strength and endurance, sensory awareness, visual and spatial awareness, and body integration (Levine, 1991).

Occupational therapy practitioners work with classroom educators to assure that the focus of the therapy is related to the academic goals of the student. The current emphasis of special education is on preparing students to function in the community and to be as independent and productive as possible (Bigge, 1991). For these students, occupational therapy may include community activities that enable them to practice entire segments of life activities—for example, becoming mobile in the community with crutches or wheelchairs, adhering to bus schedules, and getting to a destination, either for work or for a leisure activity. Such segments of life activities require planning, organization, concentration, a certain level of attention span, and memory, as well as a good self-concept, self-identity, and situational coping skills.

Occupational therapy for individuals with developmental disabilities may involve developing special adaptive devices and teaching the effective use of such devices. Orthotics and preventive measures such as positioning may be required by some developmentally delayed individuals.

Adults with developmental delay may need occupational therapy to develop their work skills and leisure skills, in addition to the needs discussed earlier. Adults with developmental disabilities may have a greater need to prepare for employment and to gain homemaking skills and community living skills, especially if they have not been included in educational programs during their youth.

THE ASSISTANT'S ROLE

Prior to 1970, few certified occupational therapy assistants (COTAs) were employed in pediatric occupational therapy departments or in school systems. In 1973, 11.0% of occupational therapists (OTRs) worked in school systems, compared to 3.6% of COTAS. In 1990, 18.6% of OTRs worked in school systems, compared to 17.0% of COTAs. School systems were the second most common employment setting for OTRs and the third most common for COTAs (AOTA, 1991).

The COTA, under the supervision of an OTR, provides direct service to schoolchildren. The exact role assumed by the COTA depends upon the school system, the school population, other staff members, and the supervising OTR. The types of service provided in school settings are reviewed in Bigge (1991) and Linder (1993).

SUMMARY

A developmental disability is a severe, chronic disability that includes many diagnostic categories. The Education for All Handicapped Children Act made it possible for individuals 3 through 21 years of age with developmental disabilities to receive free public education. Amendments to the original act provided for educational opportunities for persons from birth to 22 years of age in a variety of settings.

Occupational therapy services were included in the original act as a service related to education. Special education systems are the third largest employers of COTAs.

REVIEW QUESTIONS

1. Define , *developmental disability*, as stated in P.L. 95-602, Section 503 (b) (7) (E), p. 3005. How long does such a disability last?
2. Of the seven areas of life activities in which functional limitation may require lifelong care for the individual with developmental disability, list those areas most likely to be treated by occupational therapy.
3. Name at least three diagnoses that can result in a developmental disability.
4. What skills are required to be able to perform most life activities?
5. What was the number, name, and effective date of the first law that provided free public education to all handicapped children?
6. What is the stated role of occupational therapy in the foregoing law?
7. List 10 of the 11 categories of handicapping conditions covered by the aforesaid law.
8. Write the words for the abbreviations IEP and IFSP.
9. What is P.L. 102-119, and what services are provided under this law?

ANSWERS

1. According to P.L. 95-602, a developmental disability is a severe, chronic disability of a person attributed to a mental or physical impairment or a combination of mental and physical impairment that was manifest before age 22 years. The disability is likely to continue indefinitely. The diagnosis of developmental disability is given when there is substantial functional limitation in three or more of the major life activities.

2. Self-care, receptive and expressive language, learning, mobility, self-direction, independent living, and economic self-sufficiency.
3. Mental retardation, autism, cerebral palsy, learning disabilities, language delay.
4. Integration of intelligence, language and communication, sensorimotor skills, and adaptive skills.
5. P.L.94-142, the Education for All Handicapped Children Act of 1975, was enacted October 1, 1977.
6. Occupational therapy is a service related to education. This means that occupational therapy is needed in order for the student to progress academically. Occupational therapy must be related to the IEP of the student.
7. deaf, deaf-blind, hard of hearing, mentally retarded, multihandicapped, orthopedically impaired, other orthopedically impaired, other health impaired, seriously emotionally disturbed, specifically learning disabled, speech impaired, and visually handicapped.
8. Individualized educational program and I individualized family service plan.
9. P.L. 102-119 identifies and tracks children at risk of having developmental delays, encourages family participation in various developmental services and supports, encourages services to be provided in natural environments, and includes assistive technology services and devices.

ADDITIONAL LEARNING ACTIVITIES

1. Visit a classroom that includes students with developmental disabilities. Find out how students with different diagnoses and different needs are integrated into classes with regular schoolchildren.
2. Write or call your state association chairperson for information on the developmental disabilities special-interest section in your state. Learn how you would benefit by selecting developmental disabilities as your special-interest group when you apply for a student membership in the AOTA.
3. Volunteer at a summer camp or center for the developmentally delayed, a cerebral palsy center, or some other facility for children.

REFERENCES

American Occupational Therapy Association, Research Information Division. (1991). *Member data survey: Summary report.* Bethesda, MD: Author.

Bigge, J. L. (1991). *Teaching individuals with physical and multiple disabilities* (3rd ed.). New York: Macmillan Publishing Company.

Farnighetti, R. (Ed.). (1994). *The world almanac and book of facts, 1995.* Mahwah, NJ: Funk & Wagnalls Corporation.

Gallagher, J., Harbin, G., Eckland, J., Clifford, R., & Fullagar, P. (1992). Policy implementation of services for infants and toddlers with developmental delays. *OSERS News in Print.* Washington DC: U.S. Department

Hightower-Vandamm, M. D. (1979). Developmental Disabilities Act: An historical perspective, Part 11. *American Journal of Occupational Therapy, 33*(7), 421-423.

Levine, K. J. (1991). *Fine motor dysfunction: Therapeutic strategies in the classroom.* Tucson, AZ: Therapy skill builders.

Linder, T. W. (1993). *Transdisciplinary play-based intervention: Guidelines for developing a meaningful curriculum for young children.* Baltimore: Paul H. Brookes Publishing Co., Inc.

Johnston, R. B., & Magrab, P. R. (1979). *Developmental disorders assessment, treatment, education.* Baltimore: University Park Press.

U.S. Bureau of the Census. (1995). *Statistical abstract of the United States; 1995* (115th ed.). Washington, DC: Author.

U.S. Department of Education, Office of Special Education Programs. (1991). *Mark-up of the Individuals with Disabilities Education Act.* Washington, DC: Author.

SUGGESTED READINGS

Decker, B. (1992). Comparison of the individualized education plan and the individualized family service plan. *American Journal of Occupational Therapy 46*(3), 247-252.

Hightower-Vandamm, M. D. (1979). Developmental Disabilities Act: An historical perspective, Part 1. *American Journal of Occupational Therapy, 33*(6), 355-359.

Huebner, R. A. (1992). Autistic disorder: A neuropsychological enigma. *American Journal of Occupational Therapy, 46*(6), 487-501.

McCormick, L., & Lee, C. (1979). Public Law 94-142: Mandated partnership. *American Journal of Occupational Therapy, 33*(9), 586-588.

McHale, K., & Cermak, S. A. (1992). Fine motor activities in elementary school: Preliminary findings and provisional implications for children with fine motor problems. *American Journal of Occupational Therapy, 46*(10), 898-903.

McInerney, C. A., & McInerney, M. (1992). A mobility skills training program for adults with developmental disabilities. *American Journal of Occupational Therapy, 46*(3).

Ottenbacher, K. (1982). Occupational therapy and special education: Some issues and concerns related to Public Law 94-142. *American Journal of Occupational Therapy, 36*(9), 81-84.

Restall, G. & Magill-Evans, J. (1994). Play and preschool children with autism. *American Journal of Occupational Therapy, 48*(2), 113-120.

SUGGESTED LISTENING/VIEWING

Hanft, B., & Marsh, D. (1993). *Getting a grip on handwriting: A self-guided video and manual.* Bethesda, MD: American Occupational Therapy Association, Inc. (videocassette, 30 minutes).

MENTAL RETARDATION

The prevalence, definition, causes, and management of mental retardation are given. The range of occupational therapy services provided is summarized.

LEARNING OBJECTIVES

At the end of this section, you should be able to:

1. State the 1973 American Association on Mental Deficiency (AAMD) definition of mental retardation.
2. Explain the meanings of *intellectual functioning, adaptive behavior,* and *developmental period,* in reference to the definition of mental retardation.
3. Name the commonly used classifications of mental retardation.
4. Name and discuss four genetic causes of mental retardation.
5. Discuss prenatal, perinatal, and postnatal causes of mental retardation.
6. Discuss the effect of integrating persons with mental retardation into the community.
7. Discuss occupational therapy services needed for persons with mental retardation.

Mental retardation can occur in both sexes and in every race, religion, and nationality. Parents in every educational, social, and economic group have had children with mental retardation.

PREVALENCE OF MENTAL RETARDATION

In 1982, the Association for Retarded Citizens estimated that 6 million persons, or 3% of the population of the United States, was mentally retarded. Each year, approximately 100 thousand babies are born who have

213

the potential to become mentally retarded. Actual numbers are unavailable, because the data on individuals with mental retardation is inadequate, even though most state laws require infants with birth defects and disabilities to be registered with the state department of health. It is believed that the number of children from birth to 4 years of age with mental retardation is undercounted (New Jersey Developmental Disabilities Council, 1985). One reason for the lack of exact numbers is that many individuals who are mentally retarded have other conditions and may be listed under another diagnosis (Jacobson & Janicki, 1983; Martini & MacTurk, 1985).

In a 1992-1993 annual report to Congress, the Office of Special Education of the U.S. Department of Education stated that the total number of students receiving special education of one kind or another was 5,110,653, of which 11.3% were mentally retarded. The students with mental retardation were the third largest group of students served (U. S. Bureau of the Census, 1995).

DEFINITION

Mental retardation refers to significantly subaverage general intellectual functioning, existing concurrently with deficits in adaptive behavior manifested during the developmental period. The American Association on Mental Deficiency (AAMD) adopted this definition in 1973. The definition reflects the deletion of the "borderline" category found in earlier definitions (Grossman, 1983).

Mental retardation, as currently defined, indicates the person's existing level of performance. The cause of the retardation is not under consideration. It is possible that a variety of diagnoses includes mental retardation as a secondary diagnosis. The developmental period stated in the definition refers to the period from birth to 18 years.

Adaptive behavior is the individual's ability to meet the standards of personal independence and social responsibility expected at given ages. Since these standards vary with each age group, guidelines are established by the AAMD for those charged with making diagnoses of mental retardation.

The person who is mentally retarded does not have the ability to think, reason, calculate, or remember as well as someone who has an average or higher range of intelligence. In addition to this intellectual dysfunction, the mentally retarded individual has difficulty performing tasks and adapting his or her behavior to that expected of a person of the same age in a similar social, economic, and cultural setting.

CLASSIFICATION

Intelligence is measured by intelligence tests. The most frequently used such tests are the Stanford-Binet intelligence test and the Wechsler Intelligence Scale for Children (WISC). The words *significantly subaverage* in the definition of mental retardation refer to two or more standard deviations from the average (mean) of the tests. The person with mental retardation scores 68 or below on the Stanford-Binet test and 70 or below on the WISC test. Low scores alone, however, are not used to diagnose mental retardation. The levels of retardation and their respective scores are as follows:

Intelligence Quotient (IQ)

Level of Mental	Stanford-Binet	Wechsler Scales
Retardation	(standard deviation = 16)	(standard deviation = 15)
Mild	52-68	55-70
Moderate	36-51	40-54
Severe (Extrapolated)	20-35	25-39
Profound (Extrapolated)	19 and below	24 and below

Intelligence quotient (I.Q.) scores are obtained by dividing the score obtained on the given test (the mental age) by the chronological age (the actual age) and multiplying by 100 (Grossman, 1983).

The words *mild, moderate, severe,* and *profound* retardation are used to classify the given range of IQ scores. In educational settings, an additional set of classifications—*educable, trainable, severely mentally retarded,* and *profoundly mentally retarded*—is used to place students in designated classrooms.

ASSOCIATED PROBLEMS

In 1975, the President's Committee on Mental Retardation conducted a study of residential facilities and found that, of 105,442 residents reported to have mental retardation, at least 50.5% had one other handicapping condition. More than one handicapping condition was reported in 34%. In addition to mental retardation, 37.0% also had epilepsy, and 36.5% also had cerebral palsy or other neurological conditions. Emotional disturbance, lack of vision, and lack of hearing were other handicapping conditions reported.

ETIOLOGY

More than 200 causes have been identified as resulting in mental retardation (Gellis & Feingold, 1968). Any condition that hinders or interferes with optimal development of the fetus or the child after birth may cause mental retardation.

Genetic Causes

Biochemical abnormalities. A number of diseases that result in mental retardation have been traced to inborn errors of metabolism. These errors are passed on to the fetus by a hereditary trait. Following are some examples of biochemical causes of mental retardation:

Cretinism is a deficiency in or complete lack of thyroid hormone. In addition to mental retardation, the individual has stunted growth, coarse hair, and dry skin (Gellis & Feingold, 1968).

Tay-Sachs disease is due to faulty metabolism of fat. The body cannot assimilate certain fats. The child has general weakness and progressive loss of vision. Symptoms can begin anytime from 3 months to 18 years. Death follows shortly after the onset of the symptoms. Most children with Tay-Sachs disease die by the third year of life (Association for Retarded Citizens, 1982; Grossman, 1983).

Phenylketonuria (PKU) is the result of abnormal metabolism of amino acids. The individual lacks the enzyme phenylalanine hydroxylase. Early detection is possible by the Guthrie test, developed in the 1960s. Most states require the test to be administered to a newborn the second day after birth. If PKU is present, a proper diet started immediately may prevent mental retardation (Gellis & Feingold, 1968; Grossman, 1983). If mental retardation is prevented, the individual can lead a normal life. Women of childbearing age are advised to maintain a proper diet to prevent giving birth to a child with PKU.

Chromosomal abnormalities. Research findings suggest that practically all parts of the chromosomes are capable of affecting intelligence. Any upset in the general genetic balance can have harmful effects on both physical and mental traits.

The most familiar kind of mental retardation due to chromosome abnormality is *Down syndrome.* The syndrome is named for Dr. J. Langdon Down, who described it in 1866. In 1959, Lejeune and colleagues discovered that what in persons without Down syndrome was the chromosome pair 21 was in persons with the syndrome a trio of chromosomes (Pueschel, 1978). Down syndrome is therefore also referred to as trisomy 21. An estimated 1 per 600 to 700 births are of infants with Down syndrome (Association for Retarded Citizens, 1982; Gellis & Feingold, 1968). Associated problems of heart disease, respiratory conditions, and motor development will affect the progress of individuals with Down syndrome. Education and training opportunities can enable those who are not severely mdically, cognitively, and clinically challenged to care for their personal needs and to work in the community if they have appropriate supervision from the family or are in a community living setting.

Other chromosomal abnormalities have since been discovered. In the *cri du chat syndrome* (the infant's cry resembles the cry of a cat), the short arm of chromosome 4 or 5 is deleted. In the *translocation* chromosomal abnormality, all 46 chromosomes are present, but part of one is broken, and the broken part is fused to another chromosome (Gellis & Feingold, 1968; Grossman, 1983).

Prenatal Causes

The prenatal period is the period from conception to birth. Certain conditions during the prenatal period may cause mental retardation. Proper prenatal care may decrease the incidence of mental retardation by early detection and treatment of possible causes.

Rubella, commonly referred to as German measles, if contracted by the mother during the first 3 months of pregnancy, may cause the child to develop mental retardation and microcephaly, as well as congenital heart disease, cataracts, glaucoma, deafness, and an enlarged liver or spleen.

Incompatibility of the Rh factor in the blood between the mother and fetus can result in death or severe brain damage. Syphilis, meningitis, and other serious diseases in the mother during the prenatal period may result in mental retardation in the child. Certain drugs taken during the prenatal period may result in mental retardation, as well as physical congenital deformities. Physical malformation of the brain or other organs and inadequate oxygen in the developing fetus are also causes of mental retardation.

Perinatal Causes

The perinatal period refers to the period immediately preceding birth and the birth process itself. Birth-related injuries resulting in mental retardation have decreased in recent years due to increased knowledge and improved delivery techniques. Lack of oxygen during the perinatal period may cause mental retardation. Abnormal positions of the umbilical cord or twisting or kinking of the cord may prevent the infant from receiving adequate amounts of oxygen. Prematurity and low birth weight are considered serious threats to a newborn, although these factors are not causes of mental retardation.

Postnatal Causes

The postnatal period is the period after birth and during the developmental years of the child. Viral infections that cause inflammation of the central nervous system may cause mental retardation. Meningitis (inflammation of the meninges) has been known to cause deafness, blindness, and, sometimes, mental retardation. Accidents that cause damage to the brain may result in mental retardation. Near drowning, which interrupts the normal supply of oxygen, and the ingestion of lead and certain chemicals may result in mental retardation, cerebral palsy, seizures, or death. It has been suggested that improper nutrition and !ack of adequate stimulation are factors that contribute to an individual developing mild mental retardation.

PRIMARY CAUSES OF MENTAL RETARDATION

According to the AAMD, the most frequently listed cause of mental retardation is "unknown prenatal influence." The next highest causes are trauma or a physical agent, an environmental influence, infections, and intoxication. Other causes are chromosomal abnormalities, gestational disorders, gross brain disease, metabolic or nutritional disorders, and mental retardation following psychiatric disorder.

SETTINGS FOR THE MENTALLY RETARDED

The President's Committee on Mental Retardation reported in 1975 that, in the United States, many individuals who were mentally retarded lived in institutions or community care facilities. An institution is a public or private residential facility providing a variety of professional services on a 24-hour basis. The institution is usually located apart from the general community. The professional services are directed toward care, treatment, habilitation, and rehabilitation. The institution continues to provide a residence and care for many individuals with mental retardation who grew up in such a facility.

There are three categories of institutions serving persons who are mentally retarded: public facilities for the developmentally delayed, public facilities for the mentally ill where persons with mental retardation are among the resident population, and private residential facilities for individuals with mental retardation.

A variety of community care facilities were developed to meet specific needs of the mentally retarded population. 1) Group homes, boarding homes, and halfway houses enable individuals with mental retardation to live within the community. The residential facilities operate 24 hours a day to provide services to small groups of individuals—for example, five adult males. Individuals are supervised by the staff of the facility. Training in activities of daily living, such as dressing, hygiene, caring for personal belongings and the sleeping area, and mealtime behavior, may be done in the residential setting. When an individual has the potential for developing work skills, he or she is evaluated, a plan is developed, and the individual is usually scheduled to receive training at a designated work site in the community. 2) Foster homes are arranged for children and adults who are dependent and cannot live with their own families. 3) Nursing homes serve as a community residence for mentally retarded individuals who meet the criteria for acceptance into the facility. 4) The individual's natural home is still considered the best choice for most mentally retarded persons. Before the 1960s, parents were frequently advised to place the child in an institution. 5) Short periods of respite have become more readily available to families that need to be separated from their mentally retarded relatives for whom they provide care (President's Committee on Mental Retardation, 1975).

Beginning in 1985, increased numbers of community-based, state-operated facilities were developed to serve individuals with mental retardation. In 1993, the settings reported were foster homes, group residence, semiindependent facilities, and state institutions. The 1993 census showed a decline in the number of residents in state-operated facilities, with 140,230 at the end of 1980 and 69,760 at the end of 1993. There was an increase in the number of residents in private facilities, from 115,032 in 1982 to 229,279 in 1993 (U. S. Bureau of the Census, 1995).

Normalization of the mentally retarded, advocated in the United States during the 1960s, continues to be emphasized in the management of individuals with mental retardation. The idea of normalization originated in Scandinavia. The aim of normalization is to provide services in the least restrictive environment to meet the person's needs and to improve the quality of his or her care. Normalization efforts helped to decrease admissions to, and increased discharges from, state institutions.

TREATMENT

The United States began to focus on the needs of individuals with mental retardation in the 1960s. In the 1970s, the nation began to provide appropriate education for children of school age diagnosed with mental retardation.

Mainstreaming, a concept to integrate handicapped and nonhandicapped persons in the same service structure, became a new focus in special education. More individuals with mental retardation began attending classes held outside the institutional framework. Many were bussed to a community classroom during school hours and bussed back to the institution after classes. Mainstreaming and the acceptance of mentally retarded children in the classroom encouraged many parents to keep their children at home rather than place them in an institutional setting. Attitudes about mental retardation began to change as individuals who were believed to lack potential for learning developed new skills and behaviors after participating in special education programs.

Individuals with mental retardation received limited occupational therapy services, and today they continue to have many unmet needs. This is partly due to the lack of services for this population until the late 1960s. Many institutional settings where occupational therapy programs had not existed were not considered desirable employment settings by most occupational therapy practitioners. The shortage of occupational therapy personnel was another reason for the early limited service and continues to be a factor even now. Most individuals who reside in state facilities have conditions that make a transition to the community difficult. In long-term residential facilities for individuals with mental retardation, many of the problems that need intervention are severe and chronic.

Residents of public and private community residential facilities for individuals with mental retardation receive occupational therapy services if they attend a school system or a training program in which an occupational therapy practitioner is employed and occupational therapy is included in their intervention plan. Occupational therapy may be provided on a consultative basis in many situations because of the shortage of practitioners. Since regulations mandate educational and training programs for individuals with mental retardation, the current need for occupational therapy services greatly exceeds the available personnel.

The needs of individuals with mental retardation are extensive. Treatment and training are needed in all categories of activities of daily living, including, but not limited to, feeding, eating, mealtime behavior, toilet care, oral hygiene, bathing, dressing, grooming, functional communication, functional mobility, sexual expression, and socialization. Individuals with mental retardation usually need a longer time to learn preemployment skills, such as clothing care, time management, safety procedures, money management, making purchases in a store, eating in a restaurant, and other skills needed to function in the community. Work-related skills such as arriving on time, attending to a task for a given period without distracting others, asking the appropriate person questions at appropriate times, and behaving appropriately during lunch time and at other times when not working are all behaviors that need to be learned if the individual is to be a successful employee. All of these skills should be included in occupational therapy intervention programs. Many individuals with mental retardation have difficulty planning and participating in leisure activities. Watching television at home or in the residential setting or wandering the streets of the city are frequently how free time is spent. Play and leisure skills are not developed automatically and need to be included in intervention programs for individuals with mental retardation.

The occupational therapy practitioner can help individuals learn new behaviors and skills through a variety of techniques. Behavior modification has been successfully used to develop skills in all occupational performance areas. Sensory integrative techniques have been used to change behaviors, as well as develop gross- and fine-motor skills. Neurodevelopmental techniques have resulted in oral motor control for eating, as well as postural and motor control of the body. Orthotics, therapeutic equipment, and technology enable individuals with mental retardation and physical disabilities to participate in many life activities. Occupational therapy services can be extensive if staff is available.

THE ASSISTANT'S ROLE

The certified occupational therapy assistant (COTA) works under the supervision of the occupational therapist (OTR) in evaluation, program planning, intervention, and discharge planning. In any setting, intervention may include behavior modification techniques, as well as sensory stimulation to change behaviors. Intervention can be for any occupational performance area. Programs range from teaching activities of daily living skills to training in leisure skills to learning how to make the transition to a community living setting. In a school setting, the COTA may help the student learn academic-related handwriting, dressing, leisure, work, or social skills, as well as skills needed to function in the community. The COTA's role will depend upon the knowledge and skills he or she possesses, the predilections of the supervising OTR, the client's goal, and the mission and focus of the setting.

SUMMARY

Mental retardation is a developmental disability. The mentally retarded individual will need lifelong supervision. The occupational therapy service needs are numerous and diverse, require knowledge and skills in many areas, and provide a challenge for practitioners. Training in self-care, work, and leisure skills are included in the occupational therapy program. The role of the COTA can vary, depending on the client's goal, the preferences of the supervising OTR, the roles of other staff members, and the mission of the facility. Both direct treatment of individuals and consultative services will continue to be needed.

REVIEW QUESTIONS

1. The definition of mental retardation states that (1) the general intelligence of an individual with the condition is_____, (2) the person has deficits in_____ behavior, and (3) the condition was apparent during the_____ period.

2. Explain, in your own words, the meanings of *intellectual functioning*, *adaptive behavior*, and *developmental period*, as these terms are used in the definition of mental retardation.
3. What words are used to classify levels of mental retardation, and what scores on the Wechsler Intelligence Scale for Children (WISC) are associated with the various classifications?
4. Name four genetic causes of mental retardation, and state the potential for development with each.
5. Explain what is meant by *prenatal*, *perinatal*, and *postnatal* causes of mental retardation.
6. Discuss the effect of integrating persons with mental retardation into the community.
7. Name at least four skills needed by a student with mental retardation that might require occupational therapy.

ANSWERS

1. Subaverage, adaptive, developmental.
2. Intellectual functioning is the carrying out of the ability to think, reason, calculate, or remember, as measured on standardized tests.

   Adaptive behavior occurs when the individual effectively meets the standards of personal independence and social responsibility expected of his or her age and cultural level. Since these standards vary with age, each person's appropriate adaptive behavior must be separately evaluated.

   The developmental period stated in the definition of *mental retardation* is the period from birth to 18 years.
3. Mild retardation is evidenced by an IQ score of 55 to 70 on the Weschler Intelligence Scale for Children (WISC).

   Moderate retardation is diagnosed by an IQ score of 40 to 54 on the WISC.

   Severe retardation is manifested by an IQ score of 25 to 39 on the WISC.

   Profound retardation is diagnosed by an IQ score of below 25 on the WISC.
4. Tay-Sachs disease: The person has a poor potential for living beyond 3 years.

   Phenylketonuria (PKU): If treated and monitored with the proper diet, the person has good potential for a normal life.

   Down syndrome: Mental retardation will continue. The ability to be trained in self-care and work skills varies with the individual because of associated conditions such as heart disease and personality.

   Cri du chat: Mental retardation will likely continue.
5. The prenatal period is the period from conception to birth. The fetus

can be affected with mental retardation, depending on the health of the mother. The perinatal period is the period during which the birth process is going on. The infant can be affected with mental retardation if the mother has active herpes or if there are unusual birth conditions, such as a kinking of the umbilical cord that prevents the infant from having needed oxygen during birth. Injuries due to poor delivery methods are not as common today as they were in previous decades. The postnatal period is the period after birth and during the developmental years of the child. Viral infections, accidents, poor nutrition, and poor environmental conditions can cause mental retardation during this period.

6. When individuals are in the community in small-group homes, foster homes, or their own homes, there is more opportunity for normal stimulation and experiences. Individuals with mental retardation will have more opportunities for learning needed skills and behaviors in normal settings.

7. Occupational therapy may be needed to teach the student dressing skills, handwriting skills, social interaction skills, community safety behaviors, and work readiness skills.

ADDITIONAL LEARNING ACTIVITIES

1. Make an appointment to visit a state institution to observe programs for the mentally retarded. Among the questions you may want to ask are the following: How many residents reside in the facility? What is the age range of the residents? How many employees are on staff to provide direct care? Do residents participate in community activities? How many occupational therapy practitioners are employed at the institution?

2. Make an appointment to visit a group home. How many individuals with mental retardation reside in the home? How many staff members work throughout the day? What responsibilities do the staff members have for training the residents? How do the residents spend their usual day? What do they do on weekends and holidays?

3. Look in the blue pages of your community phone book for agencies that provide services for individuals with mental retardation. Inquire about visiting a vocational training center or day program for adults with mental retardation.

REFERENCES

Association for Retarded Citizens. (1982). *The truth about mental retardation.* Arlington, TX: Author.

Gellis, S. S., & Feingold, M. (1968). *Atlas of mental retardation syn-*

dromes. Washington, DC: Superintendent of Documents, U.S. Government Printing Office.

Grossman, H. J. (Ed.). (1983). *Manual on terminology and classification in mental retardation.* Washington, DC: American Association on Mental Deficiency.

Jacobson, J. W., & Janicki, M. P. (1983). Observed prevalence of multiple developmental disabilities. *Mental Retardation, 21,* 87-94.

Martini, L., & MacTurk, R. H. (1985). Issues in the enumeration of handicapping conditions in the United States. *Mental Retardation, 23,* 182-185.

New Jersey Developmental Disabilities Council. (1985). *New Jersey state plan for services to persons with developmental disabilities: 1985 update.* Trenton, NJ: New Jersey Department of Human Services.

President's Committee on Mental Retardation. (1975). *Mental retardation: The known and the unknown.* Washington, DC: Superintendent of Documents, U.S. Government Printing Office, DHEW Publication No. (OHD) 76-21008.

Pueschel, S. M. (Ed.). (1978). *Down syndrome: Growing and learning.* Kansas City, MO: Andrews and McMeel, Inc.

U. S. Bureau of the Census. (1995). *Statistical abstract of the United States; 1993* (115th ed.). Washington, DC.

SUGGESTED READINGS

Bigge, J. L. (1991). *Teaching individuals with physical and multiple disabilities* (3rd ed.). New York: Macmillan Publishing Company.

Copeland, M., Ford, L., & Solon, N. (1976). *Occupational therapy for mentally retarded children.* Baltimore: University Park Press.

Hirama, H. (1989). *Self-injurious behavior: A somatosensory treatment approach.* Baltimore: CHESS Publications, Inc.

Linder, T. W. (1993). *Transdisciplinary play-based interventions: Guidelines for developing a meaningful curriculum for young children* (rev. ed.). Baltimore: Paul H. Brookes Publishing Co., Inc.

SUGGESTED LISTENING/VIEWING

Howell, A., & Jackson, M. (Writers). (1978). *The handicapped child: Infancy through preschool.* Irvine, CA: Concepts Media. (3 hrs., 37-minute videotape).

Newman, K. L., & Moledom, B. (1981). *Adaptive equipment positioning.* Kent, OH: Portage Physical Therapists, Inc. (34-minute videotape).

Newman, K. L., Vogler, J., & Aronholt, S. (1981). *Feeding the multiply handicapped child.* Kent, OH: Portage Physical Therapists, Inc. (37-minute videotape).

19

CEREBRAL PALSY

Cerebral palsy is defined and described. Causes of, and words commonly used in discussing, cerebral palsy are given.

LEARNING OBJECTIVES

At the end of this chapter, you should be able to:

1. State the definition of cerebral palsy.
2. List five possible causes of cerebral palsy.
3. Correctly spell and define the following words:

agnosia	epilepsy	paraplegia
asymmetrical	hemiplegia	quadriplegia
athetosis	hypertonus	somatosensory
diplegia	hypotonus	spasticity
dysarthria	monoplegia	strabismus
dyspraxia	nystagmus	

4. Describe characteristics of spastic cerebral palsy.
5. Describe characteristics of athetoid cerebral palsy.
6. Describe the role of the occupational therapist and the occupational therapy assistant in the treatment of cerebral palsy.

Cerebral palsy is a disorder of movement and posture. The condition was first reported by Dr. W. J. Little early in the 19th century and was named Little's disease. A history of the disease and a description and the names of the different types of cerebral palsy can be found in Hardy (1983).

INCIDENCE

It is difficult to estimate the incidence of cerebral palsy because of the difficulty in diagnosing the condition in general and because the current criteria for classifying a developmental disability are based on an individual's level of functioning (Hansen & Atchison, 1993). In the late 1950s, an estimated 1 to 2 children per thousand between 5 and 15 years of age had cerebral palsy (Bobath, 1959). In the late 1980s, approximately 5 thousand babies were born in Britain with some kind of central nervous system damage (Bobath & Bobath, 1975). In the United States, according to an estimate by the United Cerebral Palsy Association, 2 to 3 of every thousand live births show central nervous system disorders that result in cerebral palsy (cited in Hansen & Atchison, 1993). An additional 2 thousand children acquire cerebral palsy in the first few years of life.

DEFINITION

Cerebral palsy is defined in *Melloni's Illustrated Medical Dictionary* (Dox, Melloni, & Eisner, 1993) as a condition marked by disturbance of voluntary motor function caused by damage to the brain's motor control centers. *Melloni's* states further that the condition is characterized by spastic paralysis or incoordination.

The term *cerebral palsy* refers to a group of conditions resulting from injury or abnormal development of the brain that occurred before age 3. The central nervous system lesion is nonprogressive, but interferes with the ability to assume and maintain normal postures and perform normal movements (Bobath, 1959; Hardy, 1983).

CLASSIFICATION

The various causes of cerebral palsy and the individual differences manifested make a precise classification of the disease difficult. A classification based on the type of motion problems the individual has and the location of involvement of the disease is used.

The most frequently encountered types of motion problems are 1) spasticity, which is displayed by increased tone or muscle contractions that cause stiff, awkward, uncoordinated, and involuntary movements; 2) athetosis, which is displayed by fluctuations in muscle tone, causing slow, irregular, twisting, uncoordinated, involuntary movements; 3) rigidity, which is displayed by increased muscle tone, causing very stiff movements and posture; and 4) ataxia, which is displayed by fluctuations between low and normal muscle tone, resulting in an inability to voluntarily direct or limit motion. A problem with postural balance is usually seen in ataxia. Other classifications and subtypes can be found in Hardy (1983) and Illingworth (1987).

Bobath (1959) proposed classifying cerebral palsy according to the bodily distribution of the handicap, together with the type of abnormal muscle tone. Bobath's classification is as follows:

1. *Diplegia.* The whole body is affected, with the lower extremities more affected than the upper. The distribution is generally symmetrical. Most children with spastic cerebral palsy are diplegic.
2. *Quadriplegia.* As with diplegia, the whole body is affected. However, in quadriplegia, the extremities are equally affected, or the upper extremities are more affected than the lower extremities. A large number of children diagnosed as spastic or athetoid are in this group. Rigidity, ataxia, flaccidity, and mixed characteristics are also seen in the group.
3. *Hemiplegia.* One side of the body is affected. The muscle tone is usually spastic.
4. *Paraplegia.* The lower trunk and lower extremities are affected.
   Bobath stated that most children with paraplegia actually have diplegia, and the upper extremities are so mildly affected that they appear normal.
5. *Monoplegia.* Only one extremity is affected. It is believed that most children diagnosed with monoplegia actually have hemiplegia. Bobath stated that the other extremity or extremities are so mildly affected that they may be overlooked.

In most diagnoses and discussions of individuals with cerebral palsy, both the motion problem and the distribution of the handicap is stated. Spasticity and athetosis are seen most frequently in cerebral palsy.

ASSOCIATED PROBLEMS

In addition to motor problems, defects in vision, hearing, and speech in varying degrees of severity are frequently associated with cerebral palsy. Perceptual dysfunction, mental retardation, and epilepsy may also be seen in children with cerebral palsy.

An estimated 50% of all cases of cerebral palsy have some motor defect of the eyes. Blindness, however, is rare. More common visual problems are an inability to focus properly, internal and external squint, an inability to move the eyes independently of the head, strabismus, nystagmus, defects in visual fields, and partial visual agnosia.

An estimated 20% of children with cerebral palsy have some hearing defect. The most common hearing defects are high-frequency deafness and auditory agnosia.

Hearing defects may be responsible for delays in speech development. Pure aphasia is rare in cerebral palsy; dysarthria, an impairment in the articulation of speech, and dyspraxia, an inability to select and organize speech elements, are more common.

Somatosensory disturbances, such as hand or finger agnosia and impairment in body image, may be present. These disturbances may be due partly to the child's inability to use the hands to reach out and manipulate objects and to explore the body.

Mental retardation is considered to occur in 50% of cerebral palsy cases. Epilepsy is also common and may be of any type (Bobath, 1959).

CAUSES

The origin of cerebral palsy may occur during the prenatal, perinatal, or postnatal period. It is generally believed that, out of 100 cases of cerebral palsy, 60 are of perinatal origin, 30 are of prenatal origin, and 10 are of postnatal origin (Bobath, 1959). Bobath stated that prematurity and neonatal asphyxia are the most frequent causes of cerebral palsy.

Prenatal causes of cerebral palsy include infection, anoxia, cerebral hemorrhage, metabolic disturbance, or blood incompatibility. Perinatal causes include obstetrical problems—in particular, anoxia, trauma, or hemorrhage. Prematurity and hemorrhagic disease of the newborn may also cause cerebral palsy. Postnatal causes include trauma, infections, toxins, vascular accidents, anoxia, and late developmental defects. In many cases, no definite prenatal, perinatal, or postnatal cause can be found.

DESCRIPTION OF CEREBRAL PALSY

The individual diagnosed with cerebral palsy frequently has sensory or perceptual disturbances, mental retardation, and/or epilepsy in addition to postural and motor disturbances. The resultant symptoms can range from severe to mild. An individual with severe cerebral palsy can be nonverbal, nonambulatory, and confined to a bed, dependent upon another for all personal care and movement. Another individual with mild cerebral palsy can lead a normal life, with the only visible evidence of the disease being minimal incoordination of one upper extremity.

All children with cerebral palsy show incoordination and abnormal muscle tone, the latter of which is either too high (hypertonic) or too low (hypotonic) to enable the child to perform movements in a normal fashion. The muscle tone may in fact fluctuate from hypertonicity to hypotonicity, especially in children with athetosis, making coordinated movements impossible (Bobath & Bobath, 1975; Illingworth, 1987).

Abnormal muscle tone may occur in response to a stimulus provided by the position of a body part with respect to other body parts. For example, turning the head to one side while the child is supine may result in flexion of the extremities on the skull side and in extension of the extremities on the face side. This reflexive response is called the *asymmetrical tonic neck reflex* (ATNR). The *symmetrical tonic neck reflex* (STNR) is also seen. It is elicited when the neck is extended when in the midline position. The reflexive response to extending the neck is extension of the upper extremities and flexion of the lower extremities. When the neck is flexed, the opposite occurs, the upper extremities flexing and the lower extremities extending (Bobath, 1959).

Abnormal muscle tone also may occur in response to the position of the body with respect to the earth's gravitational force. When the child is prone, the flexor muscles dominate, and extension may be difficult or impossible. By contrast, when the child is supine, the extensor muscles dominate, and flexion may be difficult or impossible. This reflexive flexion or extension response is called the *tonic labyrinthine reflex* (TLR) (Bobath, 1959).

Finally, abnormal muscle tone may occur in response to an outside force acting on the body of the child. For example, lifting a child with spastic cerebral palsy by holding the child under the axilla usually results in extensor hypertonicity of the trunk and lower extremities and flexor hypertonicity of the upper extremities. Also, the child's spine and neck will usually undergo hyperextension, the legs will rotate internally with the toes pointing downward, and the upper extremities will be tightly flexed with the fingers fisted. Another example of abnormal muscle tone due to an outside force can be seen when a child with athetosis is held upright and his or her feet are bounced on the floor. The child's whole body usually becomes stiff, and any movements made will be disorganized (Bobath & Bobath, 1975; Finnie, 1975).

The spastic and athetoid types of cerebral palsy are seen more frequently than any other types.

THE CHILD WITH SPASTIC CEREBRAL PALSY

Characteristic of the child with spastic cerebral palsy is lack of movement. The abnormally high muscle tone is apparent even when the child lies awake in bed. The body posture is rigid, the legs may be stiffly extended with the toes pointing down, and the fingers may be tightly clenched. The child with severe spastic cerebral palsy maintains one position because of the inability to move into another position. Contractures will occur if the child is not positioned and handled properly.

The child's mouth may be tightly closed due to the high muscle tone. The development of speech and language will depend upon the oral structure, degree of neuromotor involvement, intellectual capacity, and treatment.

If the child is able to walk, he or she will often walk on the toes. The child may appear awkward due to the inadequate equilibrium reactions, spasticity, and reflex activity.

Detailed descriptions of the child with spastic cerebral palsy can be found in Bobath (1959), Bobath (1967), Bobath and Bobath (1975), Hardy (1983), and Illingworth (1987).

THE CHILD WITH ATHETOID CEREBRAL PALSY

Characteristic of the child with athetoid cerebral palsy are disorganized body movements. The child with athetosis experiences frequent fluctuations in muscle tone, which make coordinated movements impossible. Precise or directed movements cannot be made because the child lacks the necessary fixation of the trunk and joints to support the moving body part. Head control also is poor. Children with athetoid cerebral palsy rarely develop contractures, because of their continual movement.

The mouth may be held open, with the tongue out or with the tongue thrusting in and out. Drooling is frequently seen. Speech and eating may be particularly difficult for the child with athetosis. Speech production and language development will depend upon the oral structure, degree of neuromotor involvement, intellectual capacity, and treatment.

If the child is able to walk, the walk is characterized by a lurching, stumbling manner, with a great deal of uncoordinated movement in the upper extremities.

Deafness to high-frequency sounds is common in the child with athetosis. Auditory problems should be suspected when there is a speech delay.

Children with athetoid cerebral palsy will differ according to the bodily distribution and severity of the problem.

As with the child with spastic cerebral palsy, detailed descriptions of the child with athetosis can be found in Bobath (1959), Bobath (1967), Bobath and Bobath (1975), Hardy (1983), and Illingworth (1987).

TREATMENT

The generally approved approach to treating children with cerebral palsy is to inhibit their abnormal postural reflexes and facilitate normal tone and movements. Treatment is based on an evaluation of each individual. Therapists qualified to provide intervention for children with cerebral palsy usually have knowledge and experience beyond that of an entry-level therapist. The knowledge is gained through special formal courses and continuing education courses. Detailed principles of treatment can be found in Bigge (1991), Bobath (1967), Bobath and Bobath (1975), Finnie (1975), Kramer and Hinojosa (1993), and Linder (1993).

The child with spastic cerebral palsy has difficulty moving isolated parts of the body, as well as the body as a whole. Opportunities should be provided to engage in active movements. The child will have difficulty exploring play objects and the environment, so the senses should be stimulated. Sensory stimulation to the body receptors and the opportunity for movement should be carefully graded for each child's need and tolerance. The child should experience a variety of normal movements during treatment. Static positions for long periods are not recommended.

The child with athetoid cerebral palsy experiences too many disorganized movements. Such a child needs to experience postural stability, after which movement should occur. For example, the child should have a feeling of stability in sitting or standing before engaging in activities that require movement from that position. The child with athetosis should be handled more slowly than the child with spasticity, in order to enable the athetoid child to feel the fixation of the trunk and joints. The child with athetosis also should be maintained in a position of normal postural tone long enough to feel the normal posture and normal muscle tone. The child should gain controlled movements in the midrange first and then proceed to the outer ranges. Movements should be done slowly, until control is achieved. The child needs a sense of organization and stability.

THE ASSISTANT'S ROLE

Treatment to inhibit abnormal postural tone and to facilitate normal tone and movements in a child with cerebral palsy requires knowledge and experience beyond the entry level of practice. The occupational therapist (OTR) with specific postgraduate education and training in treating cerebral palsy evaluates the patient and plans and usually carries out the treatment program, rather than delegating aspects of treatment to a certified occupational therapy assistant (COTA). When the COTA has worked with an OTR in the treatment of cerebral palsy or has completed a special course for COTAs, responsibility for parts of the intervention may be given to the COTA.

The OTR determines the COTA's role in the treatment of cerebral palsy. The COTA's duties may include preparation of the treatment area for appropriate visual and auditory stimulation, play objects, and equipment. The COTA may provide cognitive stimulation or assist the child in manipulating objects while the OTR positions and handles the child. The COTA may aid in undressing and dressing the child, may stimulate language, or may escort the child to the treatment area and the next activity. The role of the COTA will depend upon the OTR's background and orientation to treatment and the COTA's background, interests, and potential. The actual duties assumed may be greater than, less than, or entirely different from those just mentioned.

SUMMARY

Cerebral palsy is one of the diagnostic categories listed under developmental disabilities. Cerebral palsy is a complicated neurological condition that requires specialized treatment. COTAs may assist OTRs in all aspects of treatment and may receive special training from the OTR while on the job. COTAs may also attend continuing education classes that focus on their role in the treatment of cerebral palsy.

REVIEW QUESTIONS

1. Cross out the incorrect words and phrases before or after each slash to make the following paragraph correct:

    Cerebral palsy is a progressive/nonprogressive disorder of movement, posture/joint range of motion, and muscle strength due to damage or abnormal development of the brain. Cerebral palsy is a single condition/group of conditions. Frequently associated with cerebral palsy are abnormal muscle tone, muscle incoordination, blindness/visual defects, deafness/loss of high-frequency hearing, mental retardation, epilepsy, dysarthria/depression, and perceptual dysfunction.

2. List five possible causes of cerebral palsy.

3. Circle the letter of the answer that makes the best complete statement about cerebral palsy:
   1) Diplegia involves
      a. one side of the body.
      b. the lower trunk and both lower extremities.
      c. the whole body.
      d. the whole body, with the legs more than the arms.
   2) Paraplegia involves
      a. one side of the body.
      b. the lower trunk and both lower extremities.
      c. the whole body.
      d. the whole body, with the legs more than the arms.
   3) Hemiplegia involves
      a. one side of the body.
      b. the lower trunk and both lower extremities.
      c. the whole body.
      d. the whole body, with the legs more than the arms.
   4) Quadriplegia involves
      a. one side of the body.
      b. the lower trunk and both lower extremities.
      c. the whole body.
      d. the whole body, with the legs more than the arms.

4. Circle the correct word in brackets:
   The [spastic/athetoid] child has abnormally high muscle tone and finds movement difficult. Because of the inability to change body positions spontaneously, the severely affected child may develop contractures unless he or she is properly handled and treated.

5. Circle the correct word in brackets:
   The [spastic/athetoid] child has uncoordinated, disorganized movements due to fluctuations in muscle tone. There is poor head control,
   the mouth may remain open, and drooling is frequently seen.
   Contractures rarely develop.
6. Describe some general roles the COTA might play in intervention for
   the child with cerebral palsy.

ANSWERS

1. Cerebral palsy is a nonprogressive disorder of movement and posture
   due to damage or abnormal development of the brain. Cerebral palsy
   is a group of conditions. Frequently associated with cerebral palsy are
   abnormal muscle tone, muscle incoordination, visual defects, loss of
   high-frequency hearing, mental retardation, epilepsy, dysarthria, and
   perceptual dysfunction.
2. prematurity
   lack of oxygen
   viral infection
   blood disease
   trauma
3. d., b., a., c.
4. spastic
5. athetoid
6. Generally, the occupational therapist evaluates, plans, and carries out
   the treatment program for each child. The COTA assists the therapist
   in all aspects of the treatment program. Depending upon his or her
   training and experience, the COTA may or may not be involved in
   direct care, such as assisting with dressing and undressing, providing
   sensory stimulation during play periods, assisting with feeding, and
   performing similar activities.

ADDITIONAL LEARNING ACTIVITIES

1. Make an appointment to visit the local United Cerebral Palsy center.
   Ask the occupational therapist to identify different classifications of
   cerebral palsy. Observe treatment and the COTA's role if possible.
2. Make an appointment to visit a special education class that includes
   students with cerebral palsy. Observe some of the special adaptive
   and technical devices used by the students.

REFERENCES

Bigge, J. L. (1991). *Teaching individuals with physical and multiple disabilities.* New York: Macmillan Publishing Company.

Bobath, B. (1967). The very early treatment of cerebral palsy. *Developmental Medicine and Child Neurology, 9*(4), 373-390.

Bobath, B., & Bobath, K. (1975). *Motor development in the different types of cerebral palsy.* London: William Heinemann Medical Books Ltd.

Bobath, K. (1959). The neuropathology of cerebral palsy and its importance in treatment and diagnosis. *Cerebral Palsy Bulletin, 1*(8), 13-33.

Dox, I., Melloni, B. J., & Eisner, G. M. (1993). *Melloni's illustrated medical dictionary.* Baltimore: The Williams and Wilkins Company.

Finnie, N. R. (1975). *Handling the young cerebral palsied child at home.* New York E. P. Dutton and Company.

Hansen, R. A., & Atchison, B. (1993). *Conditions in occupational therapy: Effects on occupational performance.* Baltimore: Williams and Wilkins.

Hardy, J. C. (1983). *Cerebral palsy.* Englewood Cliffs, NJ: Prentice Hall.

Illingworth, R. S. (1987). *The development of the infant and young child: Normal and abnormal.* Baltimore: The Williams and Wilkins Company.

Kramer, P., & Hinojosa, J. (1993). *Frames of reference for pediatric occupational therapy.* Baltimore: The Williams & Wilkins Company.

Linder, T. W. (1993). *Transdisciplinary play-based intervention: Guidelines for developing a meaningful curriculum for young children.* Baltimore: Paul H. Brookes Publishing Co.

SUGGESTED READINGS

Lilly, L. A., & Powell, N. J. (1990). Measuring the effects of neurodevelopmental treatment in the daily living skills of two children with cerebral palsy. *American Journal of Occupational Therapy, 44*(2), 139-145.

SUGGESTED LISTENING/VIEWING

Mortola, P., & Walsh, P. (Producers). (1991). *Children with cerebral palsy.* (VHS, 25 min.). Bethesda, MD: American Occupational Therapy Association, Inc.

20

SPINAL CORD INJURY

An injury to the spinal cord can result in physical and neurological damage. An introduction to the conditions related to, and complications of, spinal cord injuries is presented.

LEARNING OBJECTIVES

At the completion of this section, you should be able to:

1. Name four causes of spinal cord injury.
2. Explain the basic reason a completely severed spinal cord results in total paralysis below the level of the injury.
3. Correctly spell and use the words *paraplegia* and *quadriplegia*.
4. Name the major spinal cord segment classifications, and give the correct number of segments in each classification.
5. State one reason that patients with spinal injuries show differences in physical and neurological damage and in recovery when the spinal cord is not completely severed.
6. Name seven possible complications of spinal cord injuries.
7. State the procedure to follow when symptoms of blood pooling occur.
8. State the procedure to follow when symptoms of autonomic dysreflexia occur.
9. Discuss the importance of a collaborative approach in treating spinal cord injury.

The spinal cord is the lower elongated portion of the central nervous system. The spinal cord is covered by meninges and is protected by cerebrospinal fluid and the vertebral column that surrounds the cord. The spinal cord contains the vital neural tracts through which various parts of the body send and receive messages from the brain (Pick & Howden, 1977).

STRUCTURE OF THE SPINE

The vertebral column consists of 33 vertebrae (bones) named according to their location in the body. The vertebral column has seven cervical vertebrae, beginning at the base of the skull. Below the cervical vertebrae are 12 thoracic, 5 lumbar, 5 sacral, and 4 coccygeal vertebrae. The coccygeal vertebrae are fused as one. Each vertebra is identified with a letter and number. C1 refers to the first vertebra at the base of the skull. Below C7 (the last cervical vertebra) is T1, below T12 (the last thoracic vertebra) is L1, and below L5 (the last lumbar vertebra) is S1 (Netter, 1989; Pick & Howden, 1977) S1-S5 refer to the 5 fused sacral vertebrae plus the 4 fused coccygeal vertebrae.

The spinal cord is divided into 31 segments, grouped into the foregoing four classifications. There are 8 cervical spinal cord segments, 12 thoracic segments, 5 lumbar segments, and 5 sacral segments (Netter, 1989; Pick & Howden, 1977) (Figure 20.1). Because the vertebral column grows more rapidly than the spinal cord, the numbers identifying the vertebrae, the spinal cord segments, and the spinal nerves originating from each segment do not match exactly in their horizontal locations. The adult spinal cord ends at approximately the L1 vertebral area (Sine, Liss, Roush, Holcomb, & Wilson, 1988).

The spinal cord and the nerves within the vertebral column are important to sensorimotor functioning. Detailed explanations of specific muscles and body functions affected by injury at particular locations of the spinal cord can be found in Hansen and Atchison (1993), Pedretti and Zoltan (1990), and Wilson, McKenzie, Barber, and Watson (1984).

CAUSES OF INJURY

Trauma to the spine that causes spinal cord injury occurs most frequently among active adolescents and young adult males. The most common age for incurring such injuries is 19.0 years, with males comprising 82.3% of those injured (Umphred, 1995). Motor vehicle accidents have consistently been listed as the leading cause of spinal cord injury (Hansen & Atchison, 1993; Sine et al., 1988; Umphred, 1995). Whether or not the added safety devices and laws for operating a motor vehicle are changing the numbers of spinal cord injuries is yet to be reported. Spinal cord injury can result from contact sports such as football, as well as from noncontact sports such as surfing, skiing, and horseback riding. Diving is reported to be the highest sport-related cause of spinal cord injury (Hansen & Atchison, 1993). Accidents and homicides are among the top 10 causes of death in the nation (Farnighetti, 1994). Often, if death does not result from severe physical assault, a bullet, or a knife wound to the body, spinal cord injury does. Gunshot wounds and accidental falls are among

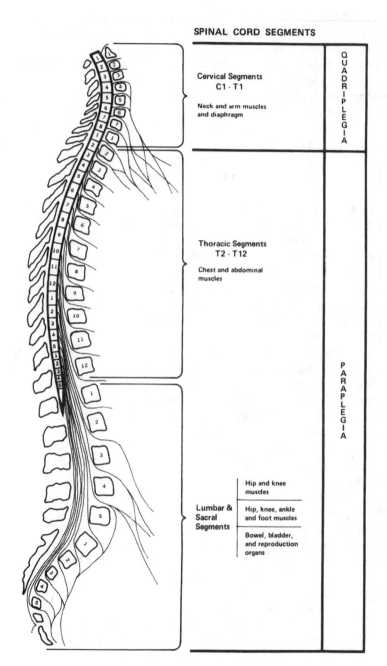

SPINAL CORD SEGMENTS

Cervical Segments
C1 - T1

Neck and arm muscles
and diaphragm

Thoracic Segments
T2 - T12

Chest and abdominal
muscles

Lumbar &
Sacral
Segments

Hip and knee
muscles

Hip, knee, ankle
and foot muscles

Bowel, bladder,
and reproduction
organs

QUADRIPLEGIA

PARAPLEGIA

FIGURE 20.1

SIDE VIEW OF THE SPINAL COLUMN AND THE SPINAL CORD

the top causes of spinal cord injury, with falls the leading cause in the elderly. The spinal cord also can be damaged by diseases such as tumors, spina bifida, scoliosis, and other conditions.

The lasting effects of spinal cord injury require enormous emotional and physical adjustment from the patient, family, and treatment team. Physical rehabilitation, counseling, and emotional support are needed not only for those who acquire a spinal cord injury at their most active stage of life, but for any person of any age who becomes less functional because of spinal cord damage.

RESULTS OF INJURY

A spinal cord injury is diagnosed as complete or incomplete. If the spinal cord is completely severed, there will be no sensation or voluntary motor ability in the area served by spinal nerves below the injury. Because the spinal nerves serve both sides of the body, damage results to both sides and is called *bilateral*. A spinal cord injury at level T2 or lower would result in paralysis of both lower extremities (paraplegia). A spinal cord injury at level T1 or above would result in paralysis of both upper and both lower extremities (quadriplegia) (Pedretti & Zoltan, 1990; Umphred, 1995). (See Figures 20.2 and 20.3.)

The American Spinal Injury Association (ASIA) prefers the word *tetraplegia* to *quadriplegia*. Tetraplegia is an impairment or loss of motor and/or sensory function in the cervical segment of the spinal cord. Impairment of function in the arms, trunk, legs, and pelvic organs results. With paraplegia, depending on the level of injury, the trunk and pelvic organs, as well as the legs, may be affected (ASIA & International Medical Society of Paraplegia, 1992).

Yarnell (cited in Sine et al., 1988, p. 10) states that the *Frankel* classification system was developed to communicate more precisely the degree of impairment resulting from spinal cord injuries. The classification is from the most severe impairment, *Frankel Class A,* indicating that the patient has no motor or sensory function below the neurological level of the injury, to *Frankel Class E,* indicating full recovery. The ASIA has modified the Frankel scale as follows to grade the degree of impairment:

A = Complete. No sensory or motor function is preserved in the sacral segments S4 and S5.

B = Incomplete. Sensory, but not motor, function is preserved below the neurological level and extends through the sacral segments S4 and S5.

C = Incomplete. Motor function is preserved below the neurological level, and the majority of key muscles below the neurological level have a muscle grade less than 3.

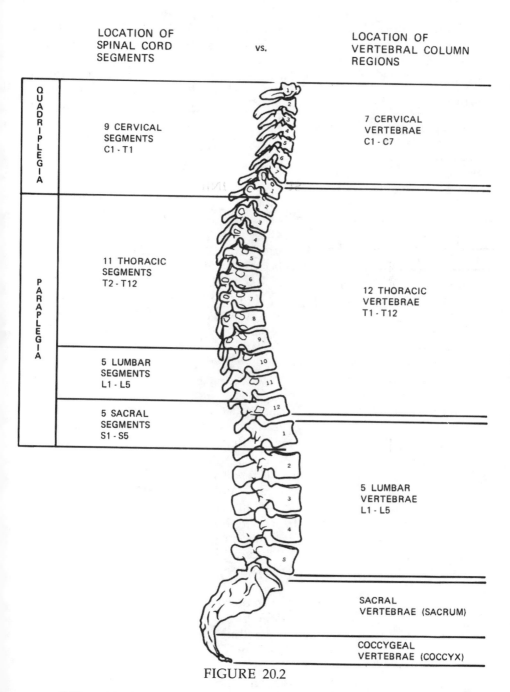

LOCATION OF
SPINAL CORD   VS.
SEGMENTS

LOCATION OF
VERTEBRAL COLUMN
REGIONS

QUADRIPLEGIA

9 CERVICAL
SEGMENTS
C1 - T1

7 CERVICAL
VERTEBRAE
C1 - C7

PARAPLEGIA

11 THORACIC
SEGMENTS
T2 - T12

12 THORACIC
VERTEBRAE
T1 - T12

5 LUMBAR
SEGMENTS
L1 - L5

5 SACRAL
SEGMENTS
S1 - S5

5 LUMBAR
VERTEBRAE
L1 - L5

SACRAL
VERTEBRAE (SACRUM)

COCCYGEAL
VERTEBRAE (COCCYX)

FIGURE 20.2

RELATIONSHIP OF VERTEBRAL COLUMN REGIONS TO
SPINAL CORD SEGMENTS

DIAGRAM OF SPINAL CORD INJURY

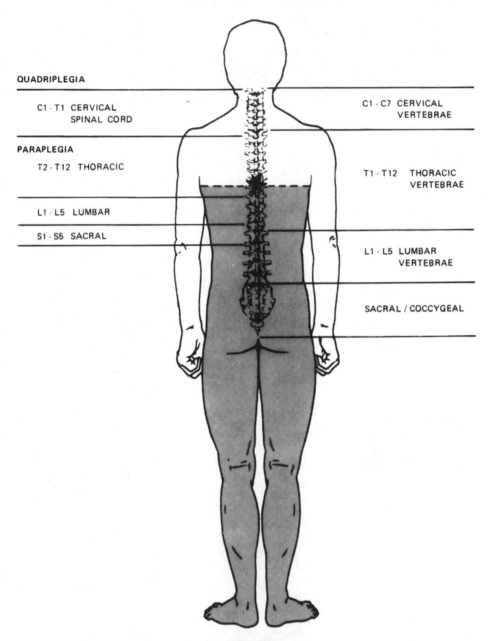

QUADRIPLEGIA

C1 · T1 CERVICAL
           SPINAL CORD

C1 · C7 CERVICAL
           VERTEBRAE

PARAPLEGIA

T2 · T12 THORACIC

T1 · T12 THORACIC
            VERTEBRAE

L1 · L5 LUMBAR

S1 · S5 SACRAL

L1 · L5 LUMBAR
           VERTEBRAE

SACRAL / COCCYGEAL

FIGURE 20.3

SHADED AREA INDICATES AFFECTED AREA RESULTING FROM
DAMAGE TO SPINAL CORD SEGMENT T10

D = Incomplete. Motor function is preserved below the neurological level, and the majority of key muscles below the neurological level have a muscle grade greater than or equal to 3.

E = Normal. Sensory function and motor function are normal.

This revised classification is an effort to establish uniform standards that incorporate research findings and to aid accurate communication between clinicians and researchers (ASIA & International Medical Society of Paraplegia, 1992; Umphred, 1995).

In most cases of injury, the spinal cord is not completely severed, because the bony vertebral column provides protection. In some accidents, the bony protective structure is crushed, damaged, or displaced and causes compression of the spinal cord and nerves. The compression accounts for some of the variations in the results of spinal cord injury and in the recovery from injury. When the spinal cord injury is incomplete, there will be some voluntary movement and/or sensation below the level of the injury. Current medical evaluations provide detailed information about the injury, and closer approximations regarding recovery can be made. However, many factors influence each patient's response to treatment and recovery. The medical literature, as well as personal accounts of individuals who have had a spinal cord injury, report unexpected recovery following such injury.

Prior to 1970, individuals with spinal cord injuries at the C1 to C4 levels rarely survived the initial trauma, and rehabilitation was seldom attempted for those who did survive. Since the 1970s, new information in medicine, engineering, and technology has increased the survival rate and made it possible to stabilize the body systems so that patients can participate in rehabilitation programs (Garber, 1985; Latham, Gregorio, & Garber, 1985).

Although there are increasing numbers of accounts of greater-than-expected recovery from spinal cord injury, many cases result in permanent, serious loss of sensation and motor ability. Predictions regarding the results of injury and recovery of function are well established from thousands of prior cases. Illustrations of injury sites with the muscles and nerves affected, the loss of function, and the expected gains from treatment can be found in many texts (e.g., Hansen & Atchison, 1993; Pedretti & Zoltan, 1990; Umphred, 1995; Wilson et al., 1984).

COMPLICATIONS OF SPINAL CORD INJURY

An incomplete spinal cord injury may involve several segments of the cord in which some functioning below the level of the injury is possible. The following references provide additional information about each of the complications mentioned next: Hansen & Atchison (1993); Pedretti

& Zoltan (1990); Sine et al. (1988); Umphred , (1995); Wilson et al. (1984).

In spinal cord injuries at the T12 or lower levels, normal respiration can be expected. In spinal cord injuries above the T12 level, breathing and coughing pose a problem and may result in respiratory tract infections, reduced energy, and a diminished tolerance for activities of daily living. A person with a complete spinal cord injury above the C4 level is usually dependent upon a respirator.

Pressure sores and decubitus ulcers are potential complications of spinal cord injury due to the loss of sensation and the prolonged sitting or lying without movement. Patients are taught to inspect areas of their bodies that are prone to pressure sores.

Osteoporosis of the lower extremities may result from disuse. Fractures of the bones in the lower extremity also become a possibility. Patients are encouraged to stand daily to prevent or delay the degeneration of the long bones.

Autonomic dysreflexia may occur in patients with spinal cord injury above the T6 level. In this condition, a reflex action in which the blood pressure rises in response to some stimulus causes perspiration, nausea, chilling, flushing, a severe headache, and irregularity in pulse rate. The stimulus is frequently pressure on the bladder or bowel, a urinary tract infection, or decubitus ulcers. Autonomic dysreflexia requires immediate medical attention. The patient should be placed in an upright position to lower the blood pressure. The catheter should be unclamped so that the bladder is draining. Immediate nursing care should be provided (Pedretti & Zoltan, 1990).

Postural hypotension is a condition that results from *decreased* blood pressure. The reduced muscle tone in the trunk and legs following a spinal cord injury results in blood pooling in the lower extremities. Normal muscle tone and muscle contractions maintain normal circulation of the blood, even during periods of inactivity. When a patient with spinal cord injury attempts to sit up after a long period of bed rest, the reduced blood pressure can result in lightheadedness, dizziness, weakness, unresponsiveness, and fainting. These are all symptoms of postural hypotension. To prevent them from occurring, the patient can be instructed to assume an upright position slowly. Other preventative measures are to have the patient wear antiembolism hosiery and abdominal binders. When symptoms of postural hypotension occur, one should help the patient to assume a semireclining or horizontal position until the symptoms are no longer evident and the patient responds.

Involuntary hypertonicity (spasticity) results below the injury level. If the spasticity differs from the usual spasms seen in some patients with spinal cord injury, its cause should be investigated. Among the causes of increased spasticity are infections, pressure sores, positioning, and emotional problems. A variety of treatment techniques are used to control hypertonicity; however, if the increased spasticity is painful or begins to result in contractures, medical or surgical intervention may be needed.

The loss of range of joint motion, muscle strength, and general endurance that follows a severe spinal cord injury may result in deformity of the joints and further weakening of musculature. Therapeutic exercises and activities, as well as orthotic measures, are used to prevent deformity and weakness.

Bowel and bladder control will not be voluntary. Urinary tract infections, constipation, and diarrhea are possible complications. A proper diet with adequate fluid intake and assistive devices are needed for bowel and bladder function. Monitoring and attending to warning signs of infections can help prevent serious problems.

Sexual sensation is absent in a person with a complete spinal cord injury, but it may be present in those with an incomplete injury. Persons with complete or incomplete spinal cord injury are able to participate in sexual activities, as well as become parents, if other factors do not intervene. Sexual counseling should be available for all persons with spinal cord injury.

TEAM APPROACH TO TREATMENT

The services of many disciplines are needed to treat the patient with spinal cord injury. When a traumatic spinal cord injury occurs, often the individual was in control of his or her body and had special life goals. After the injury, not only is the person suddenly placed in a dependent role, but achieving the goals suddenly appears impossible. The questionable extent of the subsequent recovery and the permanent results of the injury place a tremendous psychological burden upon the patient, family, friends, and medical staff. The psychological and neurophysiological effects of the injury require physicians, nurses, social workers, psychologists, and occupational, physical, respiratory, and speech therapists, as well as family, spiritual, and other support staff, to work together to treat and rehabilitate the person. . A collaborative approach ensures that the team members are aware of all of the various techniques and methods that are being used, because not all persons with a spinal cord injury respond in the same way. For example, a person with a spinal cord injury at the C6 level may be able to perform a task by using a method commonly used by a person with a C5 or a C7 lesion (Hill, 1986). In such a case, team discussions may focus on whether or not the performance of the task and the neurophysiological and psychosocial effects of the performance using a particular method are appropriate.

OCCUPATIONAL THERAPY GOALS

Occupational therapy practitioners play a vital role as members of the team that treats spinal cord injuries. An evaluation of the patient's daily-life activities is necessary to assess the impact of the injury and to evaluate the effects of the treatment. The Functional Independence Measure (FIM) (Hamilton & Fuhrer, 1987) is recommended by ASIA as an instrument that will estimate the disabilities resulting from the injury as they affect the patient's safety and dependence on others and on technological devices. The FIM evaluates six areas of functioning: self-care, sphincter control, mobility, locomotion, communication, and social cognition. The self-care area comprises eating, grooming, bathing, dressing the upper body, dressing the lower body, and toileting. The FIM score describes the patient's functional independence on a 7-point scale. A score of 7 indicates complete independence, a score of 6 modified independence. Scores from 5 down to 1 place the patient in an increasingly dependent category, meaning that human supervision or physical assistance is more and more required.

The goals of occupational therapy will depend upon the goals of the treatment team and the level and severity of the spinal cord injury. Generally, the occupational therapy goals focus upon self-care, the individual's tolerance to work, the use of adaptive devices, the prevention of complications, and psychological support (Hansen & Atchison, 1993; Pedretti & Zoltan, 1990; Wilson et al., 1984). The cognitive capabilities, the emotional status, and the motivation of the patient will greatly affect the goals of intervention.

THE ASSISTANT'S ROLE

The certified occupational therapy assistant (COTA) who works with persons with spinal cord injury in an acute care or rehabilitation setting is supervised by an occupational therapist (OTR) and is a member of the treatment team. The COTA must have had supervised experience beyond entry-level practice before working with patients with spinal cord injury. The COTA assists the OTR in all aspects of the occupational therapy program to aid the patient in achieving preestablished goals (Hill, 1986). Following the acute phase of treatment, the COTA may be responsible for monitoring or teaching specific self-care skills and activities, with or without adaptive devices, assisting with therapeutic exercises, and assisting with the construction of splints. The therapeutic activities can have goals related to the occupational performance areas of activities of daily living, work, or leisure.

The COTA may be involved with an Independent Living Program that includes persons with spinal cord injury following their acute care and rehabilitation. In such community-based settings, the COTA receives supervision from an OTR when the state regulations specify that COTAs are to be supervised.

SUMMARY

Spinal cord injuries result in bilateral loss of motor ability and sensation in body parts served by spinal nerves below the injury to the cord. The severity of the loss depends upon the damage to the cord. Traumatic accidents account for most spinal cord injuries. A large proportion of persons with spinal cord injury are adolescents and young adults, which creates a difficult emotional situation for the patient and family. The treatment of spinal cord injury is a complicated process requiring careful team management. The COTA who is a member of a team charged with treating spinal cord injuries must have specialized knowledge and skills beyond entry-level practice and receives supervision from an OTR.

REVIEW QUESTIONS

1. The leading cause of spinal cord injury is:
   a. diving.
   b. accidental falls.
   c. gunshot wounds.
   d. motor vehicle accidents.
2. The cause of total paralysis below the site of the spinal cord injury is:
   a. a level C4 spinal cord injury.
   b. a gunshot wound damaging the cord and vertebrae.
   c. a complete severance of the neural pathways at the site of the injury.
   d. a level T1 spinal cord injury.
3. A level C4 spinal cord injury results in paralysis called _____, and a level L4 spinal cord injury results in paralysis called _____.
4. What are the designations for the spinal cord segments, and how many levels are in each designation?
5. Give one example of how complete and incomplete spinal cord injuries differ.
6. Name seven complications of spinal cord injuries.
7. What are some obvious signs of blood pooling, and what should be done when it is seen?
8. What are some signs of hyperreflexia, and what should be done immediately?
9. Why is a collaborative team approach important for the treatment of spinal cord injury?

ANSWERS

1. d.
2. c.

3. tetraplegia or quadriplegia, paraplegia
4. There are four segments: cervical (9 levels), thoracic (11), lumbar (5), and sacral (5).
5. Both incomplete and complete spinal cord injuries show bilateral loss of motor ability and sensations; however, in a complete spinal cord injury the loss is complete below the level of the injury, whereas in an incomplete spinal cord injury some sensation and voluntary movement may be evident below the level of the injury.
6. Complications can be decreased respiratory function and inability to cough, loss of bowel and bladder control with possible infections, osteoporosis due to disuse of the lower extremities, postural hypotension that can cause blood pooling and fainting, autonomic dysreflexia or hyperreflexia, pressure sores from maintaining the same body position for long periods of time, and contractures of the joints due to their decreased movement.
7. Dizziness, facial pallor, and feeling faint are obvious signs of blood pooling. When a person shows any of these signs, help him or her to assume a horizontal position with the lower extremities above the level of the heart. Stay with the person until the symptoms are no longer evident and the person can respond that he or she is feeling better.
8. Severe headache, perspiration, flushing, chilling, nausea, and an irregular pulse rate are signs of hyperreflexia. When a person shows any of these signs, request immediate nursing and medical attention, place the person in an upright position to lower the blood pressure, unclamp the catheter so that the bladder is draining, and remain with the person until the situation returns to normal.
9. A team approach in treating spinal cord injury is important because of the multiple involvement of neurological, orthopedic, medical, dietary, respiratory, emotional, cognitive, and psychosocial factors. The uncertain, but potentially permanently disabling effects of the injury require careful and long-range planning. The individual's cognitive ability remains intact, and the the person can be helped in planning strategies to work toward achieving earlier-formulated goals with the use of assistive devices and technologies.

Answer the following extra questions:

Circle the number preceding the true statements.

1. Spinal cord injury results in unilateral loss of motor ability.
2. Spinal cord injury results in bilateral loss of motor ability.
3. Traumatic accidents are responsible for most spinal cord injuries in adolescents and young adults.

4. Disease processes are responsible for most spinal cord injuries in adolescents and young adults.
5. A completely severed spinal cord at L2 would result in paraplegia.
6. A completely severed spinal cord at L2 would result in quadriplegia.
7. Bladder and bowel control is lost following a spinal cord injury.
8. When a patient with a spinal cord injury faints after being transferred from a bed into a wheelchair, the wheelchair should be locked and tilted back so that the feet are above the level of the heart.
9. Patients with spinal cord injury are unable to have sexual relationships.
10. Spasticity is involuntary excessive muscle tone.

Circle the letter preceding the word that correctly completes the statement.

1. A spinal cord injury at the C6 level results in:
   a. paraplegia.
   b. tetraplegia.
   c. hemiplegia.
   d. monoplegia.
2. A patient with paraplegia usually has difficulty with:
   a. cognition.
   b. self-feeding.
   c. ambulation.
   d. communication.

ANSWERS

True statements are numbers 2, 3, 5, 7, 8, and 10.
1. b
2. c

REFERENCES

American Spinal Injury Association and International Medical Society of Paraplegia. (1992). *International standards for neurological and functional classification of spinal cord injury, revised 1992.* Chicago: American Spinal Injury Association.

Farnighetti, R. (Ed.). (1994). *The world almanac and book of facts—1995.* Mahwah, NJ: Funk and Wagnalls Corporation.

Garber, S. L. (1985). Nationally speaking—new perspectives for the occupational therapist in the treatment of spinal cord-injured individuals. *American Journal of Occupational Therapy, 39*(11), 703-704.

Hamilton, B. B., & Fuhrer, M. J. (Eds.). (1987). *Rehabilitation outcomes: Analysis and measurement.* Baltimore: Brooks, Inc.

Hansen, R. A., & Atchison, B. (1993). *Conditions in occupational therapy: Effect on occupational performance.* Baltimore: Williams and Wilkins.

Hill, J. (Ed.). (1986). *Spinal cord injury: A guide to functional outcomes in occupational therapy.* Chicago: Rehabilitation Institute of Chicago.

Latham, P. A., Gregorio, T. L., & Garber, S. L. (1985). High-level quadriplegia: An occupational therapy challenge. *American Journal of Occupational Therapy, 39*(11), 705-714.

Netter, F. H. (1989). *Atlas of human anatomy.* Summit, NJ: CIBA-Geigy Corporation.

Pedretti, L. W., & Zoltan, B. (1990). *Occupational therapy: Practice skills for physical dysfunction* (3rd ed.). St. Louis: The C. V. Mosby Company.

Pick, T. P., & Howden, R. (Eds.). (1977). *Anatomy, descriptive and surgical by Gray, H.* (Revised American from the 15th English edition.) New York: Bounty Books.

Sine, R. D., Liss, S. E., Roush, R. E., Holcomb, J. D., & Wilson, G. B. (1988). *Basic rehabilitation techniques: A self-instructional guide.* Rockville, MD: Aspen Publishers, Inc.

Thomas, C. L. (Ed.). (1993). *Taber's cyclopedic medical dictionary* (17th ed.). Philadelphia: F. A. Davis Company.

Umphred, D. A. (Ed.). (1995). *Neurological rehabilitation.* St. Louis: The C. V. Mosby Company.

Wilson, D. J., McKenzie, M. W., Barber, L. M., & Watson, K. L. (1984). *Spinal cord injury: A treatment guide for occupational therapists* (rev. ed.). Thorofare, NJ: Slack Incorporated.

SUGGESTED READINGS

Bowen, R. E. (1994). The use of occupational therapists in Independent Living Programs. *American Journal of Occupational Therapy, 48*(2), 105-112.

21

GERIATRICS

Characteristics of persons aged 65 and older living in the United States are examined.

LEARNING OBJECTIVES

At the end of this chapter, you should be able to:

1. Define *geriatrics* and *gerontology*.
2. Discuss the delivery of occupational therapy services to the U.S. population aged 65 and older.
3. Name at least five physiological changes that occur in the aging process.
4. Name the most frequently reported chronic conditions of persons aged 65 and older.
5. Discuss the stereotyping of older persons and its effect on health care.

Geriatrics is defined as the branch of medicine concerned with the problems of aging. It includes all aspects of aging, including the physiological, pathological, psychological, economic, and sociological problems of the elderly. *Gerontology* is the scientific study of the effects of aging and of age-related diseases on the human being (Thomas, 1993).

THE OLDER PERSON IN AMERICA

In 1900, less than 4% of the total U.S. population was over 65 years of age. By 2050, 22.9% of the U.S. population (more than one in five persons) will be over 65 (Cessna, Jacobs, & Foster, 1994). The U.S. Senate Special Committee on Aging classifies the aging population in accordance with its demographic trend over the years. In its report, *Aging America: Trends and Projections,* the committee uses the term "older" to refer to age 55 and older, "elderly" to age 65 and older, "aged" to 75 and older, and "very old" to 85 and older (Vierck, 1984). These terms are not used precisely with these meanings by the general public, to whom "elderly" more frequently refers to people over 65 years of age.

In 1900, there were 772,000 people between the ages of 75 and 84 and 122,000 who were 85 and over (Cessna, Jacobs, & Foster, 1994; Vierck, 1984). Using the above terminology, in 1990 there were 31.1 million Americans who were elderly. There was a 22% increase in the elderly during the decade of the 1980s alone. In 1990, of the 31.1 million elderly, 10 million were 75 to 84 years of age, 6.9 million were 80 years or older, and 3 million were 85 or older (Farnighetti, 1993). By 2050, the 85-or-older group will make up 5.1% of the total U.S. population. In 1990, 35,808 reported being 100 years of age or older. The centenarian population more than doubled in the 1980s and is predicted to number 1.3 million by 2050 (U.S. Bureau of the Census, 1994).

Women tend to live longer than men, and an estimate indicates that elderly women outnumber elderly men 3 to 2 (Vierck, 1984). A 1991 analysis of census data reports that, of persons 65 years and older, there were 67.5 males to every 100 females. Of persons aged 65 to 74 years, there were 8,022,000 males and 10,258,000 females; of persons aged 75 to 84 years, 3,888,000 males and 6,424,000 females; and of persons aged 85 years and older, 881,000 males and 2,279,000 females. The 85-years-and-older group made up 1.3% of the U.S. population (U.S. Bureau of the Census, 1993). White males born in 1993 have a life expectancy of 72.1 years, while white women are expected to live to 78.9 years. Nonwhite males have a life expectancy of 67.4 years, and nonwhite women are expected to live 75.5 years (Farnighetti, 1994). The relatively rapid rise in the number of persons over age 65 calls for a reevaluation of our attitudes toward the elderly and an emphasis on the social, economic, environmental, and health needs of the entire U.S. population.

In 1991, California and New York had the greatest number of persons aged 65 to 74 years and 85 years and older, while California and Florida had the greatest number of persons aged 75 to 84 years. Other states with large numbers of persons over 65 years are Texas and Pennsylvania. Population projections to 2010 indicate that the 65-or-older group will continue to populate the south, midwest, and west in greater numbers (U.S. Bureau of the Census, 1995).

HEALTH STATUS

Studies suggest that many beliefs about a decline in the cognitive, physical, and sensory processes beginning at about age 50 are untrue. Researchers propose that any such decline is more likely due to pathology than to the natural aging process (Kiernat, 1991). In a 1981 survey, 8 of

10 elderly reported their health as good or excellent, and only 8% described their health as poor (Vierck, 1984).

The U.S. Bureau of the Census (1993) found that in the 1990 census the chronic conditions most frequently reported by those 65 years of age and older were arthritis, hypertension, heart conditions, hearing impairments, orthopedic deficits, and vision impairments.

Cohen (1988) reported that a loss in brain weight in an otherwise healthy older adult does not lead to a decrease in intellectual functioning. The brain seems to compensate for cell losses that occur as a person ages. The feedback mechanism in the brain serves to maintain one's functional capacities. Indications are that older individuals retain the capacity to learn, to respond appropriately to challenges, and to adapt to new situations. Older persons perform better in solving practical problems than do others in a traditional testing situation. Performance in problem-solving tasks peaks in middle years, and the level of performance of 60- to 70-year-olds is about equal to that of 20-year-olds. Cognitive activity and intellectual performance are believed to be the most important factors in maintaining mental health and satisfaction with life in older individuals. Physical illness and stress can cause a decline in cognitive functioning.

PHYSIOLOGICAL CHANGES

Functional loss in sensory and somatic functions does not generally occur until age 70 and in some individuals does not appear until 90 years of age. The heart and circulatory functions remain adequate to meet the usual demands of daily living for most people through their nineties. Changes in older individuals occur gradually and are the result of changes in the composition of the body as a whole and a decreased elasticity and pliability in the tissues and organs. The ratio of body liquid to body fat decreases, resulting in a decrease in the production of saliva, ocular lubrication, and sweat, as well as a diminution of intestinal mobility (Kiernat, 1991).

With aging comes decreased pliability of the lenses in the eyes, resulting in a diminished ability to keep objects focused on the retina. The lens becomes rigid and yellow, which affects color perception. Ninety-five percent of individuals over 70 years of age have evidence of clouding of the lens. The pupils of the eyes become smaller, leading to a diminished refractive ability. The majority of persons 75 years and older have decreased visual acuity, due to the diminished refractive ability, yellowing of the lens, and a slower reaction to light and dark. It is unknown whether the various physiological changes are due to pathology or are a part of the normal aging process (Kiernat, 1991).

Changes in auditory acuity begin in midlife. One third of individuals aged 60 to 70 years of age report significant high-frequency hearing loss.

Minor changes are reported in the gustatory sense. The ability to taste salt diminishes moderately in the older individual, while the ability to taste sweet, sour, and bitter remains intact. Dental disease, poor oral hygiene, and medications can alter the ability to taste. It is unknown why the ability to detect and identify odors and to appreciate pleasant smells diminishes with age. Because the ability to smell affects the desire to eat, as well as the ability to detect unsafe foods and unsafe environmental odors, additional research on the changes in the olfactory sense is needed (Kiernat, 1991).

The decreased capacity to evaporate moisture through sweating places the older individual at risk for heat stroke. This affliction can occur when the external temperature exceeds body temperature. The opposite, hypothermia, can occur when the external temperature is below 50° to 65° Fahrenheit. The ability to discriminate between two points on the skin of the extremities is diminished in older individuals.

Muscle strength peaks at about 30 years of age, and muscle mass and overall strength decline at a rate of about 1% per year. This decline does not affect daily activities, however, until around 70 years of age. Equilibrium and postural support depend on the individual's health and daily activities. The ability to respond to unusual demands diminishes.

CAUSES OF DEATH

In the United States, in 1980, heart disease was the number-one cause of death for all ages. For persons 65 years of age or older, heart disease, cancer, and stroke were the leading causes of death in 1980, as well as in 1993. In both of those years, among the five leading causes of death in those 65 years and older were chronic obstructive pulmonary disease and related conditions and accidents (Vierck, 1984). In 1993, heart diseases accounted for 32.6% of deaths, cancer 23.4%, stroke 6.6%, pulmonary disease 4.5%, and accidents 3.9%. The 1993 numbers show that more women than men died of heart disease (324,100 vs. 271,214) and stroke (78,760 vs. 46,722).

NURSING HOME RESIDENTS

The U.S. Bureau of the Census (1994) found that almost 1.8 million people resided in nursing homes that year (Brotman, 1980). It was estimated that, by the year 2000, 1.2 million additional nursing home beds would be required. Those most likely to need long-term care in nursing homes were the very old, the frail, and persons without families (Deutschman, 1985; Shuping, 1985). In 1991, there were 33,006 nursing homes, compared to 22,004 in 1971. By contrast, hospitals decreased in number from 7,678 in 1971 to 6,738 in 1991. The number of skilled nursing facilities grew from 4,277 in 1971 to 9,711 in 1991. These numbers indicated an increase in the elderly population and their growing need for long-term care. In the 1990s, a shift from long-term care in nursing homes to home health care began. In 1992, 75.2% of those 65 years or older received health care in their homes (U.S. Bureau of the Census, 1994).

THE STEREOTYPED OLDER PERSON

Studies by many disciplines show that numerous previously held opinions about the older person are groundless and interfere with the provision of services to them (Creecy, Berg, & Wright, 1985; Guerette & Moran, 1994; Kiernat, 1991; Larson, Zuzanek, & Mannell, 1985; Moritani & deVries, 1980). Senility was often thought to accompany aging naturally. Symptoms of confusion, forgetfulness, and an inability to concentrate, when displayed by a person 65 years or older, was humorously or seriously considered a symptom of aging and often casually referred to as senility. The older person who deviated from his or her usual cognitive functioning was often labeled senile. The attitude of the individual labeling the elderly person often indicated a feeling that the predisposition to senility was beyond treatment. When the same symptoms were seen in younger people, in-depth medical and psychological studies were expected and usually done. As physicians and gerontologists studied older people, it was learned that anxiety, pain, fatigue, or other causes can on occasion produce temporary symptoms of senility in individuals of any age. Not all elderly individuals have chronic symptoms of senility that are seen in Alzheimer's disease and other progressive conditions.

For many years, age 65 became synonymous with a retirement party, a gold watch awarded for years of service, unemployability, and eventual uselessness. A change in emphasis to better nutrition, appropriate health care, exercise, and pleasurable activities resulted in healthier elderly people who are now considered to be in the middle years, rather than the late period, of their life. Retirement age is no longer set at 65: An older age is no longer identified with the end of employment and the ability to contribute to society.

In past years, older persons were believed to be unable to adapt to or tolerate change. Dogmatic ideas and a rigid attitude often described the older person. Actually, most characteristics of an older individual are those the person had when he or she was younger. Many older people learn new skills, begin new relationships, travel, move to new locations, and adjust well to changes. The older person is a unique individual, with unique traits, just as children and younger adults have unique, individual traits. Kiernat (1991) reported that older individuals continue to develop new ways to respond to their environment, and aging does not result in rigid responses and behaviors. However, a change in the time required to respond to environmental stimuli is noted with aging.

Some care givers of the elderly tend to shield the person from daily stresses. The attitude that the elderly person has worked hard most of his or her life and should now rest is well meaning; however, without some life stresses and anxieties, the person can lose interest in living. Sitting in a rocking chair or a lounge chair for long periods is now known to be detrimental to the entire human system. Just as muscles atrophy and joints contract without exercise and use, the mind and body will deteriorate without stimulation.

A generally held inaccurate belief is that elderly persons prefer to be alone. However, this is not true of all, or even the majority of older persons. Most want to socialize and be involved in group activities of a kind and at a time of their own choosing. Frequently, older persons are alone of necessity. The U.S. Bureau of the Census (1995) reported that, of the 30.2 million civilian, noninstitutionalized men and women 65 years or older in the United States in 1994, 56.2% (16.0% men and 40.2% women) were living alone. The loss of family due to relocation or death, an inability to travel, physical or sensory losses, and limited finances are some reasons an older person may lead a solitary life. Some older persons adjust to such a life, and others do not. Changes in life-style may cause changes in the older person's behavior, which can create yet more problems.

Stereotyped beliefs result in the older person being treated in ways that are often detrimental. The older person should be treated as someone with individual capabilities, individual disabilities, and individual potentials. Although statistics may describe the average characteristics of a given group, rarely does an individual fit the exact description of that average. Each person, together with his or her unique genetic, biological, physiological, psychological, sociological, economic, and environmental background and influences, is different from every other person, regardless of many similarities.

IMPLICATIONS FOR OCCUPATIONAL THERAPY

In 1981, Tickle and Yerxa recommended a comprehensive day health care to meet the needs of at-risk older persons living in the community. Such programs, with adapted activities of daily living, devices, environments, and leisure activities, were felt to be a method of helping individuals maintain their independence in the community. Benzing (1986) recommended a community networking plan. The communication among service providers would establish a prevention program for the older individual in the community, help meet the needs of such individuals, and aid them in remaining in their homes.

In 1994, Guerette and Moran suggested that there was a need for a network of care providers with the means to communicate with professionals in each discipline about the status of at-risk individuals in the community. Although studies show that many elderly individuals would be able to perform their daily living activities independently, some chronic conditions, such as arthritis, can result in gradual impairment and permanent debilitation if the elderly person does not receive intervention. Many elderly people living in the community do not make their needs known because they are unaware of them, perhaps believing that their impairment is an inevitable process of aging, or because they do not know how or to whom to make their needs known. Often, by the time the individual contacts the primary physician about a particular medical condition, independent functioning is already impaired. Guerette and Moran (1994) suggest that early intervention by therapists, rehabilitation engineers, social workers, and the primary care physician can delay or even prevent debilitating impairments, potential hazards, and hospitalizations. These researchers recommend an assessment of the individual's level of independence in activities of daily living. Inability to perform such activities—for example, bathing and toileting—places the person at risk of losing his or her personal safety and independence. The individual's independence in regard to functioning in the community is at risk when the instrumental activities of daily living—the more complex activities that require social and environmental interactions (for example, shopping and banking)—are unable to be performed. A computerized data base is suggested as a means of sharing information with the network of professionals. The information gathered and shared will improve the quality of services offered to the elderly and reduce their rates of unmet needs for service, emergency room use, and hospital admissions, in addition to preventing or delaying losses of functional ability.

The need to lower the cost of health care and the desire of elderly individuals to remain in their homes have created alternatives to long-term residential care. Community-based day programs, health care programs in the private home, and subacute facilities were developed as means of containing costs and providing services to older individuals. All of these facilities and programs should have occupational therapy services available for those who require them.

THE ASSISTANT'S ROLE

The certified occupational therapy assistant (COTA), under general supervision or with consultation from an occupational therapist (OTR), is qualified to provide services to help individuals maintain or maximize their level of independence in all activities of daily living, as well as to enable them to remain productive and participate in leisure activities.

Treatment may include activities to increase or restore muscle strength, mobility of the joints, and gross- and fine-motor coordination. General postural stability and movement promoting the functional activities of self-care and leisure activities are emphasized in occupational therapy. The principles and special techniques of occupational therapy are described in many excellent articles and texts (e.g., Eggers, 1983; Kirchman, Reichenbach, & Giambalvo, 1982; Neustadt, 1985; Pedretti & Zoltan, 1990).

COTAs can serve as resource persons to other staff and family members in caring for the elderly person. COTAs working with the elderly individual may be able to help prevent impairment through the intervention process and by educating the patient, family members, and other care givers in proper body mechanics, joint-protection techniques, and the use of adaptive devices. On average, an older person with a disability who is living at home owns about 14 assistive devices in order to remain as independent as possible (Stone, 1994). Adapting the environment to the needs of the elderly individual and teaching the appropriate use of selected adaptive devices, orthotics, special clothing, and activities can help the patient maintain the highest possible level of independence and dignity.

Many COTAs are employed as activities directors in long-term care facilities and supervise staff in providing recreational and socialization activities to maintain the individual's general physical and mental status, as well as the desired quality of life.

SUMMARY

One out of eight persons in the United States is expected to be 75 years or older by the year 2050. One million persons are expected to be 100 years of age or older by the year 2080. Formerly held negative, stereotypical ideas about individuals aged 65 years and older are no longer valid and affect the delivery of service to this age group. The longer life span, together with an increasing number of older persons, indicates an increased need for research, new methods of health care delivery, and an increased need for occupational therapy services. COTAs can play a major role in the health care and leisure time activities of the older American.

REVIEW QUESTIONS

1. Define geriatrics and gerontology.
2. Discuss occupational therapy services for persons aged 65 years and older.
3. Name at least five physiological changes that result from the aging process.

4. Circle the chronic conditions most frequently reported by noninstitutionalized individuals aged 65 years and older in 1990.
   a. Hodgkin's disease
   b. arthritis
   c. Alzheimer's disease
   d. depression
   e. arteriosclerosis
   f. hearing impairments
   g. heart conditions
   h. rheumatoid arthritis
   i. hypertension
   j. orthopedic conditions
   k. Parkinson's disease
   l. visual impairments
5. Discuss some stereotyped beliefs that have been held about older individuals and the possible effects of those beliefs on the therapeutic process.

ANSWERS

1. Geriatrics is the branch of medicine concerned with the problems of aging. Gerontology is the scientific study of the effects of aging and of age-related diseases on the human being.
2. As studies of the elderly increased, so did the medical treatment and rehabilitation of the elderly. Not all elderly individuals require long-term nursing home care, and more elderly individuals are receiving occupational therapy services in their homes, in community programs, or on a short-term treatment basis.
3. A decrease in the following areas are seen in the majority of persons over age 70: muscle strength; elasticity of tissues; the capacity to evaporate moisture, which creates a potential for heat stroke because of the inability to regulate body temperature through sweating; auditory acuity, with high-frequency hearing loss in one third of persons over 60 years of age; visual acuity; and the ability of the lenses to accommodate to light.
4. In decreasing order of frequency, b, i, g, f, j, and l.
5. Stereotyping leads to developing preconceived ideas about what an individual can or cannot do. If our minds are set that a person will behave or function in a certain way, we may be preventing the individual from reaching a goal of therapy by our attitudes and actions. For example, believing that elderly individuals become senile, lose their memories, or develop concentration problems may prevent the therapist from reporting a behavior that may in fact be due to a reaction to medication or a change in the individual's medical condition.

Similarly, believing that elderly persons want to be alone may prevent the therapist from encouraging the elderly person to join a group activity that will be therapeutic.

ADDITIONAL LEARNING ACTIVITIES

1. Make an appointment with a social worker in a nursing home or some other long-term care facility. Ask the social worker to describe the difference in the residents of today compared to 5 years ago. What is the average age of the residents? What percentage receive weekly or monthly visitors? If there is time, ask other questions, such as How do the residents pay for their care and what is the average daily cost per person?

2. Speak to a person of approximately 60 years, another person of 70 years, and another of 80-90 years or older. What differences in mental or physical functioning did you observe in these three individuals that you attribute to their ages? What differences in attitude did you observe in these individuals, compared to young adults? Did you change your opinions about older persons and the effects of age? If you did, elaborate on your opinions.

REFERENCES

Benzing, P. (1986). Community networking: Definition, process, and implications for occupational therapy and physical therapy. *Physical and Occupational Therapy in Geriatrics,* 4(4), 15-30.

Cessna, C. B., Jacobs, N. R., & Foster, C. D. (Eds.). (1994). *Growing old in America.* Wylie, TX: Information Plus.

Cohen, G. D. (1988). *The brain in human aging.* New York: Springer.

Creecy, R. F., Berg, W. E., & Wright, R., Jr. (1985). Loneliness among the elderly: A causal approach. *Journal of Gerontology, 40,* 487-493.

Deutschman, M. (1985). Environmental competence and environmental management. *Journal of Long-Term Care Administration, 13,* 78-84.

Eggers, O. (1983). *Occupational therapy in the treatment of hemiplegia.* Oxford: Butterworth-Heinemann Ltd.

Farnighetti, R. (Ed.). (1993). *The world almanac and book of facts, 1994.*

Farnighetti, R. (Ed.). (1994). *The world almanac and book of facts, 1995.* Mahwah, NJ: Funk & Wagnalls Corporation.

Guerette, P., & Moran, W. (1994). ADL awareness. *TeamRehab Report,* 5(6), 41-44.

Kiernat, J. M. (1991). *Occupational therapy and the older adult: A clinical manual.* Gaithersburg, MD: Aspen Publishers, Inc.

Kirchman, M. M., Reichenbach, M. A., & Giambalvo, B. S. (1982). Preventive activities and services for the well elderly. *American Journal of Occupational Therapy, 36*(4), 236-240.

Larson, R., Zuzanek, J., & Mannell, R. (1985). Being above versus being with people: Disengagement in the daily experience of older adults. *Journal of Gerontology, 40*, 375-381.

Moritani, T., & deVries, H. (1980). Potential for gross muscle hypertrophy in older men. *Journal of Gerontology, 35*, 672-682.

Neustadt, L. E. (1985). Adult day care: A model for changing times. *Physical and Occupational Therapy in Geriatrics, 4*(1), 53-66.

Pedretti, L. W., & Zoltan, B. (1990). *Occupational therapy practice skills for physical dysfunction.* St. Louis: The C.V. Mosby Company.

Shuping, F. (Managing Ed.). (1985). About this issue. *Journal of Long-Term Care Administration, 13,* 73.

Stone, J. H. (1994). Aging and assistive technology. *TeamRehab Report, 5*(8), 24-27.

Thomas, C. L. (Ed.). (1993). *Taber's cyclopedic medical dictionary* (17th ed.). Philadelphia: F. A. Davis Company.

Tickle, L. S., & Yerxa, E. J. (1981). Need satisfaction of older persons living in the community and in institutions. Part I: The environment. *American Journal of Occupational Therapy, 35*(10), 644-649.

Tickle, L. S., & Yerxa, E. J. (1981). Need satisfaction of older persons living in the community and in institutions. Part II: Role of activity. *American Journal of Occupational Therapy, 35*(10), 650-655.

U.S. Bureau of the Census. (1993). *Statistical abstract of the United States; 1993* (113th ed.). Washington, DC: Author.

U.S. Bureau of the Census. (1994). *Statistical abstract of the United States; 1994* (114th ed.). Washington, DC: Author.

U.S. Bureau of the Census. (1995). *Statistical abstract of the United States; 1995* (115th ed.). Washington, DC: Author.

Vierck, E. (Coordinator). (1984). *Aging America: Trends and projections.* Washington, DC: Special Committee on Aging, United States Senate.

SUGGESTED READINGS

Hasselkus, B. R. (1992). Meaning of activity: Day care for persons with Alzheimer disease. *American Journal of Occupational Therapy, 46*(3), 199-206.

Kubler-Ross, E. (1969). *On death and dying.* New York: Macmillan Publishing Company.

Picard, H. B., & Magno, J. B. (1982). The role of occupational therapy for hospice care. *American Journal of Occupational Therapy, 36*(9), 597-598.

Tse, S., & Bailey, D. (1992). T'ai chi and postural control in the well elderly. *American Journal of Occupational Therapy, 46*(4), 295-300.

Yerxa, E. J. (1994). Dreams, dilemmas, and decisions for occupational therapy practice in a new millennium: An American perspective. *American Journal of Occupational Therapy, 48*(7), 586-589.

SUGGESTED LISTENING/VIEWING

Melvin, J. (1993). *Working with the cognitively impaired adult.* Bethesda, MD: American Occupational Therapy Association, Inc. (audio-cassette, 37 minutes).

Rabin, P. V. (1990). *What is dementia?* Baltimore: Video Press, University of Maryland at Baltimore. (videocassette, 16 minutes).

Cerebrovascular Accident

The patient who has had a cerebral vascular accident (CVA) is seen in hospitals, subacute facilities, nursing homes, private homes, and rehabilitation centers. An orientation to the condition is presented.

LEARNING OBJECTIVES

At the end of this chapter, you should be able to:

1. Correctly spell the words for which CVA is an abbreviation.
2. Explain why *stroke* is frequently used synonymously with CVA.
3. State the three most frequent causes of a CVA.
4. List the four major arteries supplying blood to the brain.
5. Describe the motor dysfunction that can result from a right CVA.
6. Describe the motor dysfunction that can result from a left CVA.
7. Spell correctly and define *flaccidity* and *spasticity*.
8. Define *hemianesthesia, hemiplegia, hemiparesis, homonymous hemianopsia, dysarthria, global aphasia, expressive aphasia*, and *receptive aphasia*.
9. Describe the various possible mental aftereffects of a stroke.
10. Describe the various possible emotional aftereffects of a stroke.
11. Explain how to prevent or alleviate edema in a stroke patient.
12. Define subluxation, and discuss its prevention and treatment.
13. State three areas in which the certified occupational therapy assistant (COTA) can assist the occupational therapist (OTR) during intervention in CVA patients.

Stroke is a common term used to denote a cerebral hemorrhage. The term is appropriate because a cerebral hemorrhage occurs suddenly without warning and results in loss of sensation and motor power in a matter of minutes. The words *cerebral vascular (cerebrovascular) accident* technically describe the stroke, that is, a sudden mishap (acci-

261

dent) to the blood vessel (vasculum) in the brain (cerebrum). The terms *stroke* and *cerebrovascular accident (CVA)* are often used synonymously (Thomas, 1993).

CAUSES

The terms *stroke* and *CVA* are frequently used to refer to the cause of organic lesions in the brain resulting from an interrupted blood flow to the organ. The lesions are believed to be due most frequently to one of the following causes of the diminished blood flow:

1. *hemorrhage*, resulting from a rupture in a weakened blood vessel that suddenly prevents normal blood flow in the vessel;
2. *embolus*, a floating blood clot that is stopped by a narrowing of the walls of a blood vessel and suddenly blocks the normal flow of blood in the vessel; and
3. *thrombus*, a blood clot on the inner wall of a blood vessel caused by a buildup of plaque, which obstructs the normal flow of blood in the vessel.

Direct trauma, tumors, abscesses, hemorrhage, infarction, arteriovenous malformation, or any agent that assaults the sensorimotor cortex or its pathways can result in symptoms of hemiplegia or hemiparesis (Sine, Liss, Roush, Holcomb, & Wilson, 1988).

ANATOMY

Four major arteries supply blood to the brain: the common carotid, internal carotid, vertebral, and basilar arteries. Textbooks on anatomy and physiology give detailed information on these arteries, and a good medical dictionary (e.g., Dox, Melloni, & Eisner, 1993; Thomas, 1993) is a quick reference to them and illustrates their distribution in the brain. The diagrams presented in either of these sources show the range of potential neuromuscular results following a stroke.

A loss of the normal blood supply to the localized areas of the brain causes damage to the brain cells and nerves serving those areas. The effects of such damage generally can be predicted; however, the intricacy of the sensorimotor cortex and its pathways and the uniqueness of each affected individual do not allow precise prognoses to be made. Extensive tests are required to determine which specific areas are damaged and to diagnose the condition. Medical science has established that motor nerves from one side of the brain cross to the opposite side before passing down the spinal cord. The motor nerves on the left side of the brain, therefore, control the motor activity of the right side of the body. A lesion on the

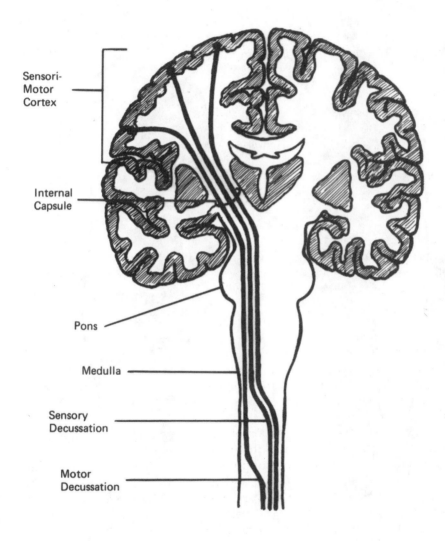

FIGURE 22.1 FRONTAL CROSS SECTION OF THE BRAIN

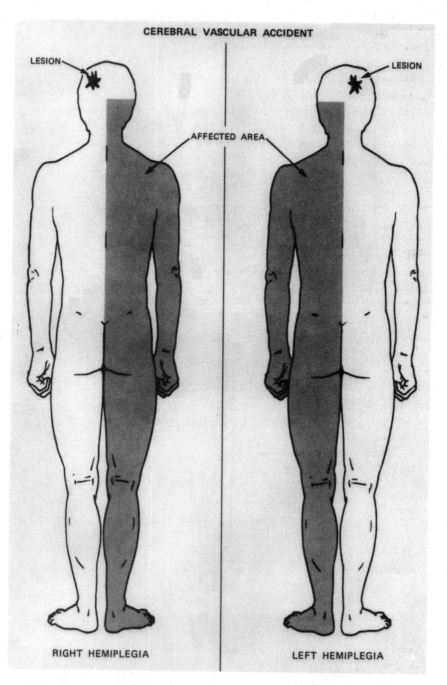

FIGURE 22.2   POSTERIOR VIEW OF AFFECTED AREA

right side of the brain, then, results in motor dysfunction on the left side of the body and vice versa. This condition has been labeled *hemiplegia*. A CVA or stroke generally results in one side (hemi) of the body developing paralysis (plegia) or weakness (paresis). The motor effects are usually seen beginning at the lower third of the face and extending down the length of the affected side of the body (Sine et al., 1988). (See Figures 22.1 and 22.2.)

Varying degrees of neuromuscular and mental dysfunction and behaviors will result from a CVA, depending upon the location and the extent of the cerebral lesion. The effect on the patient may require retraining or readjustment due to sensorimotor, perceptual, communication, or cognitive dysfunction. The occupational performance areas of activities of daily living, work, and leisure are usually affected in some manner. The immediate family may need to temporarily or permanently make adjustments in their daily life activities because of the residual effects of the CVA. Social activities and relationships may be affected. If the individual who has had a CVA was employed, the employment may be altered temporarily or permanently. The physical environment in and about the individual's residence and the employment setting also may need to be altered.

Clinical symptoms of the CVA patient are described in the next section; most patients will show some variation from these descriptions.

GENERAL PHYSICAL CHARACTERISTICS

After a CVA, any hemiplegia or hemiparesis that occurs is evident on the side of the body opposite that of the lesion in the brain. Sensorimotor effects of a left CVA will thus be evident on the right side of the body, and sensorimotor effects of a right CVA will be evident on the left side of the body.

A typical pattern of abnormal neuromusculature is evident in the hemiplegic syndrome, although individual differences may be seen. The affected lower extremity generally retains more strength than the affected upper extremity. The functioning of the lower extensors usually returns earlier than that of the lower flexors. In the upper extremity, the flexors are stronger than the extensors. Some patients recover their normal functioning without any treatment whatsoever (a phenomenon referred to as "spontaneous neurological return") within 2 to 3 months following the onset of the CVA. This phenomenon occurs more frequently in hemiplegia secondary to cerebral thrombosis.

FLACCIDITY AND SPASTICITY

Following the initial week or two of flaccidity (absent or minimal muscular tone) after a stroke, spasticity (increased muscular tone) develops in the affected extremity. The word *flaccidity*, or *hypotonia,* describes the muscle tone of the affected extremity when the patient is unable to voluntarily lift the extremity off a surface against gravitational force. The word *spasticity*, or *hypertonia*, describes the muscle tone of the affected extremity when the patient attempts to move the extremity, and either it does not move at all or any movement it does have appears stiff and awkward. The awkward movements are due to the increased tone and the inability to control movements. As regards the upper extremity, spasticity describes the muscle tone when the patient voluntarily attempts to extend the flexed elbow, and the elbow joint does not extend. Gradually and slowly trying to extend the elbow may finally achieve the desired results. However, an attempt by the patient to extend or move the elbow quickly will result in increased spasticity, and the elbow may flex even more. (Bobath, 1978; Eggers, 1983; Pedretti & Zoltan, 1990). Sine et al. (1988) cautions that, if left untreated, spasticity can promote contractures.

Flaccidity of a patient's affected upper extremity can be felt by lifting the patient's forearm off the surface and feeling the weight of the upper extremity. The patient can demonstrate the flaccidity by his or her inability to voluntarily maintain the wrist in alignment with the forearm when the latter is held parallel to the floor. Spasticity of a patient's affected upper extremity can be felt by attempting to extend the extremity when the elbow is flexed and feeling the involuntary resistance to having the extremity straightened. Resistance can also be felt in attempting to flex the elbow when the affected extremity is extended. The amount of resistance will depend on the body position that is assumed by the patient while the demonstration is being conducted, as well as on the severity of the patient's condition.

GENERAL SENSORY CHARACTERISTICS

Loss of sensation on the affected side (hemianesthesia) varies from one patient to another. The sensations may be heat, cold, touch, awareness of the spatial position of the body, and other sensations to the body surface, muscles, and joints. The loss may range from diminished tactile sensation in various areas of the affected side to total loss of sensation. In the latter case, some patients may be unaware of severely injuring a hand until they see blood from the open wound. Some patients will be unable to walk, because they lack sensation of position, even though the leg muscles are adequate. Cognitive training is important, in order to protect the patient from injury and get him or her to be as functional as possible (Pedretti & Zoltan, 1990; Sine et al., 1988).

ATTENTION

Following a CVA, patients frequently ignore the affected side of the body. In addition, objects, people, sounds, and the environment on that side are ignored. This phenomenon is referred to as "neglect" or "one-sided neglect." It has been suggested that the reason for the inattention is that the unaffected cerebral hemisphere overdirects the visual attention to the intact visual field. The head and eyes are, therefore, turned toward the intact side. Usually, they resume their normal midline position within a few days or weeks. If this does not occur, severe perceptual problems will result (Sine et al., 1988).

HOMONYMOUS HEMIANOPSIA

Homonymous hemianopsia is the loss of half of the visual field on the same side of each eye. This condition commonly occurs in hemiplegia. The result is blindness I on the hemiplegic side. This type of blindness is more disabling than complete blindness in one eye. Normally, the brain functions in a way that enables a person to focus visually on the center of the visual field. By contrast, the patient with homonymous hemianopsia sees only half of whatever is being viewed. Such patients need to be taught to turn to the affected side to gain a broader view of their environment. Safety precautions, such as discouraging a resumption of driving, need to be discussed with the patient (Pedretti & Zoltan, 1990; Sine et al., 1988).

Patients with one-sided neglect and homonymous hemianopsia have difficulty compensating for these losses. Cognitive orientation to the affected side and training are essential. Patients may need to be trained, for example, to make sure that they read an entire street sign, to eat from both sides of a plate, to wash and dress both sides of the body, and to relearn other daily life activities previously done automatically (Eggers, 1983; Pedretti & Zoltan, 1990; Sine et al., 1988).

A perceptual deficit that Sine et al. (1988) refer to as a "verticality dysfunction" may result in the patient seeing objects and spaces, such as a doorway, at a slant. Without cognitive training, patients may be unsafe in the community and behave inappropriately in social settings.

COMMUNICATION

Communication is the exchange of messages through sound, written symbols, or physical gestures. Adequate communication is dependent upon the adequacy of one person's expressions (expressive language) and the adequacy of another person's ability to receive the messages sent (receptive language). Communication is a complex process even between normal persons.

Motor ability is required for expressive language (i.e., to speak, to write, and to gesture with the hands or body). Patients who have had a

CVA may have oral motor disturbances that result in *verbal apraxia,* which is the inability to say words because of an inability to plan and carry out the necessary oral motor movements. Some patients may know what they want to say, but may be unable to plan the muscular movements or to speak the words. Some patients may have less severe motor loss resulting in difficulty in articulation (dysarthria). The severity of dysarthria and apraxia varies from one patient to another.

Motor ability is required for receptive language (i.e., to listen, to read, and to watch). Some patients who have had a CVA may hear what is said, but may not be able to process or retain what is heard, a condition called *agnosia.*

Aphasia is the loss of the ability to communicate. Aphasia may be referred to as expressive, receptive, mixed, or global. In expressive aphasia, the patient has difficulty speaking, writing, or gesturing. In receptive aphasia, the patient has difficulty recognizing, understanding, or integrating incoming messages. Mixed aphasia is a condition in which there are elements of both expressive and receptive aphasia. Global aphasia is a total aphasia, both receptively and expressively (Sine et al., 1988).

In the majority of people, the speech and language areas of the brain are in the left hemisphere. If the damage resulting from a CVA occurs in that hemisphere, the patient will very likely have a problem in communication, as well as a right hemiplegic syndrome (Pedretti & Zoltan, 1990; Sine et al., 1988). Communication problems compound an already difficult treatment program. The patient can be helped by consistency in the communication methods used by staff and family members.

MENTAL STATUS

Mental confusion can be expected shortly after the onset of a stroke. The nervous system has received a sudden shock. The individual may continue to be in a state of mental confusion and frustration due to memory loss from one day to the next. Memory loss may continue to be evident during and after rehabilitation. Loss of normal judgment may result and remain (Pedretti & Zoltan, 1990; Sine et al., 1988).

Memory loss and loss of judgment can create difficult situations for the patient and his or her family and friends. For example, an individual who frequently entertained in the past may feel able to manage to have a large party because he or she is only minimally physically affected, without realizing the cognitive and psychological limitations that come into play. The poor judgment exercised in planning and insisting on carrying out such an event can result in embarrassment, frustration, and anger for individuals involved in the event. Poor judgment in many daily life events over a period of time can lead to difficult and estranged relationships. A difficult employment situation can occur when a person with a CVA previously employed in a position with financial or legal responsibilities feels that he or she can resume the same responsibilities and does not realize the extent to which judgment and memory have been affected.

EMOTIONS

Most stroke patients have a period of reactive depression. Some may go through the stages of grief, feeling the lost use of their body. Many respond positively as they show general progress. Others may develop severe depression or psychosis. They may become emotionally unstable. Patients may suddenly start laughing or crying inappropriately. Frequently, they apologize for their behavior and state that they do not know why it happens and that they cannot control it. Reassurance and understanding need to be expressed to the patient, whose inability to control his or her emotions adds to the confusion, frustration, and loss of self-confidence and self-esteem (Pedretti & Zoltan, 1990; Sine et al., 1988).

EDEMA

Most of the normal circulation of body fluids is due to muscle contractions. In the stroke patient, problems occur when muscles become flaccid or weak. Fluid retention, or edema, is often the result of prolonged, stable body positions, especially while sitting. Elevating the arm and leg and moving or massaging the affected side with the intact extremity help prevent or alleviate edema.

SUBLUXATION

Subluxation is the incomplete separation of the bones at a joint (Thomas, 1993). Because of the flaccid affected upper extremity, there is added pressure away from the shoulder (the glenohumeral joint) when in a standing or sitting position. Slings similar to those used to immobilize and support a fracture in the arm have been used. However, these traditional slings have been shown to aggravate the situation in some cases because of the tendency of the extremity to lean into the sling. Dynamic slings that have some elasticity and are less stable have been found by some therapists to be more therapeutic for subluxation of the shoulder. Slings need to be selected individually for each patient, as no one type of sling meets the needs of all hemiplegic patients. Controversy exists over the effectiveness of slings (Botvinik, 1983). The physician, the supervising therapist, and, when appropriate, the patient need to make the final decision regarding whether to use a sling and, if so, what type.

THE ASSISTANT'S ROLE

The OTR, assisted by the COTA, evaluates the patient's needs in the occupational performance areas. The COTA, supervised by the OTR, provides intervention to develop skills needed by the patient to function in his or her daily life. The skills may be basic activities of daily living skills, such as bathing, personal hygiene, dressing, grooming, and eating, or may be cognitive and psychosocial skills needed to function in employment or social settings. How to plan and organize time, how to organize objects and materials needed for a given task, and how to set priorities are examples of cognitive skills needed for independence in such activities as dressing, preparing a meal, and planning the day's activities. The COTA may be responsible for helping the patient relearn money management, home management, shopping, how to use public transportation, and leisure and socialization skills. Special techniques and activities utilized in the intervention will depend on the practice model used by the OTR and upon the patient's goals. The activities employed during therapy may be familiar to the COTA; however, it is important that the COTA have an understanding of the practice model the OTR has in mind. The same activity may be used differently, depending upon whether the OTR is is applying a neurodevelopmental treatment model, a functional rehabilitation model, a cognitive model, an occupational adaptation model, or some other model.

The CTR evaluates the patient's need for adaptive devices. When such devices are recommended, the OTR or COTA educates the patient and others who are involved in treating the patient care about the purpose, care, and use of the devices. The OTR or COTA monitors the use of the device and, together with the patient, evaluates the appropriateness of the device to assure that the patient is satisfied with its effectiveness.

The OTR and COTA work together on occupational therapy concerns and are members of a team composed of professionals from other disciplines. The disciplines represented are usually occupational, physical, and speech therapy, psychology, social work, dietetics, nursing, and medicine. Occupational therapy services vary from one treatment center to another. In one center, a referral to occupational therapy may occur shortly after the patient has been admitted to the center, in order to train the patient in self-care activities. In another center, the nurse may have the responsibility for training the patient. In one center, the occupational therapy staff may treat the upper extremities through supervised therapeutic exercises. In another facility, the physical therapy staff may supervise all therapeutic exercises, and the occupational therapy staff may provide functional activities following physical therapy.

Occupational therapy evaluations usually include evaluations of how the patient performs various activities of daily living, muscle tests, testing of the range of motion of the joints, sensory tests, cognitive tests, and tests to determine the patient's interests. Treatment may include positioning and exercises using pulleys, inclined tables, skateboards, finger ladders, and other commercial and therapist-originated therapeutic devices. Hand splints are usually constructed by occupational therapists. In some settings, physical therapists or orthotists may be responsible for all orthotic devices.

A stroke affects the whole person, physically, cognitively, emotionally, and socially. Following a stroke, the person will need to adapt to his or her environment and future life generally and specifically. A team of specialists is required to help the individual cope with and adapt to the effects of the stroke. The special knowledge and skills necessary to treat the patient are gained through formal education and well-supervised experience, followed by continual self-education.

SUMMARY

The terms *stroke* and *CVA* are often used interchangeably. A person who has had a CVA or stroke experiences weakness or paralysis of the affected motor areas. Sensory loss, perceptual disturbances, changes in cognitive ability, and loss of emotional control also may occur. A stroke can affect the patient's social, vocational, and family roles. Early treatment, retraining in daily living skills, and coping strategies are included in occupational therapy programs for persons who have had a CVA.

REVIEW QUESTIONS

Fill in the blank spaces with the correct words.

1. *CVA* is an abbreviation for _____.
2. Why is the word *stroke* often used in place of *CVA* or what it abbreviates?
3. A stroke occurs when trauma affects the sensorimotor cortex or its pathways and a _____ results. Three causes of stroke are_____ (when the blood flows out of a torn vessel), or when an _____ suddenly blocks the flow of blood, or when a _____ obstructs the normal flow of blood.
4. Name the four major arteries supplying blood to the brain.
5. The loss of the normal blood supply to the right side of the brain results in motor and neurological dysfunction on the _____ side of the body. Visible motor signs can be _____ or
_____.
6. The loss of the normal blood supply to the left side of the brain results in motor and neurological dysfunction on the _____side

of the body. Visible motor signs can be _____ or
_____ .

7. Usually, during the acute stage following a stroke, the upper extremity of the affected side shows _____ , evidenced by _____ . After the acute stage, the extremity becomes _____ , evidenced by _____ .

8. Match each of the words of Column I with the most appropriate phrase in Column II.

Column I
____ hemianopsia
____ dysarthria
____ expressive aphasia
____ receptive aphasia
____ hemiplegia
____ hemiparesis

Column II
a. inability to speak
b. paralysis of one side of the body
c. loss of half of the visual field
d. inability to understand words
e. weakness of one side
f. difficulty in speaking

9. What are mental events may follow a stroke?
10. Name some emotional reactions that can result from a stroke.
11. Edema in an extremity can be prevented or alleviated by:
   a. including fiber in the diet.
   b. avoiding excessive use of the extremity.
   c. general exercise on a daily basis.
   d. massage and elevation of the body part.
12. What is subluxation of the shoulder joint, and how can it be prevented or treated?
13. How does the COTA play a role in the treatment of the patient who has had a CVA?

ANSWERS

1. cerebralvascular accident
2. The words *cerebral vascular accident* describe the stroke, which is a sudden accident to the blood vessel (vasculum) in the brain (cerebrum).
3. lesion, hemorrhage, embolus, thrombus
4. the common carotid, internal carotid, vertebral, and basilar arteries.
5. left, hemiplegia, hemiparesis
6. right,   hemiplegia, hemiparesis
7. flaccidity, lack of muscle tone, spastic, involuntary abnormally high muscle tone
8. c f a d b e
9. confusion, loss of memory, loss of judgment
10. Following a stroke, the person may experience a loss of control over his or her emotional expressions (such as laughing instead of crying

when feeling sad), depression, frustration, anger, loss of confidence, and lowered self-esteem.
11. d.
12. Subluxation is an incomplete dislocation of a joint. Slings have traditionally been used to treat the condition. There are differing thoughts on the type of sling that is most effective.
13. The COTA assists in all areas of intervention, under the OTR's supervision and depending upon the OTR's practice model. The COTA can monitor the patient's involvement in activities of daily living such as basic self-care, in cognitive activities such as training, in organizational and management skills such as scheduling and handling daily self-care activities, and in the use of adaptive devices.

REFERENCES

Bobath, B. (1978). *Adult hemiplegia: Evaluation and treatment.* London: William Heinemann Medical Books Limited.

Botvinik, P. L. (1983). Letter to the editor. *American Journal of Occupational Therapy, 37*(6), 415.

Dox, I., Melloni, B. J., & Eisner, G. M. (1993). *Melloni's illustrated medical dictionary.* Baltimore: Williams and Wilkins Company.

Eggers, O. (1983). *Occupational therapy in the treatment of adult hemiplegia.* Oxford: Butterworth-Heinemann Ltd.

Pedretti, L. W., & Zoltan, B. (1990). *Occupational therapy: Practice skills for physical dysfunction* (3rd ed.). St. Louis: The C. V. Mosby Company.

Sine, R. D., Liss, S. E., Roush, R. E., Holcomb, J. D., & Wilson, G. B. (1988). *Basic rehabilitation techniques: A self-instruction guide.* Rockville, MD: Aspen Publishers, Inc.

Thomas, C. L. (Ed.). (1993). *Taber's cyclopedic medical dictionary* (17th ed.). Philadelphia: F. A. Davis Company.

SUGGESTED READINGS

Siev, E., Freishtat, B., & Zoltan, B. (1986). *Perceptual and cognitive dysfunction in the adult stroke patient: A manual for evaluation and treatment* (rev. ed.). Thorofare, NJ: Slack.

Titus, M. N., Gall, N. G., Yerxa, E. J., Roberson, T. A., & Mack, W. (1991). Correlation of perceptual performance and activities of daily living in stroke patients. *American Journal of Occupational Therapy, 45*(5), 410-418.

Trombly, C. A. (1992). Deficits in reaching in subjects with left hemiparesis: A pilot study. *American Journal of Occupational Therapy, 46*(10), 887-897.

OCCUPATIONAL THERAPY
IN ADULT HEMIPLEGIA:
NEURODEVELOPMENTAL APPROACH

Neurodevelopmental treatment (NDT) is used by NDT-certified occupational therapists (OTRs) to treat patients of all ages. This chapter provides an orientation to NDT for adult patients with hemiplegia and discusses the certified occupational therapy assistant's (COTA's) role in NDT.

LEARNING OBJECTIVES

After reading this section, you should be able to:

1. Name the originators of NDT.
2. State the basic aims of NDT for the adult with hemiplegia.
3. Explain why the adult with hemiplegia is taught to use both extremities to perform self-care activities during the early stages of treatment.
4. Explain the importance of bilateral activities for the adult with hemiplegia.
5. Describe how the adult with hemiplegia with involvement of the upper extremity can engage in bilateral activities.
6. Explain the benefit to the adult with hemiplegia of bearing weight on the affected upper extremity while using the unaffected upper extremity.
7. Explain why the adult with hemiplegia whose shoulder movements and upper extremity function are returning is encouraged to continue with bilateral activities during treatment.
8. List at least five ways that the COTA can assist the NDT-certified OTR during treatment.
9. State at least three precautions that the COTA should observe when assisting the NDT-certified OTR.

ORIGIN OF NEURODEVELOPMENTAL TREATMENT

Dr. Karel Bobath, a neurologist, and his wife, Berta Bobath, a physiotherapist (the British term for physical therapist), both deceased and formerly of the Bobath Centre, London, England, developed the philosophy and guiding principles of NDT. The Bobaths viewed their approach as that of managing the patient, with an eye toward helping him or her lead a better life. They believed that such management involved helping the patient function in daily activities. In any individual, motor functioning is closely related to sensory, perceptual, and personality factors (Bohman, 1986).

Special postgraduate courses to certify therapists in NDT for adults have been given in the United States to physical therapists, occupational therapists, and speech therapists since the late 1960s. Courses for COTAs were started in the late 1980s. A certificate is granted by the NeuroDevelopmental Treatment Association upon successful completion of required course work and upon meeting specific criteria set by the association.

BASIC PRINCIPLES OF NDT

Lesions in the brain following a cerebral vascular accident (CVA) can result in motor, sensory, cognitive, emotional, and perceptual problems. Neurological involvement leads to abnormal postural tone, usually seen as flaccidity or spasticity when movement is attempted. The abnormal tone prevents normal, coordinated movements.

The involvement of one side of the body leads to changed perceptions and use of the body. The normally symmetrical body becomes asymmetrical. The asymmetry and the loss of normal movements lead to faulty perceptions of the body and the environment.

Without proper treatment, a patient will perform abnormal movements and assume abnormal postures with varying degrees of spasticity. If the patient continues to use these movements and postures, normal movements and normal postural tone become increasingly difficult to attain.

The basic aim of NDT is to change the abnormal patterns of movement (Bobath, 1978). The treatment aims to 1) facilitate movement on the hemiplegic side, 2) help the patient regain symmetry of the body, and 3) help the patient regain normal movements. Treatment procedures inhibit abnormal postures and spasticity, creating the possibility of feeling normal muscle tone, normal posture, and normal sensorimotor experiences. Active participation in bilateral movements allows the patient to feel symmetrical again. Proper positioning allows the patient to feel normal muscle tone and postures (Eggers, 1983).

The patient is taught to avoid using only the unaffected side to compensate for the affected side in performing movements. Using only one side of the body reinforces asymmetry and results in faulty perceptions.

OCCUPATIONAL THERAPY ASSESSMENT FOR NEURODEVELOPMENTAL TREATMENT

The goal of assessment is to determine the functional ability of the patient in order to plan a treatment and management program. Since the aim of occupational therapy is to aid the patient in the performance of activities of daily living, information is needed about the patient's cognitive level, gross-motor and fine-motor function, sensation, and perception. Information about the patient's living quarters, work situation, and social life contribute to planning treatment (Eggers, 1983).

Testing should correspond with the aims of occupational therapy. Practical information, such as whether the person can hold a fork and make necessary movements for independent feeding, is best obtained from functional motion tests, rather than from tests of individual muscle strength. Movements—especially their quality and how they are made—are of utmost importance in planning treatment.

GROSS-MOTOR FUNCTION

The following gross-motor functions are evaluated prior to planning occupational therapy (for a valid assessment, any spasticity of the upper extremity should be inhibited prior to assessing functional ability):

1. The ability to roll over, move, and sit up in bed.
2. The ability to get into a sitting position and maintain balance while in that position.
3. The ability to stand and maintain balance in the standing position.
4. The ability to move from one location to another.
5. The general functioning of the affected upper extremity.
6. The ability of the affected upper extremity to bear body weight.
7. The ability of the affected hand to touch various parts of the body, e.g., both knees, the opposite elbow, the top of the head, the mouth, and the back of the neck. These movements are needed for personal hygiene and dressing.
8. The ability of the affected hand to grasp and release objects of various shapes and sizes.
9. The ability to perform various coordination activities with both hands.

FINE-MOTOR FUNCTION

The following fine-motor functions are assessed when the patient is minimally affected or has made sufficient recovery after having been moderately or severely affected:

1. *Finger dexterity.* Test the patient's ability to handle and use coins, cards, keys, pens, and similar objects. The ability to pick up small objects, such as pins and matches, and the ability to control the grasp and release of objects are examples of finger dexterity.
2. *Speed of movement and functions.* Test the patient's ability to make rapid, successive alternating movements (diadochokinesia) with the fingers, hands, and wrist. Examples of daily living activities requiring such movements are pouring liquid from a bottle and turning a doorknob or key, as well as many movements used in dressing, eating, and other routine activities.
3. *Automatic reactions.* Test movements needed for automatic reactions, such as catching an orange that is about to roll off the table.
4. *Coordination.* Test the patient's ability to use both hands in a coordinated manner during two-handed activities.

SENSATION

Sensation should be assessed before the treatment program is planned and at intervals during the program. The following sensations are tested:

1. *Superficial (exteroceptive) sensation.* This is sensation felt by receptors in the skin and includes touch, pressure, heat, cold, and pain. To test this sensation, stimuli are applied to the surface of the body. Pressure with the finger, a light touch with a cotton ball, and sharp and dull stimuli using a safety pin are possible tests to measure the patient's superficial sensation. The patient's sensation of heat and cold can be tested by filling four small glass containers with water heated to specified temperatures. Pinching different areas of the body may be a way of testing for sensation of pain.
2. *Deep (proprioceptive) sensation.* This is the sensing of positions and movements of the body by receptors located in the muscles, joints, tendons, and periosteum. Changes of movement and position are tested in the shoulder, elbow, wrist, and fingers. Without visual aid, the patient describes the movements and positions felt as the therapist moves the upper extremities.
3. *Stereognosis.* Objects familiar to the patient and that the patient can manipulate, such as scissors, a coin, a key, and a pen, are successively placed in the hand to be tested. Without visual aid, the patient tries to identify the object by tactile perception.

4. *Perception of form.* Geometric shapes are included in the stereognosis test.
5. *Weight differentiation.* Identical containers with different weights are used to test the patient's ability to differentiate between heavy and light objects.

When sensation tests require eliminating visual aids, do not use blindfolds on the patient or have the patient close both eyes, as the patient may become insecure and perform inadequately, and the patient-therapist relationship may suffer. For some testing, a plain cardboard can be held over the patient's hands. To test for stereognosis, a miniature bench with a curtain covering the open ends can be placed on the table. The patient's hand is positioned under the bench, and the therapist can place objects in the hand while the curtain obstructs the patient's view.

PERCEPTION

Assessing perception includes assessing the patient's memory, ability to perceive spatial relationships, ability to concentrate, and praxis, that is, the ability to plan and execute movement.

ADDITIONAL ASSESSMENT

The following information is essential for planning occupational therapy intervention:

Vision and hearing. What visual problems are present? How severe is any hemianopsia, or double vision? Do any auditory problems exist? Is it possible to train the individual cognitively to compensate for any loss, so that safety and independence are maintained? How will any loss that cannot be compensated for affect all other aspects of daily living?

Interests and motivation. What interests did the individual have? What was his or her previous motivational level? Was the individual active or sedentary? What perception do people who know the patient have about the patient's personality and needs?

Home and environment. What are the physical aspects of the patient's home and immediate environment? What architectural barriers exist that should be modified if the patient needs to use a cane, crutches, walker, or wheelchair upon discharge? Are others living in the home? What is the patient's relationship to them?

Work. Is the patient expected to return to the previous work situation? Can the former duties be carried out? Can the homemaker carry out responsibilities independently? Will adaptive devices aid the patient's independence in homemaking responsibilities? Will orthotics or special work techniques help the individual return to the job? Will the patient need retraining?

The above and related questions need to be answered as early as possible in order to plan for discharge. The OTR can evaluate the home and work situation and help the individual and his or her family make realistic plans. The OTR can evaluate the need for adaptive devices and techniques, help to develop them, and train the patient and family in their use should a need for them be indicated. Such devices and techniques may make the difference between dependence and independence.

Deficits and abilities in motor, sensation, and perceptual functioning are reassessed as the patient progresses. In the NDT approach, the OTR must reassess and modify the treatment during each session. For this reason, the treatment should be carried out by an individual who understands its principles and has had supervised experience using the NDT approach.

TREATMENT

The OTR who uses the NDT approach does not try to teach the patient how to compensate for the results of hemiplegia by using only the uninvolved side. The basic aim of early treatment is to help the patient facilitate movement on the hemiplegic side, regain symmetry of the body, and regain normal movements. Thus, the aim of treatment is to inhibit abnormal postures, abnormal movements, and abnormal tone.

The patient is an active participant in the treatment. The OTR serves as motivator, facilitator, and teacher. The patient is taught how to handle the affected extremity and use bilateral movements for self-care and other functional activities. These activities, properly guided by the OTR, give the patient an opportunity to feel normal postures, normal movements, and normal tone.

During the initial stages of treatment, the OTR guides the movements of the patient to prevent abnormal patterns of movement. The OTR helps the patient to assume specific positions that will inhibit spasticity and abnormal movements and facilitate normal movements. When the patient demonstrates the ability to control basic postures and movements within those positions, additional movements and postures are gradually introduced.

Recovery of upper extremity function in the adult with hemiplegia usually progresses from proximal to distal and from gross movements to fine movements. Eggers (1983) organized the recovery process into four stages and developed treatment goals according to each stage. Her text contains clear illustrations of treatment activities, with explanations and precautions.

Davies (1985) emphasizes the individual differences in patients. She cautions that no prescription suits every patient. Treatment of the adult with hemiplegia should include a sequence of activities tailored to the individual to prepare him or her for actual functioning in daily living.

TREATMENT GOALS DURING STAGES OF RECOVERY

The following summary of Eggers's (1983) stages of upper extremity dysfunction and treatment goals will serve to orient the COTA to the course of recovery from hemiplegia. Keep in mind that it is a partial description of a complex and comprehensive condition.

During the first stage of recovery, the patient will have little or no function in the involved upper extremity. Occupational therapy will be concerned with proper postural movements during transfers, with adapting the wheelchair to fit for proper positioning of the upper extremity, and with engaging the patient in bilateral activities.

Movement of the affected extremity is needed to facilitate the return of function. Initially, the OTR will be moving the affected extremity and teaching the patient how to move it together with the unaffected extremity. To avoid abnormal tone and abnormal movements, the patient's body, including the hands and fingers, must be properly positioned.

Under supervision, the COTA may engage the patient in tabletop activities. An activity such as pushing a block or ball back and forth involves flexion and extension of the upper extremity joints. The patient can be helped to perform such activities with clasped hands, with the involved thumb on top and the forearms and hands midway between supination and pronation.

The hands can also be positioned with the affected palm flat on the table and the unaffected hand over the dorsum of the affected hand, with the fingers of the unaffected hand abducting the fingers of the involved hand. Abducting the fingers helps to inhibit spasticity. Movements should be slow and carefully supervised by the OTR. Sudden, quick movements should be avoided, as these may elicit increased muscle tone.

In Stage 2, the patient has slight shoulder movement, and arm function is possible, but no hand function is present. In this stage, individuals have a tendency to use the unaffected body part exclusively. To avoid overuse of the unaffected extremity, bilateral activities are continued. With some movement available proximally in the involved extremity, therapy may include unilateral activities.

Activities performed on the floor with the patient seated in a chair are suggested. An example is to have the patient bend forward and use the affected extremity to move a ball forward toward a target. Table activities that involve a transfer of weight in the extremities are encouraged. These activities not only facilitate movement of the affected extremity, but also facilitate balance while sitting, symmetry, and attention to the affected side.

In Stage 3, the patient is able to lift the arm above the horizontal level, and gross grasp is possible. Treatment includes facilitating the grasp by having the patient pick up a variety of objects placed in front of and to the side of the body opposite the affected arm and moving and releasing the objects.

In Stage 4, the patient has arm function, grasp, and release, but lacks fine-motor coordination, dexterity, and rapid movements. Treatment aims are to develop fine-motor coordination, thumb opposition, diadochokinesis, and automatic reactions.

Examples of activities used in treating hemiplegia include playing games (e.g., board games involving small objects and card games), imitating upper extremity movements, performing work activities (e.g., assembling nuts and bolts and using tools such as a screwdriver), performing home care activities (e.g., polishing silverware and washing dishes), and doing other daily tasks involving forearm supination and pronation, as well as the prehension patterns.

THE ASSISTANT'S ROLE IN NDT

Neurodevelopmental treatment theory and practice are not normally included in the curriculum of the student who aspires to be a COTA. Nor does the entry-level role of the COTA, as currently defined, include competency in NDT evaluation and treatment. Nonetheless, because NDT approaches are often used by OTRs and experienced COTAs in the treatment of adult patients with hemiplegia, it is worthwhile to present them in this chapter. There have also been studies on task-oriented approaches that challenge treatment based on traditional developmental theories (e.g., Mathiowetz & Haugen, 1994; Umphred, 1995). These approaches are an attempt to search for the best possible treatment of central nervous system dysfunction.

During the initial stage following a cerebral vascular accident, the COTA may or may not be involved in the patient's treatment, depending on the COTA's education and experience. During the latter stages of treatment, the COTA may assist the OTR in various aspects of therapy. Both the COTA and the OTR need to assume responsibilities for their roles. The COTA should seek guidance and information; the OTR should assume a supervisory role and assign responsibilities within the COTA's capabilities.

Upon completion of special courses on NDT for COTAs, or with experience working with an NDT-certified OTR, the COTA may be responsible for assisting the OTR in the following ways:

1. Preparing the treatment area.
2. Assisting in teaching and monitoring self-care skills.
3. Teaching the patient to participate in games and activities.
4. Teaching the patient to perform specific fine-motor activities as di-

rected, monitoring the activities in order to correct errors, and providing verbal reinforcement to help the patient maintain interest and motivation.

5. Designing or assisting with the design and construction of equipment and activities used for treatment.

6. Maintaining data during treatment or during any activity, as requested by the OTR.

PRECAUTIONS DURING THERAPY

The following precautions are suggested for the COTA when assisting the OTR using the NDT approach:

1. The COTA should receive close supervision from the OTR, since the COTA does not conduct NDT independently.

2. Specific parts of the treatment program for one patient should not be taken out of context and tried with another patient.

3. Observation and monitoring should be done continuously to prevent abnormal postural tone and abnormal movements.

4. Directions should be carried out explicitly when participating in an activity with a patient.

5. Improper sequences of movements must be avoided, since unwanted associated reactions can result.

6. The COTA should remain alert to asymmetry and abnormal postures in the patient and help the patient avoid these.

7. The COTA should report to the OTR any evidence that the patient is in pain.

SUMMARY

The neurodevelopmental treatment (NDT) of adult patients with hemiplegia, developed by Dr. Karel Bobath and Mrs. Berta Bobath, emphasizes active participation by the patient and the attainment of the functional skills needed for daily living. The basic aims are to regain normal movement and symmetry, to avoid abnormal postures, abnormal tone, and abnormal movement, and to help the individual manage to live a productive, satisfying life.

REVIEW QUESTIONS

In Questions 1-6, circle the letter preceding the most appropriate ending to the given expression:

1. Neurodevelopmental treatment evolved out of knowledge, careful observations of treatment results, and the dedication of:

    a. Karel Bobath.
    b. Carol Slezak.
    c. Ortrud Eggers.
    d. Patricia Davies.
    e. Karel and Berta Bobath.

2. The basic aim of neurodevelopmental treatment for adult hemiplegia is to:
    a. Increase tactile and proprioceptive stimulation to the extremities in order to regain sensations.
    b. Teach the patient to become independent by using the unaffected side.
    c. Regain movement through a set pattern of rolling, crawling, and then walking.
    d. Teach the patient how to function by having the patient repeat movements used in each developmental stage.
    e. Regain symmetry, normal postural tone, and normal movements.

3. The adult with hemiplegia in which the upper extremity is affected is taught to perform as many self-care activities as possible with both extremities because:
    a. Cognitive attention is given to the affected extremity.
    b. Movement on the affected side is facilitated by the active movements of the unaffected side.
    c. Sensory stimulation is provided to the affected extremity.
    d. Functional movements are encouraged.
    e. All of the above.

4. The patient with hemiplegia who is seated and who uses both hands to grasp objects placed near his or her affected side and carry them across to the unaffected side is probably increasing:
    a. Trunk rotation.
    b. Visual motor perception.
    c. Sitting balance.
    d. Body symmetry.
    e. All of the above.

5. Suppose an adult with hemiplegia in which the upper extremity is affected plays checkers while standing at a table, bearing weight on the affected upper extremity and playing with the unaffected extremity. This adult receives the benefits of:
    a. Maintaining equilibrium reactions.
    b. Social and psychological stimulation.
    c. Visual-perceptual and cognitive stimulation.
    d. Inhibiting spasticity of the involved extremity.
    e. All of the above.

6. The adult with hemiplegia frequently wants to perform activities as independently as possible and as soon as possible by ignoring the

hemiplegic side and using only one hand. This is discouraged during the early stage of therapy because:
a. Asymmetry is emphasized.
b. Inattention to the hemiplegic side increases.
c. Abnormal tone is more likely to occur.
d. Abnormal postures and movements are predictable.
e. All of the above.
7. How can an adult with hemiplegia in which the upper extremity is affected position his or her hands to bilaterally perform 1) a self-care activity and 2) a leisure activity?
8. State five ways that an experienced COTA might assist the OTR who uses the NDT approach.
9. State three precautions to observe when assisting the OTR who uses the NDT approach.

ANSWERS

1. e
2. e
3. e
4. e
5 e
6 e
7. 1) Place the affected hand on a sponge or folded washcloth, and place the unaffected hand over the dorsum of the affected hand to wash as much of the body as possible.
2) Clasp the hands with the digits of the unaffected hand, abducting the digits of the affected hand with the thumb on top and the forearms midway between pronation and supination. Tabletop activities and games can be adapted using a ball, beanbag, or other objects, and activities such as painting with a large-handled brush, stencil painting, or block printing with a dowel handle attached to the block can be done with clasped hands.
8. 1) Prepare the treatment area and the patient to begin treatment.
2) Supervise a patient in self-care activities, and cue the patient to perform proper body position and movements, as directed by the OTR.
3) Report any observed asymmetry and abnormal tone during the patient's tabletop activities.
4) Teach the patient the rules and procedures of games and crafts he or she will engage in during treatment.
5) Collect data during treatment, as requested by the OTR.
9. 1) When in doubt, clarify instructions with the OTR.
2) Do not encourage the patient to exert excessive effort (that is likely to increase tone) to complete an activity.

3) Do not encourage the patient to work on tasks with only the unaffected body parts when the patient states that he or she can do the task more easily with one extremity than by using both extremities. When only unaffected body parts are used, asymmetry will result.

REFERENCES

Bobath, B. (1978). *Adult hemiplegia: Evaluation and treatment* (2nd ed.). London: William Heinemann Medical Books Ltd.

Bohman, I. (1986). The philosophy and evolution of the neurodevelopmental treatment (Bobath approach). *NeuroDevelopmental Treatment Association Newsletter,* May, 1-3.

Davies, P. M. (1985). *Steps to follow: A guide to the treatment of adult hemiplegia.* Berlin: Springer-Verlag.

Eggers, O. (1983). *Occupational therapy in the treatment of adult hemiplegia.* Rockville, MD: Aspen Publishers, Inc.

Mathiowetz, V., & Haugen, J. B. (1994). Motor behavior research: Implications for therapeutic approaches to central nervous system dysfunction. *American Journal of Occupational Therapy, 48*(8), 733-743.

Umphred, D. A. (Ed.). (1995). *Neurological rehabilitation.* St. Louis: The C. V. Mosby Company.

OCCUPATIONAL THERAPY FOR ARTHRITIS

The patient who has arthritis is seen in hospitals, long-term care facilities, rehabilitation centers and school systems. The physical and psychosocial effects that can occur are presented.

LEARNING OBJECTIVES

At the end of this chapter, you should be able to:

1. Correctly spell words that describe common arthritic conditions.
2. State the approximate age of onset of arthritis.
3. Describe physical symptoms of arthritis.
4. State potential psychosocial effects of arthritis.
5. Explain why arthritis is considered a chronic condition.
6. Relate the word *remission* to arthritis.
7. State general medical goals in treating arthritis.
8. State general occupational therapy goals in treating arthritis.

The word *arthritis* combines the Greek-derived prefix *arthro,* meaning "pertaining to the joints," with the Greek-derived suffix *itis,* meaning "inflammation of" (Thomas, 1993). The word is used in reference to more than 100 different disorders of the joints and connective tissues. Some of the conditions classified as arthritis cause pain in the joint, but do not actually involve inflammation.

Rheumatism is a word that is used in reference to acute and chronic conditions involving inflammation, stiffness of muscles, and pain in joints. The term includes arthritic conditions. *Rheumatism* is used in Great Britain as the general word encompassing the conditions that in the United States are referred to by the word *arthritis* (Arthritis Foundation, 1978).

Rheumatologists are medical doctors and researchers who specialize in the study of diseases of the joints and supporting structures and inflammatory diseases of the blood vessels. *Rheumatology* is the division of medicine devoted to the study of rheumatic diseases (Thomas, 1993).

INCIDENCE

The National Institutes of Health's National Institute of Arthritis and Musculoskeletal and Skin Diseases (NIH/NIAMSD) stated that 37 million Americans have one or more of the rheumatic diseases. An additional 25 million Americans have osteoporosis. An estimated 16 million persons have osteoarthritis, a degenerative joint disease that is the most common of all the rheumatic diseases. By age 65, an estimated 75% of the population shows X-ray evidence of osteoarthritis in at least one of the commonly affected joints (NIH/NIAMSD, 1993). Arthritis affects more individuals who are 65 years of age and older than any other chronic condition and is the number-one cause of disability in older people. Arthritis was reported by 533.3 of 1 thousand persons between the ages of 65 and 74 years and by 583.2 of 1 thousand persons who were 75 years of age and older (U.S. Bureau of the Census, 1995). The NIH/NIAMSD (1986) and the Harrington Arthritis Research Center (n.d.) estimate that more than 2 million persons are afflicted by rheumatoid arthritis. Other major forms of arthritis are gout, which afflicts 1 million persons, systemic lupus erythematosus, with an estimated 500,000 persons affected, ankylosing spondylitis, and juvenile rheumatoid arthritis, which affects 250,000 children. One in seven persons in the United States is reported to have arthritis, with an estimated 1 million new cases diagnosed each year.

ETIOLOGY

The cause of arthritis in its many forms is unknown. It is hypothesized that organisms, not yet specifically identified, invade the body, lie dormant, and periodically attack the particular joint structure or other parts of the body. Because the onset is usually reported as mildly painful with minimal inflammation and is short lived, the individual rarely seeks medical diagnosis or intervention. The condition frequently occurs during a period of emotional and physical stress and may be minimized by the person affected. Recurring symptoms often occur during psychological stress and lead researchers to consider stress as a possible cause of arthritis.

Heredity is believed to be a significant factor in arthritis. The focus of current research is on genetics, the immune system, and the application of molecular biology techniques to gain a greater understanding of risk factors for developing rheumatic and musculoskeletal diseases and disorders. The research effort is aimed at developing specific preventative measures and treatments for these conditions (NIH/NIAMSD, 1993).

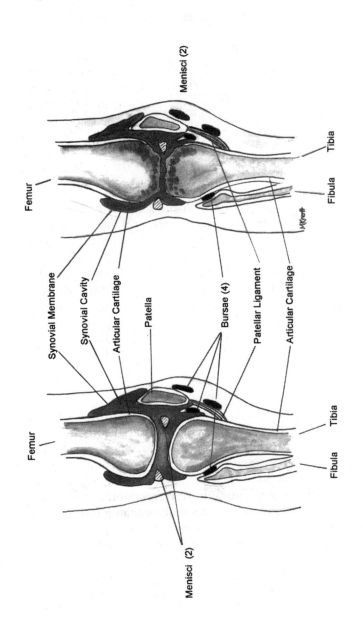

FIGURE 24.1.

COMPARISON OF A NORMAL JOINT AND AN ARTHRITIC JOINT

(illustration by Monica Knott)

ANATOMY

A joint is the location in the body where two bones meet. In normal joints, cartilage, a cushioning material, covers the juncture ends of the two bones. Cartilage enables bones to slide smoothly against each other. The entire joint is enclosed in a capsule that is lined by a membrane called the *synovium*. The synovium releases drops of *synovial fluid* into the spaces between the bones to nourish the cartilage and lubricate the joint. The synovial fluid makes movement smooth and easy. Muscles, tendons, and ligaments provide support to the bones and help the bones to move in the correct position. A *tendon* is a fibrous connective tissue that attaches muscles to bones and other parts. A *ligament* is a band or sheet of fibrous connective tissue that connects the articular ends of bones and binds them together to facilitate or limit motion. A *bursa* is a padlike sac in connecting tissue, usually located around joints, that is lined with synovial membrane and filled with synovial fluid. Bursa act to reduce friction between tendon and bone, between tendon and ligament, or between other structures where friction is likely to occur (Thomas, 1993).

The synovial membrane is the primary site of inflammation. The membrane lines joint capsules, tendon sheaths, and bursae throughout the body. The current theory is that when the synovial membrane becomes inflamed, an excess of synovial fluid is produced, and the drainage mechanism becomes inadequate, trapping the fluid within the capsule. The result is a fusiform-shaped swelling at the affected joint. If the inflammation is prolonged, the synovial cells proliferate and the membrane thickens.

GENERAL SYMPTOMS

Most inflammatory joint diseases involve the entire body. Every cell in the body is affected, even though the person's attention on the inflamed joint or joints suffices to ignore other systems of the body. The generalized effect on the body may include malaise, weakness, fatigue, depression, decreased libido, and anorexia. When systemic symptoms become acute, low-grade fever occurs and can be accompanied by myalgia, arthralgia, and stiffness.

The Arthritis Foundation (1978) gives the following general warning signs:

1. Pain and stiffness upon arising from sleep or after being in one position for a period of time.
2. Pain, tenderness, or swelling in one or more joints.
3. Swelling in one or more joints.
4. Recurrence of pain, stiffness, swelling in more than one joint.

5. Pain and stiffness, especially in the neck, elbows, lower back, knees, and other joints.
6. Tingling sensations in the fingertips, hands, and feet.
7. Unexplained weight loss, fever, weakness, or fatigue.

Medical attention is recommended when pain, stiffness, or swelling in the joints is experienced for 2 or more weeks. Early diagnosis and proper management of the symptoms may prevent deformities and debilitation (Morrow, 1995).

COMMON TYPES OF ARTHRITIS

Osteoarthritis, rheumatoid arthritis, ankylosing spondylitis, systemic lupus erythematosus, and gout are the most frequently encountered forms of arthritis. Details and current research on these and additional arthritic conditions can be found in medical journals and books on arthritis and rheumatology. Occupational therapy for the arthritis patient is discussed in texts such as Hansen &, Atchison, 1993; Melvin, 1989; and Pedretti & Zoltan, 1990.

Osteoarthritis

More individuals have osteoarthritis than any other type of arthritis. In the United States, the peak onset years are from 45 to 50 years of age, with 75% of people over 65 showing signs of the disease. A common prediction is that everyone who lives to an advanced age will develop osteoarthritis. Current estimates are that 16 million people in the nation have osteoarthritis with symptoms that cause problems, and another 30 million show signs of osteoarthritis, but do not report problems. Under age 45, twice as many women as men are affected; however, both sexes are equally affected in the 65-years-and-older age group (Eisenbeis, Sutton, Stabenow, & Banwell, 1986; NIH/NIAMSD, 1993).

Osteoarthritis is a chronic disease that results in damage to the cartilage and other tissue around a joint, causing pain and limitation of movement in the joint. Any joint can be affected, but some are more prone to attack. Weight-bearing joints—that is, the hips, knees, and spine—are most frequently affected. The distal and proximal joints of the fingers and the proximal joint of the thumb and big toe are frequently affected. Inflammation of the joint is not always present, even though the word *osteoarthritis* implies that some inflammation is present.

In osteoarthritis, degeneration of the cartilage in the joints occurs. The degeneration may result in cracks, frays, loss of elasticity, or complete wearing away of the cartilage. As the cartilage wears away, the bone ends start to thicken, and spurs may develop. The surrounding ligaments begin to thicken as well. The burden placed on the muscles surrounding the joint makes the muscles and joint react to the changing cartilage, ligaments, and bone by becoming tense, stiff, and painful.

The term *degenerative joint disease* is sometimes used synonymously with *osteoarthritis,* as are the terms *arthrosis* ("pertaining to the joints" + "condition"), *osteoarthrosis* ("having a relationship to a bone" + "pertaining to a joint" + "condition"), and *hypertrophic* ("excessive" + "concerned with nourishment") *arthritis.* The term *trophic* applies particularly to a type of efferent nerves believed to control the growth and nourishment of the parts they innervate (Thomas, 1993).

Less frequently affected by osteoarthritis are the proximal joints of the fingers and the joints of the wrists, elbows, shoulders, and ankles, unless these joints were subjected to previous disease, injury, or stress. For example, football players are more likely to have osteoarthritis of the knee, baseball players the elbow of the dominant upper extremity, and ballet dancers the ankles. Osteoarthritis resulting from "wear and tear" is referred to as *secondary osteoarthritis.* If no apparent cause can be determined, the osteoarthritis is referred to as *primary.*

Secondary osteoarthritis is believed to result from the stress and strain placed on joints as people perform their daily routine and thus is expected to occur later in life. However, if injury to a joint occurs, osteoarthritis can begin at any age.

A defective gene that weakens the cartilage is believed to be a predisposing factor in the occurrence of osteoarthritis. Another possibility is that a virus affects members in the same family. Other theories are that chemical abnormalities exist and that structural imperfections in the joints cause it to wear out sooner.

Pain is usually the first symptom reported in osteoarthritis. Because of pain, individuals engage in less physical activity and movement involving the affected joints. Less physical activity and reduced mobility result in weakness of the muscles surrounding the joint.

Rheumatoid arthritis

There are an estimated 2 million individuals with rheumatoid arthritis in the United States. This form of arthritis is considered the most serious because of its possible crippling results (NIH/NIAMSD, 1993).

Rheumatoid arthritis is a chronic disease and affects the joints, but can also affect the lungs, heart, blood vessels, spleen, eyes, muscles, and skin. In fact, the entire body can be affected. More severe pain is reported by individuals diagnosed with rheumatoid arthritis than by those with other types of arthritis.

Women are affected with rheumatoid arthritis three times as often as men. The age of onset peaks at about 30 to 40 years (Eisenbeis et al., 1986; Schumacher, 1988).

The onset of rheumatoid arthritis is gradual, with general malaise and slight tenderness usually beginning in the small joints of the fingers, wrist, and feet. Early symptoms are frequently minimized and attributed to the weather or to engaging in an activity that placed stress on the muscles and joints that are painful and stiff. The symptoms subside, and the individual feels reassured that they are of no major importance. The symptoms may reappear, usually more noticeably, with increased pain, swelling, weakness and fatigue, loss of appetite and weight, and perhaps even fever, but again disappear after a few days. Each time the symptoms recur, damage to the area remains, even though the individual does not see or feel the damage. The symptoms may disappear for months or years. One percent of individuals with rheumatoid arthritis may have complete remission—that is, their symptoms never recur. However, most will have recurrent symptoms after periods of remission.

In those who have them, the recurring symptoms can range from mild to severe. The course of the disease can vary greatly from one person to another. Since the entire body is vulnerable, the person with rheumatoid arthritis can develop fatigue and anemia and lose weight due to loss of appetite. The lymph glands and spleen can become enlarged. More joints and more parts of the body can become affected with each episode. One person in five with rheumatoid arthritis develops rheumatoid nodules, usually at the elbows. These nodules are small lumps under the skin.

Since the cause of rheumatoid arthritis is unknown, there is currently no known cure for the disease. Treatment is aimed at the symptoms. The goals of treatment are to relieve pain, reduce inflammation, keep the joints mobile and functional, and prevent damage and deformity to the joints. Psychotherapy may be included in the treatment, to relieve emotional stress. Surgery may be needed for joints that are severely damaged and deformed.

Children who develop juvenile rheumatoid arthritis usually do so before age 16. Females are affected three times as often as males. The peak age of onset of the condition for females is around 2 to 3 years of age. For males, there is a peak around 2 and another around 9 years of age. The onset in children can be sudden, with high fever, a rash resembling that found in measles, and very little involvement of the joints, or the symptoms can resemble adult rheumatoid arthritis.

Ankylosing spondylitis

Ankylosing spondylitis is also called *Marie-Strumpell disease.* The spine is affected with inflammatory arthritis. The cause is unknown, although there appears to be a hereditary predisposition to the disease. This form of arthritis affects males more often than females. Its onset is in the teens or early adulthood. The affected individual may complain of pain in the lower back and legs, as the small joints of the spine and the sacroiliac joints are usually affected first. The hips and shoulders may become involved as the disease progresses. If complications occur, they may include inflammation of the eyes. Loss of mobility of the spine may result due to fusion of the affected spinal joints. Curvature of the spine with a resultant stooped posture can ensue if preventative measures are not taken. The condition is difficult to diagnose in its early stages, and when it is finally diagnosed, permanent damage has usually occurred.

The disease may subside after a number of years, leaving stiffness, but minimal pain, so that affected individuals can lead relatively normal lives with early diagnosis, treatment, exercise, postural training, and orthopedic correction (NIH/NIASM, 1993).

Systemic lupus erythematosus

Systemic lupus erythematosus (*systemic*—"pertaining to the whole body"; *lupus*—"chronic, progressive, usually ulcerating, skin disease"; *erythema*—"redness over the skin") affects the connective tissues (Thomas, 1993). The condition is sometimes referred to as *SLE* or, simply, *lupus.*

As is implied in the name, systemic lupus erythematosus is a systemic, as opposed to localized, condition. The disease can inflame, change, or damage organs throughout the body. The kidneys, heart, lungs, blood vessels, nervous system, brain, and skin can be affected. Remission is common, but the condition is chronic. The remissions and recurrences of symptoms are unpredictable. Any combination of the following symptoms can appear: fatigue, loss of energy, loss of weight, fever, weakness, anemia, pain in the joints, rash, and kidney problems. A butterfly-shaped rash over the cheeks and nose is sometimes observed on individuals with systemic lupus erythematosus.

Those most frequently affected with lupus are women 15 to 35 years of age, although the disease can occur at any age. The cause is unknown. Treatment for the symptoms of systemic lupus erythematosus is individualized, since the condition affects each person differently (Arthritis Foundation, n.d.; NIH/NIAMSD, 1993).

Gout

An estimated 1.6 million individuals have gout. Men are affected more frequently than women, and symptoms usually begin in middle age. Women compose 5% of those with gout, with symptoms appearing after menopause. Gout is rare in children.

Gout is classified as a form of arthritis because inflammation of the joints is a common symptom. The joints and kidneys are affected by a buildup of excess uric acid in the tissues. Uric acid that is normally discharged from the body, mostly in the urine, either is excreted in inadequate amounts or is overproduced by the body. Salt crystals of uric acid form in the joints, causing inflammation and severe pain. The first joints

affected are usually the knee and foot, but the big toe is the most frequently affected joint. Usually, a single joint is the focal point during
each attack of gout, although any joint can be affected. Symptoms generally begin at night.

Gout is not considered hereditary, although the chemical defect in the
body is hereditary, and a familial tendency for the disease exists.

There is no known cure for gout. Proper diet, drugs to control painful
symptoms, and medication to increase the excretion of uric acid through
the kidneys and prevent overproduction of the uric acid can control the
disease enough to enable an individual to lead a normal life. Occupational therapy is usually not needed for gout (Arthritis Foundation, n.d.;
NIH/NIAMSD, 1993).

TREATMENT GOALS

Currently, there is no single treatment for any form of arthritis. Treatment is directed toward reducing the symptoms of the disease and over-
coming the limitations caused by stiffness and pain in specific joints. In
addition to taking medication to relieve pain and inflammation, patients
are educated about the disease and helped to have a positive attitude and
remain actively involved in their daily activities. Educational efforts include alerting patients to false promises of a cure. The Arthritis Foundation (n.d.) states that for every dollar spent in legitimate arthritis research,
25 dollars will be spent on quackery. Although there is no cure, specialists can help individuals cope with the condition and function maximally in their daily lives. Treatment usually includes a program of medication, rest, exercise, protection of the joints, and rehabilitation measures
to relieve pain, reduce inflammation, prevent damage and deformities in
the joints, and keep the joints mobile.

The goals of occupational therapy in treating the symptoms of arthritis depend on the chronicity of the condition and the patient's responsiveness to medication. The goal of early treatment is to preserve the
integrity of the musculoskeletal system during flare-ups of the disease
and to enable the patient to have optimal functioning during periods of
remission.

Melvin (1989) outlined the treatment for diseases of the joints during
their various phases. She states that, during the acute and subacute phases,
when the symptoms of pain and inflammation are first diagnosed as
being due to arthritis, and the patient experiences alternating periods of
remission and exacerbation of symptoms, basic treatment should focus
on reducing pain and inflammation, maintaining the range of motion
and integrity of the joints, maintaining strength and endurance of muscles,
providing emotional support to the individual, engaging the individual
in appropriate activities, and helping the affected person learn about the
disease and how to manage it.

Melvin states that patients are more active after they have had arthritis for a number of years (the chronic phase of the disease) than during the acute or subacute phase. In the chronic phase, the affected joints are stiff and synovitis is present, making the supporting joint structure vulnerable to deformity. The treatment is the same as described for the acute and subacute phases, but with a different emphasis, namely, on protecting the joints. Assistive equipment, exercise, and orthotics become important modalities during this phase, in order to maintain the integrity of the joints. In children, a series of casts to correct contractures may be needed.

Goals during the chronic phase of arthritis are to improve muscle strength, increase range of motion, manage stress, maintain the feet in proper condition (using orthotics if necessary), provide vocational counseling if work is a factor, and teach independent living skills.

Modalities and techniques of treatment include rest, muscle relaxation, the application of heat or ice, range-of-motion exercises, positioning, work simplification, energy conservation, and engagement in activities of daily living and appropriate leisure activities. The patient should be helped to express his or her feelings and be provided emotional support. Each technique and modality must be used judiciously and specifically for the individual patient. The exact application of the techniques is not within the scope of this text and can be found in other occupational therapy textbooks and courses.

THE ASSISTANT'S ROLE

Under the supervision of the occupational therapist, the certified occupational therapy assistant (COTA) may be given the responsibility of training patients in methods of protecting joints, energy conservation, work simplification, wearing and taking care of splints, and using a variety of assistive devices (Melvin, 1989; Pedretti & Zoltan, 1990; Sine, Liss, Roush, Holcomb, & Wilson, 1988). With such training, patients can manage their activities of daily living, work or productive activities, and leisure activities as independently as possible. The COTA may be a member of the treatment team (Eisenbeis et al., 1986) responsible for providing intervention from a patient's initial diagnosis to discharge from a health care facility. The COTA may continue to help the patient by evaluating the home environment and providing services to enable the patient to function maximally in daily living activities in his or her home.

SUMMARY

The etiology of the more than 100 common conditions listed under the encompassing term *arthritis* is yet unknown. Currently, there is no known method of prevention or cure for arthritis. Research continues on the condition said to be the number-one crippling disease in the United States. Treatment consists of managing symptoms with medication to reduce pain and inflammation, and rehabilitating patients to help them learn various strategies and techniques to function as independently as possible in carrying out their daily life tasks and activities. The goals of occupational therapy are to educate the individual about the condition, various energy conservation, work simplification, and joint-protection techniques, adaptive devices, and stress reduction activities in order to enable the patient to lead the most productive and desired life-style possible. The COTA plays a major role in this educational process.

REVIEW QUESTIONS

1. In the blank spaces, write the correctly spelled arthritis conditions that best complete the statement:

    An arthritic condition that affects the connective tissues is_____. The largest number of people with arthritis have_____. The arthritic condition considered most serious because of its potential crippling effects is_____._____is due to the buildup of excess uric acid in the tissues.

2. Circle the letter preceding the best answer that relates age to the given condition:

    1) Systemic lupus erythematosus primarily affects:
        a) women 15 to 35 years of age.
        b) middle-aged men.
        c) children from 5 to 16 years of age.
        d) men and women over age 60 years.

    2) Osteoarthritis is usually diagnosed by X ray in 97% of:
        a) women 30 to 40 years of age.
        b) middle-aged men.
        c) children from 5 to 16 years of age.
        d) men and women over age 60 years.

3. Circle the letter preceding the best answer that relates to symptoms of the given arthritic condition.

    1) *Arthritis* means:
        a) inflammation of a joint.
        b) swelling and pain.
        c) chronic limitation of movement.
        d) inflammation and deformity.

    2) Osteoarthritis usually affects:
        a) weight-bearing joints.
        b) connective tissues.

    c) the spine of adolescents and young adults.
    d) visceral organs and the brain.
  3) Systemic lupus erythematosus affects:
    a) weight-bearing joints.
    b) connective tissues.
    c) the spine of adolescents and young adults.
    d) visceral organs and the brain.
  4) Ankylosing spondylitis affects:
    a) weight-bearing joints.
    b) connective tissues.
    c) the spine of adolescents and young adults.
    d) visceral organs and the brain.
  5) In arthritis, the primary site of inflammation is:
    a) the bones of the joint.
    b) the joint capsule.
    c) the distal bones.
    d) the synovial membrane.
4. What are the potential psychosocial effects of arthritis?
5. Explain why arthritis is considered a chronic condition.
6. Relate the word *remission* to arthritis.
7. State the general goals of medical treatment for arthritic conditions.
8. State the general goals of occupational therapy for arthritic conditions.

ANSWERS

1. systemic lupus erythematosus, osteoarthritis, rheumatoid arthritis, Gout.
2. 1) a, 2) d.
3. 1) a, 2) a, 3) b, 4) c, 5) d.
4. reduced social activities because of pain, discomfort, and fatigue; depression; anorexia.
5. The arthritic condition generally remains in the person, and symptoms can return, usually when the individual experiences mental or physical stress.
6. *Remission* means that the symptoms subside and the individual may not feel any effects of the arthritic condition for a period of days, weeks, months, or years. After that period, the symptoms recur. Usually, the effects of each episode remain in the system. Remission of symptoms may be spontaneous, unpredictable, or complete.
7. Current medical treatment is to relieve the patient of symptoms of pain and swelling. In gout, medical treatment and diet together can control the condition.
8. The general goals of occupational therapy in treating arthritic conditions are 1) to educate the patient in order to reduce symptoms, overcome limitations, and prevent contractures; 2) to help the patient main-

tain mobility in the joints through active and passive exercises, and 3) to teach the patient joint-protection and work simplification techniques and the use of adaptive devices so as to conserve energy and function as independently as possible in daily life activities. Other goals of occupational therapy are to help the patient learn coping strategies, to engage the patient in stress reduction activities, and to provide psychological support when needed.

ADDITIONAL LEARNING ACTIVITIES

1 Inquire at local rehabilitation hospitals about support groups or swimming programs for people with arthritis, and request a visit to the hospitals. If a swimming group exists, it may welcome your volunteer assistance if you meet its requirements.
2. Request a visit with the activities director of a long-term care or rehabilitation facility to observe individuals with arthritis engaging in cooking or recreational activities.

REFERENCES

Arthritis Foundation. (1978). *Arthritis: The basic facts.* Atlanta: Author.

Arthritis Foundation. (n.d.). Various brochures: *About gout. Arthritis quackery and unproven remedies. Arthritis surgery information to consider. Systemic lupus erythematosus.* Atlanta: Author.

Eisenbeis, C. H., Sutton, J., Stabenow, C., & Banwell, B. F. (1986). *Arthritis: Multi-disciplinary team approaches.* Pittsburgh: American Rehabilitation Educational Network.

Hansen, R. A., & Atchison, B. (1993). *Conditions in occupational therapy: Effect on occupational performance.* Baltimore: Williams and Wilkins.

Harrington Arthritis Research Center. (n.d.). *The verdict—arthritis. The sentence?* Phoenix: Author.

Melvin, J. L. (1989). *Rheumatic disease in the adult and child: Occupational therapy and rehabilitation* (3rd ed.). Philadelphia: F. A. Davis Company.

Morrow, S. (1995). Arthritis 101. *Arthritis Today, 9*(3), 18-21, 24.

National Institute of Arthritis and Musculoskeletal and Skin Diseases. (1986). Arthritis Institute established. *Memo/National Arthritis and Musculoskeletal and Skin Diseases Information Clearinghouse.* Bethesda, MD: Author.

National Institutes of Health, National Institute of Arthritis and Musculoskeletal and Skin Diseases. (1993). *An overview of arthritis and related disorders.* Bethesda, MD: Office of Scientific and Health Communication.

National Institutes of Health, National Institute of Arthritis and Musculoskeletal and Skin Diseases. (1993). *1993 research highlights: Arthritis, rheumatic diseases, and related disorders.* Washington, DC: Department of Health and Human Services.

Pedretti, L. W., & Zoltan, B. (1990). *Occupational therapy: Practice skills in physical dysfunction.* St. Louis: The C. V. Mosby Company.

Schumacher, H. R. (Ed.). (1988). *Primer on the rheumatic diseases* (9th ed.). Atlanta: The Arthritis Foundation.

Sine, R. D., Liss, S. E., Roush, R. E., Holcomb, J. D., & Wilson, G. (Eds.). (1988). *Basic rehabilitation techniques.* (3rd ed.). Rockville, MD: Aspen Publications, Inc.

Thomas, C. L. (1993). (Ed.). *Taber's cyclopedic medical dictionary* (17th ed.). Philadelphia: F. A. Davis Company.

U.S. Bureau of the Census. (1995). *Statistical abstracts of the United States; 1995* (115th ed.) Washington, DC: Author.

SUGGESTED READINGS

Barnes, M. R., & Crutchfield. (1984). *The patient at home: A manual of exercise programs, self-help devices, and home care products* (2nd ed.). Thorofare, NJ: Slack, Inc.

Hansen, M., Ritter, G., Gutmann, M., & Christiansen, B. (1990). *Understanding stress: Strategies for a healthier mind and body.* Bethesda, MD: American Occupational Therapy Association, Inc.

Platt, J. V., Begun, R., & Murphy, E. D. (1992). *Daily activities after your total knee replacement.* Bethesda, MD: American Occupational Therapy Association, Inc.

Platt, J. V., Hahn, R., Kessler, S., & McCarthy, D. Q. (1990). *Daily activities after your hip surgery.* Bethesda, MD: American Occupational Therapy Association, Inc.

Rosenfeld, M. S. (1993). *Wellness and lifestyle renewal.* Bethesda, MD: American Occupational Therapy Association, Inc.

SUGGESTED LISTENING/VIEWING

Jaffer, A. (1989). *Arthritis: Self-help, exercise and joint protection.* La Jolla, CA: Medical Impact, Inc. (VHS, 55 minutes).

Marx, H., & Lumsden, R. M. (1988). *Arthritis: Best use of the hands.* Phoenix: Video Education Specialists. (VHS, 20 minutes).

25

PSYCHIATRY

This introduction to psychiatry includes a brief history of psychiatry in the United States and some indicators of mental health and mental illness. Classifications of selected mental disorders and treatment techniques, as they relate to adults, are briefly described.

LEARNING OBJECTIVES

At the end of this chapter, you should be able to:

1. Correctly spell and match each of the following words with its definition: *psychiatry, psychiatrist, psychotherapy.*
2. Correctly spell and match each of the following disorders with its definition or primary symptoms: *organic mental syndromes and disorders, psychoactive substance use disorders, schizophrenia, mood disorders, anxiety disorders, somatoform disorders, personality disorders.*
3. Correctly spell and match each of the following words with its use in occupational therapy: *affect, ambivalence, anxiety, apathy, blocking, delusion, depersonalization, depression, euphoria, flight of ideas, grandiose, hallucination, hypochondriasis, perception, phobia, psychotic.*
4. State at least four indicators of mental health.
5. State at least four indicators of mental disorder.
6. Name and briefly describe three psychiatric treatment procedures.
7. Name at least four settings in which mental disorders are treated.
8. State at least three goals of occupational therapy for patients with psychiatric diagnoses, and give an example of an activity that can be used with such patients.

Psychiatry is that branch of medicine which deals with the origin, diagnosis, prevention, and treatment of mental disorders. A *psychiatrist* is a medical doctor with additional years of study in psychiatry. A psychiatrist specializes in the treatment of individuals with mental disorders (Thomas, 1993). Mental disorders are manifestations of diseases that are primarily behavioral or psychological. Psychiatry was the last specialty to be included within the medical profession (Kaplan & Sadock, 1988). *Psychotherapy* is a method of treating disease—especially nervous disorders—by mental rather than physical means (Thomas, 1993).

INCIDENCE

One out of four Americans is estimated to have some form of mental or emotional disorder. More patients in hospitals receive treatment for mental disorders than for any other problem.

PREVALENCE

The passage of the Community Mental Health Centers Act of 1963, which advocated deinstitutionalization of patients and cessation of treatment provided in community mental health clinics, drastically reduced the numbers of patients in institutions (Kaplan & Sadock, 1988). The shift to community outpatient treatment became evident in statistics from the National Institute of Mental Health (NIMH). A 1967 study showed 367,000 resident patients in public hospitals for the mentally ill. By 1973, the number had dropped to 186,000. The total number of psychiatric inpatients in state, county, and private mental hospitals, general hospitals, Veterans' Administration hospitals, and other facilities was 405,500 in 1971 and fell to 230,200 in 1979. Concomitantly, patient care episodes in community mental health centers totaled 753,000 in 1971 and rose to 2,249,000 in 1979 (Kaplan & Sadock, 1988). The two trends are continuing in the 1990s, as state psychiatric institutions lower their populations and more psychiatric conditions are treated in the patient's community.

HISTORY

Throughout most of recorded history, fear and superstitious beliefs surrounded mental illness. Some people believed that the mentally ill were touched by God, some believed that the moon caused mental illness, and still others believed that the mentally ill were subhuman. Early treatment of the mentally ill included banishment from the city, resulting in death from starvation or being killed by wild animals. Using chains to restrain people whose behaviors were viewed as evidence of mental illness, confining such people in dungeons, or even killing them was common practice.

In 1792, Dr. Philippe Pinel, a psychiatrist in France, began a movement for the humane treatment of the mentally ill. Those who were confined were unchained. Citizens expected the worst, such as being hacked to death by "madmen." But this did not occur. Americans were encouraged by Pinel's successful treatment and began to have a change in attitude about mental illness.

In the early 1800s, Dr. Benjamin Rush, the most famous American physician of his time and a signer of the Declaration of Independence, published the first general book on psychiatry in America. He organized the first course in psychiatry in the United States, at the Pennsylvania Hospital in Philadelphia. He advocated activity, recreation, and exercise, as well as decent, clean living quarters in the hospital, for psychiatric patients. In the same decade, Amariah Brigham supervised patient activity programs and wrote about the influence of mental activity on health. In the mid-1900s, Adolph Meyer published his views on mental illness. Meyer saw the mentally ill patient as a biological and psychological unity who would benefit from community-based psychotherapy coupled with mentally integrated activity. Kaplan and Sadock (1988) present the fascinating history of psychiatry, from Hippocrates of Cos (ca. 450-355 B.C.) to 1980, outlining the major contributors to the field and their contributions.

World Wars I and II added to the public's knowledge of mental illness. Federal and state governments began funding programs for research, training, and services for the mentally ill. The National Mental Health Act of 1946 provided for the establishment of the NIMH, where researchers seek to find ways to prevent and treat mental illness (NIMH, 1972).

INDICATORS OF MENTAL HEALTH

Behavior that is normally accepted by society helps set guidelines for recognizing mental disorders and abnormal behavior. Mental health and normal behavior are dependent upon many factors. The timing of the behavior, the appropriateness of the behavior, its quality, and the way the behavior is perceived by others influence the determination of normal behavior. Following are some commonly accepted indicators of mental health (King, 1985):

1. The ability to tolerate the daily stresses of living without persistent physical or psychological symptoms.
2. The ability to judge reality accurately.
3. The ability to take a long-term, rather than short-term, view of things.
4. The ability to have sustained relationships.
5. The ability to love and receive love.
6. The ability to work with enjoyment and productivity.
7. The ability to live within a realistic code of ethics.
8. The ability to satisfy one's own personal needs without harming anyone else or anyone's valued possessions.

INDICATORS OF MENTAL DISORDERS

Frequently, the individual with a mental disorder seems unaware of the symptoms. Family members and friends may observe that the person is "different" or behaving "strangely." The following persistent behaviors or symptoms may suggest that an evaluation of an individual's mental or medical condition should be considered (National Association of Private Psychiatric Hospitals, 1979):

1. Extreme elation or depression. Extreme elation may be expressed by loud laughter and increased verbal and motor activity from a normally quiet, sedate person. Extreme depression may be a persistent decreased energy level or loss of interest in usual activities and may be so severe that the person does not talk, move, or attend to his or her own care (*disturbed affect*).
2. A change in cognitive ability, such as being unable to recall or utilize previously stored, commonly used information.
3. A sudden or gradual disturbance in orientation as to time, place, and people. The person may even become confused in formerly familiar places and situations (*confusion*).
4. Memory loss—that is, the inability to recall past experiences (*amnesia*).
5. Difficulty verbalizing thoughts or ideas or difficulty taking them to their logical conclusions (*blocking*).
6. Hearing, seeing, smelling, or tasting things that do not exist in the person's vicinity (*hallucinations*).
7. Remaining awake for hours (*insomnia*) or sleeping more than usual for no apparent physical reason.
8. A drastic change in life-style. For example, a relatively casual, relaxed person may suddenly become compulsively neat and rigid.
9. A change in one's relationship to people. For instance, a shy, quiet person may become loud and aggressive, or a friendly person may avoid people.
10. A feeling of strangeness or detachment about one's body or body parts (*depersonalization*).
11. Believing that what is patently false is true (*delusion*) and an inability to accept logic or evidence showing that it is false.

CLASSIFICATIONS OF MENTAL DISORDERS

Classifications of mental disorders are not fixed or agreed upon by all professionals who work in psychiatry (Greben, Rakoff, & Voineskos, 1985; Kaplan & Sadock, 1988). In the United States, the American Psychiatric Association (APA) classification of mental disorders is generally used for clinical and research purposes. In 1994, the *Diagnostic and Statistical Manual of Mental Disorders, Fourth Edition* (*DSM-IV*ä) was adopted for use. *DSM-IV* is expected to be published in the 1990s to coincide with the 10th edition of the World Health Organization's *International Classification of Diseases* (APA, 1987).

The *DSM-IV*ä lists 18 major classifications of mental disorder and more than 200 specific disorders (APA, 1994). The next section summarizes some of the mental disorders that are most likely to be encountered from information from the *DSM-IV*ä and general texts on psychiatry. The current edition of the *DSM* and current journals and texts are most useful because reclassifications occur as a result of research findings and legislative changes in society. For example, some earlier categories of mental disorder reflect cultural biases. Also, terminology may change or be deleted from current official classifications, although the terms may still be used by clinicians (Kaplan and Sadock, 1988).

It is important to keep in mind that, to make a diagnosis of mental disorder requires specialized training which includes a body of knowledge and clinical skills. Occupational therapy practitioners do not have the specialized training to make such a diagnosis. The information that follows provides an introduction to some of the current major classifications of mental disorders.

SUBSTANCE-RELATED DISORDERS

A psychoactive substance is defined as a substance that can alter one's consciousness or state of mind when taken into the body. Such a substance may be legal, as, for example, alcohol and drugs prescribed by physicians, or illegal, as, for instance, heroin and cocaine. Psychoactive substances can result in either psychological dependence, which is a craving for the drug in order to avoid the expected generalized feeling of anxiety if one does not ingest the drug, or physical dependence, which is the need to take the substance to prevent withdrawal symptoms. In a given instance, dependence can be both psychological and physical. Drug abuse is the illegal use of a drug.

Psychoactive substance-related disorders concern the pattern of use of the substance and the resultant impairment. A pattern of pathological use involves behavior such as the inability to reduce the amount of or stop using the substance, intoxication throughout the day, using the substance nearly every day for at least a month, and periodically taking an overdose of the substance that results in impaired functioning. Impairment is often manifested in behaviors such as fights with family members and friends, the loss of job, and legal problems. Among the references that detail the effects of specific substances on the central nervous system are APA (1987) and Kaplan and Sadock (1988).

A diagnosis of psychoactive substance-related disorder is based on a pattern of pathological use, impairment in social or occupational functioning caused by the use of the substance, and a disturbance lasting at least 30 days. The prevalence of psychoactive substance-related disorders varies with the wide range of substances involved.

The symptoms of psychoactive substance-related disorders vary with the individual, the substance, and the length and amount of use. Euphoria, grandiosity, hallucinations, paranoid ideation, suspiciousness, ritualistic behavior, and changes in one's sleep pattern and motor activity may occur. Hospitalization is required for severe disorders. The treatment varies with the cause (Kaplan & Sadock, 1988).

SCHIZOPHRENIA

Patients with schizophrenia seem to have a biological vulnerability to the condition; however, psychosocial factors are considered to affect the development and course of the disorder. Every symptom seen in schizophrenia is seen in other psychiatric and neurologic disorders. An estimated 20 to 30% of individuals with schizophrenia are able to lead somewhat normal lives. About 50% remain significantly impaired. (APA, 1994; Kaplan & Sadock, 1988; Keith & Mosher, 1981).

Five types of schizophrenia are listed in the *DSM-IV*ä (APA, 1994):

1) *Disorganized type*. In the disorganized type of schizophrenia, previously called hebephrenia, the individual is frequently incoherent, the delusions are disorganized, contact with reality is poor, and the person displays a silly, inappropriate affect and may burst out laughing for no apparent reason. Motor activity is frequently aimless.

2) *Catatonic type*. The catatonic schizophrenic may have a reduction in motor activity or show rigidity, posturing, or purposeless motor excitability. There can be a rapid alteration from excited behavior to stupor. Supervision is recommended during both periods of excitement and periods of stupor to prevent the patient from injuring him- or herself or others. Mutism may occur.

3) *Paranoid type*. The paranoid schizophrenic may have delusions of being persecuted, delusions of grandeur, or delusional jealousy. Hallucinations may be of any of these delusional varieties. The typical patient with a diagnosis of paranoid schizophrenia usually functions adequately socially. His or her intellectual functioning will be maintained in areas not affected by delusions. There is less regression of mental functioning, emotional response, and behavior than in other types of schizophrenia. The patient's behavior is often tense, guarded, and reserved and may become hostile and aggressive.

4) *Undifferentiated type*. The person with undifferentiated schizophrenia has prominent delusions and hallucinations, is incoherent, or

behaves in a disorganized fashion, without fitting the criteria of other types of schizophrenics.

5) *Residual type.* In the residual type of schizophrenia, the individual has had at least one previous episode of schizophrenia with psychotic symptoms. The patient continues to show symptoms of the disorder.

Prevalence

Anywhere from 0.2% to 2.0% of the population of the United States is estimated to have schizophrenia. The onset for men is usually between age 15 and 25, and for women it is between 25 and 35. Studies show no difference in the prevalence of schizophrenia between males and females. The onset of schizophrenia before age 10 or after age 50 is rare. An estimated 50% of patients with schizophrenia have attempted suicide, and 10% are reported to have succeeded within a 20 year follow-up period. For reasons unknown, persons with schizophrenia have a high mortality rate from natural causes. An estimated 50% of all mental hospital beds

of the hospitalization stay has decreased, but the number of admissions has increased, and readmission within 2 years after the first hospitalization is estimated at 40 to 60% (Kaplan & Sadock, 1988).

In industrialized nations, schizophrenics are more frequently reported in the lower socioeconomic groups. This tendency may be due to the personality of the schizophrenic, which predisposes the individual toward fewer relationships. As the person's mental capabilities decline, he or she is placed in menial jobs or becomes unemployed, which may prevent the individual from moving out of the lower socioeconomic classes. (Kaplan & Sadock, 1988).

Etiology

The etiology of schizophrenia is unknown. It is likely that a variety of disorders with similar behavioral symptoms are diagnosed as schizophrenia. The diagnosis is made on the basis of the psychiatric history of the person and an examination of his or her mental status, since no laboratory test exists to confirm schizophrenia. Constitutional, biochemical, genetic, neurological, and psychosocial theories of the disorder are currently being examined (APA, 1994; Cohen, 1993; Kaplan & Sadock, 1988; Pardes, 1981).

Symptoms

In schizophrenia, there may be reduced or excessive emotional responsiveness. A reduction in affective expression may be shown by a monotonous voice and an expressionless face. Feelings of omnipotence may be expressed. Sudden outbursts of anger may be observed. Disorderly thought processes may be evidenced by a poverty of speech, blocking of thoughts, perseveration or increased speech, loose association of ideas, and incoherent speech. Thoughts may be characterized by delusions, which may be paranoid in nature. The delusions are often supported by perceptual distortions. Hallucinations may occur in any of the sensory modalities, but are usually auditory in the person with schizophrenia. Tactile hallucinations involving tingling or burning sensations may be expressed. The delusions and hallucinations are pervasive. Memory is usually intact, as is orientation to person, time, and place (APA, 1994; Kaplan & Sadock, 1988).

It is estimated that 20 to 30% of those patients diagnosed with schizophrenia can lead a fairly normal life. Patients who remain significantly impaired for their entire lives are estimated at 40 to 60% (APA, 1987; Kaplan & Sadock, 1988).

For patients who remain moderately or severely symptomatic, impairment in goal-directed activity is common. Ambivalence regarding various courses of action may result in diminished activity. Purposeful motor activity may decrease noticeably. Peculiar body movements such as rocking, pacing, or stereotyped gesturing may occur. There is a tendency to withdraw from the external environment. A preoccupation with thoughts of self and fantasies dominate the person's life. The individual's appearance may become disheveled or unclean and his or her behavior eccentric. The deterioration in the level of functioning may occur in areas of work, social relations, and self-care (Kaplan & Sadock, 1988).

MOOD DISORDERS

Normally, individuals have a wide range of moods and emotional expressions appropriate for any given situation. Persons with mood disorders show a disturbance of mood, lose control over their emotions, and express a feeling of distress. *Mood* refers to the individual's internal emotional state. *Affect* refers to the individual's expression of emotions. (Kaplan & Sadock, 1988).

When only major depressive episodes are evident, the individual is said to have major depressive disorders, or *unipolar depression.* The probability of developing unipolar depression is estimated at 20% in women and 10% in men. The mean age of onset is about 40 years, with a range of 20 years to 50 years. When both depressive episodes and mania are evident, the disorder is called *bipolar disorder.* The probability of developing bipolar disorder during one's lifetime is estimated at 1% in both men and women. The mean age of onset is about 30 years, although the range is from childhood to 50 years. *Hypomania, cyclothymia,* and *dysthymia* are additional categories of mood disorders (APA, 1994; Kaplan & Sadock, 1988).

The etiology of mood disorders is unknown. Biological rhythms and biochemical, genetic, and psychosocial factors have been studied, but the studies are inconclusive. Current theories hypothesize that bipolar disorder is the severe expression of unipolar depression, as well as s that mania and depression are two ends of a continuum of emotional expression (APA, 1994; Cohen, 1993; Corfman, 1979; Greben et al., 1985; Kaplan & Sadock, 1988; Rowe, 1984; Sargent & Swearingen, 1981; Yahraes, 1978).

Details of symptoms seen during mania and major depressive episodes can be found in special texts and journals on the subject. The following is an overview of the subject based on the APA's (1987) *DSM-III-R* and the writings of Kaplan & Sadock (1988):

A pathological manic condition is suspected in an individual when his or her response to an idea or situation is an exaggerated feeling of well-being and elation (euphoria) and yet is accompanied by hyperactivity and irritability. A pathological depressive condition is suspected when the individual's response to an idea or situation is abnormal sadness and is accompanied by somatic and psychological impairments.

Major affective disorders involve either a manic episode or a significant depressive episode. The mood during a manic episode is elevated, expansive, or irritable. There may be an unusual increase in activity, such as organizing and planning many activities, calling friends and acquaintances without regard to the time of day or night, ordering people to perform in certain ways to carry out unrealistic activities, or making large numbers of purchases without regard to their cost. Extreme feelings of mental and physical well-being and grandeur may be expressed, together with increased physical activity, increased and rapid speech during which the general train of thought can be diverted by chance stimuli from the environment (called *flight of ideas*), and a decreased need for sleep. The individual is usually unaware of his or her intrusive, demanding behavior.

During a major depressive state, the person is in a sad, despairing mood with a sense of hopelessness and uselessness. Guilt, shame, and anxiety may be expressed. Interest in oneself and the environment decreases. Family, friends, and hobbies are neglected. If the person continues to work, he or she does so with little enthusiasm for the job. Making a minor decision may take hours, and concentration is difficult.

Physical complaints may become prominent. Headaches, back and limb pain, and gastrointestinal complaints are expressed. Loss of appetite and weight may occur. Some patients eat for comfort and hence may gain abnormal amounts of weight during a depressive state.

Insomnia can become marked. If the person falls asleep, the sleep may be fragmented or short. Some patients, on the other hand, may sleep excessively. Complaints of fatigue and exhaustion are common.

The individual's posture may be slumped. Sighing and crying may occur sporadically. Motor activity may decrease noticeably and become so slow that the individual appears mute and immobile. By contrast, a depressed person can also show signs of restlessness, agitation, and inability to sit still.

ANXIETY DISORDERS

Anxiety is a normal reaction that is a way to alert the individual to possible danger. Nonetheless, even when anxiety is normal, the feeling is unpleasant. The individual feels helpless and vulnerable because of the inability to predict exactly what will occur, the difficulty of planning exact actions, and the physical reactions that accompany anxious feelings. Normal anxiety implies that the individual is cognitively and psychosocially alert and is able to perceive impending physical danger or senses the need to be mentally and physically alert in order to react to a potentially unpleasant social situation.

The *DSM-IV*ä gives complete information on anxiety disorders. Those which will be briefly described here are panic disorder, agoraphobia, social phobia, simple phobia, obsessive-compulsive disorder, posttraumatic stress disorder, and generalized anxiety disorder (APA, 1994).

A *phobia* is an intense fear of an object, activity, or situation. The individual consciously limits his or her activities in order to avoid the phobic reaction. *Agoraphobia* is a fear of being unable to escape a crowded situation. It is considered the most severe phobic disorder.

Social phobia is a persistent fear of situations in which the person may be closely observed and judged. There is a fear of humiliation and embarrassment. The individual realizes that the fear is unreasonable, but still tries to avoid such situations.

Simple phobia is an irrational fear of certain kinds of objects or situations. The objects feared may be spiders, animals, or other objects. The situations feared may be closed spaces (*claustrophobia*), heights (*acrophobia*), or other situations, such as storms, illness, injury, and death.

An *obsession* is a reoccurring thought, feeling, idea, or sensation that is intrusive. A *compulsion* is a reoccurring behavior that is consciously performed. Two examples of compulsions are to count and recount items and to check several times before leaving the house that the burners on the stove are turned off. The obsessive, compulsive, or obsessive-compulsive behavior is considered a disorder if it causes distress to the person or interferes with his or her daily routine, employment, or relationships with others.

Those who have experienced traumatic events that would normally be stressful for anyone may experience *posttraumatic stress disorder.* This disorder includes reexperiencing the traumatic event in dreams and in thoughts while awake, feeling numb to other life experiences, including relationships, and associated symptoms of autonomic instability, depression, and cognitive difficulties, such as the inability to concentrate.

Generalized anxiety disorder is a chronic disorder in which the individual is unrealistically worried about two or more life circumstances. The condition lasts longer than 6 months. Individuals with this disorder seem to be anxious about many things.

Two to three percent of the general population are estimated to have anxiety disorders. Hospitalization is rarely required if the phobia is unrelated to medical conditions or to severe psychopathological disorders. Treatment such as systematic desensitization is usually given on an outpatient basis (Kaplan & Sadock, 1988).

SOMATOFORM DISORDERS

Somatoform disorders include a group of disorders in which the symptoms presented suggest physical disorders, although there are no organic causes. The *DSM-IV* categorizes six types of somatoform disorders, as follows (APA, 1994; Kaplan & Sadock, 1988).

Somatization disorder is a common subtype of somatoform disorders. The individual has numerous physical complaints and may seek medical attention from one or more physicians. The physical complaints may include cardiopulmonary and gastrointestinal symptoms and visual and auditory problems, as well as pain in the extremities, back, and chest.

Conversion disorder is uncommon. The condition is diagnosed when physical malfunctioning, such as paralysis, suggests a physical disorder, but no physiological reason is found. Symptoms usually involve parts of the body that are under voluntary control and are apparently due to psychological needs or conflict.

Somatoform pain disorder is a condition in which there is severe and prolonged pain for which no physical reason can be found. The pain can be low back pain, a headache, atypical facial pain, and pelvic pain, as well as other kinds of pain.

Hypochondriasis is diagnosed when the individual shows excessive preoccupation with his or her health. The person makes faulty interpretations of physical signs or feelings and expresses a concern that he or she has a serious disease. The fear of the condition persists, despite medical examinations and evidence that no disease exists. The body parts of most frequent concern are the head and neck, the abdomen, the chest, and the back.

PERSONALITY DISORDERS

Personality traits are those unique, individual ways a person perceives himself or herself and the environment and relates to others and the environment. When personality traits become rigid and cause the person difficulty in adapting to personal, social, or work situations, a disorder exists (APA, 1994).

There are many subclassifications of personality disorders, but all can be placed into three clusters. The first cluster includes the paranoid, schizoid, and schizotypal personality disorders. Individuals with these disorders are perceived as odd and eccentric. The second cluster includes the histrionic, narcissistic, antisocial, and borderline personality disorders. These individuals are perceived as overly dramatic, emotional, and erratic. The third cluster includes persons perceived as anxious or fearful and who have dependent, obsessive-compulsive, or passive-aggressive personality disorders.

Disturbances in mood, depression, and anxiety are common complaints of those with personality disorders. Such individuals are not likely to seek psychiatric treatment. If treatment is suggested, they probably will refuse it, as they tend to deny their problems. The prevalence of personality disorders is unknown. Genetic factors are believed to contribute to their etiology, according to results from a study of 15 thousand pairs of American twins. Hospitalization is rare. (Kaplan & Sadock, 1988).

TREATMENT

The major models of psychiatric treatment are the psychotherapies, the behavior therapies, the somatic therapies, and social and environmental therapy. Rowe (1984) grouped psychiatric treatment into eight broad divisions: individual psychotherapy, group psychotherapy, family therapy, adjunctive or activity therapy, somatic therapy, pharmacotherapy, behavioral therapy, and humanistic therapy. Kaplan and Sadock (1988) classified psychiatric treatment into two major categories: the psychotherapies and the biological therapies. For these researchers, the psychotherapies include psychoanalysis and psychoanalytic psychotherapy, brief dynamic psychotherapy and crisis intervention, group psychotherapy and combined individual and group psychotherapy, psychodrama, family therapy and marital therapy, behavioral medicine and biofeedback, behavior therapy, hypnosis, and cognitive therapy. The biological therapies include psychopharmacology, that is, drugs used to treat psychosis, depression, bipolar disorder, anxiety, and insomnia; electroconvulsive therapy; and other organic therapies, such as psychosurgery, light therapy, acupuncture, and acupressure.

Following are introductory comments on some of the aforementioned psychiatric treatments. The references at the end of the chapter and current textbooks and journals on the subject give more detailed information on the various treatments used by psychiatrists.

Individual psychotherapy. The patient enters into an agreement with the psychotherapist to interact with him or her in a prescribed way, usually for an approximate, but predetermined, length of time.

Group therapy. The patient becomes a member of a group of patients receiving psychotherapy. The interactions among the group members are part of the therapy.

Combined individual and group psychotherapy. The patient is seen both individually and in a group setting by the therapist.

Family therapy. The patient receives group therapy in which the family constitutes the group.

Pharmacotherapy. The patient is treated with drugs that affect the central nervous system. Pharmacotherapy is used when it is felt that the psychiatric disorder involves defective functioning of the central nervous system. The specific drug or combination of drugs and their dosage are dependent upon many factors and must be prescribed by the patient's

Electroconvulsive therapy (ECT). ECT is considered by some psychiatrists to be one of the most effective treatments for major depression (Cohen, 1993; Kaplan & Sadock, 1988) and for certain conditions such as acute, catatonic, or affective symptoms of schizophrenia and mania.

Behavioral medicine and biofeedback. These therapies are used mostly in disorders considered to be within the area of self-control. Among such disorders are obesity and psychoactive substance use disorders.

Behavior therapy. Therapeutic techniques based upon principles of learning may be effective in treating certain mental disorders. Systematic desensitization was developed by Joseph Wolpe to treat anxiety disorders. Aversion therapy, behavior modification, and cognitive therapy may be effective behavior therapy techniques for specific patients.

Humanistic therapy. This kind of therapy is based on the principle that each individual is capable of achieving his or her potential. Each person is believed to be responsible for choosing his or her own treatment. The role of the therapist is to provide understanding and acceptance of the person's choices. Humanistic therapy includes client-centered therapy, existential analysis, and gestalt therapy.

Adjunctive therapy. In some settings, this term is used to denote therapy not directly carried out by psychiatrists or psychotherapists. This kind of therapy may include psychodrama, art, music, and occupational, recreational, and vocational therapy, as well as other forms of therapy.

TREATMENT SETTINGS

Psychiatric treatment is most frequently provided in psychiatrists' offices, community settings, mental health or psychiatric units of general hospitals, private psychiatric hospitals or rehabilitation centers, state psychiatric hospitals, military hospitals, or Department of Veterans' Affairs medical centers. Outpatient treatment, in which the patient receives treatment and returns to his or her place of residence the same day, usually occurs in the psychiatrist's office or a community setting; however, it can occur in any other setting where outpatient psychiatric treatment is available. The patient is usually treated on an outpatient basis when the condition is not considered a severe disorder and the patient does not pose a danger to him- or herself or others. Some disorders that might be treated on an outpatient basis are anxiety disorders, personality disorders, somatoform disorders, and some psychoactive substance use disorders. Other disorders, such as mood disorders, schizophrenia, and organic brain disorders, are often characterized by periods during which the disorder can be treated on an outpatient basis, in addition to periods that require hospitalization.

When the patient requires close supervision of treatment and a variety of treatments, he or she may need to be admitted as an inpatient. Admission may be to a private psychiatric hospital or rehabilitation center, a general hospital psychiatric unit, or a military or Department of Veteran's Affairs hospital, depending upon the individual's medical benefits and hospitalization insurance coverage. The initial admission as an inpatient may be short term. If the patient's condition is diagnosed as chronic, longer term hospitalization in a state institution or a Department of Veteran's Affairs hospital may be needed. Kaplan and Sadock (1988) report that most patients with chronic mental disorders now live in their community rather than in institutions; however, a clear picture of their progress is not available because of insufficient methodological follow-up studies.

Despite the passage of the 1963 Community Mental Health Centers Act, and the intent to provide psychiatric treatment in the community with an emphasis on prevention and maintaining the individual in the community, lack of funds and a dearth of qualified personnel curtailed the growth of the program. The community mental health programs were proposed as total programs, including emergency services, outpatient services, partial hospitalization, inpatient services, and consultation-education services. The service team was to include psychiatrists, child psychiatrists, clinical psychologists, psychiatric social workers, psychiatric nurses, administrative and clerical staff, and occupational and recreational therapists for inpatient and partial hospitalization programs. Continuity of care was to occur through the sharing of information with agencies in order to follow through with the needed programs for patients (Kaplan & Sadock, 1988).

THE ASSISTANT'S ROLE

Occupational therapy is frequently prescribed for psychiatric patients. The particular setting and the specific skills of the occupational therapy staff often determine the emphasis of the programs. The occupational therapist (OTR) is assisted by the certified occupational therapy assistant (COTA) in evaluating the patient's performance and in planning an intervention program based on the patient's goals. The COTA, with supervision from the OTR, conducts individualized or group intervention programs to help the patient maximize his or her daily living skills. The general goal of occupational therapy is to motivate the patient to function to the best of his or her ability in the occupational performance areas of daily living, work, and leisure activities. To help the patient achieve occupational therapy goals, the COTA engages the patient in sensorimotor, cognitive, and psychosocial activities to improve self-care, communication, socialization, and work-related skills. Some examples of goals are helping an employable woman dress appropriately for a particular work setting, helping a student learn verbal and nonverbal communication skills to improve his or her participation in a group, and helping a young adult to follow procedures outlined as appropriate for a work setting or a game.

To achieve the particular occupational therapy goal, the COTA engages the patient in specific occupations such as creative arts, crafts, music, horticulture, homemaking, or other normal daily life activities that relate to the patient's interests and goals. These activities provide occasions for successful experiences that will motivate the patient to work toward achieving his or her goals. Group activities are structured in such a manner as to aid the patient in developing group interaction skills. A variety of normal activities are used to reinforce normal aspects of the patient's functioning and to overcome dysfunctional behavior. Self-identity, coping with various situations, sensory integration, bodily integration, cognitive integration, and self-management are all goals that can be aided by occupational therapy (Allen, 1985; Barris, Kielhofner, & Watts, 1983; Cottrell, 1993; Early, 1993; King, 1985; Mosey, 1973).

SUMMARY

Mental disorders are treated by a variety of techniques. Pharmacotherapy, behavior therapy, and psychotherapy continue to be most frequently used. Combining pharmacotherapy with cognitive and psychosocial treatment is common. The *DSM-IV*ä and other psychiatric textbooks give detailed information on psychiatric terminology and classification.

REVIEW QUESTIONS

1. Place a T in front of the true statements.
    1) _____Psychiatrists are medical doctors.

   2) _____A psychiatrist is permitted to dispense drugs for medication.

   3) _____A clinical psychologist with a Ph.D. is a psychotherapist.

   4) _____Psychiatrists are not licensed to practice general medicine.

   5) _____A clinical psychologist with a Ph.D. is a psychiatrist.

2. Circle each number preceding a true statement.

   1) Alzheimer's disease is considered an organic mental disorder.

   2) Schizophrenia is a syndrome of organic mental disorder.

   3) Phobia is classified under somatoform disorders.

   4) Major depression is a mood disorder.

   5) Schizophrenia is caused by hallucinations.

   6) An individual who is dependent on cocaine has a somatoform disorder.

   7) A person with a personality disorder usually requires hospitalization.

   8) Individuals with somatoform disorders frequently seek treatment from medical doctors.

   9) An individual with repeated cycles of a period of unusually high energy and happiness, then a period of normal levels of energy and feelings, followed by a period of unusual lack of energy and depressed feelings, may have bipolar disorder.

   10) Sustained false beliefs about events and misperceptions of sensory stimuli that affect the individual may be due to a schizophrenia disorder.

3. Circle each number preceding a true statement.

   1) A person who receives auditory messages from a gold filling in a molar is probably having delusions.

   2) A patient who believes that he tastes a bitter poison in any egg sandwich when there is no bitter taste or poison is said to have a delusion.

   3) A person's expression of her emotions is referred to as affect.

   4) A person who has an intense fear of insects may have an anxiety disorder.

   5) A person who cannot give a reason for his fear of leaving home each day to go to work may have agoraphobia.

   6) A person who reports hearing verbal instructions "whispered in my right ear" when no one is around to do so may be having hallucinations.

   7) A person who believes that the CIA, FBI, and IRS are attempting to get her fired from a job when there is no evidence to verify the belief probably has a delusion.

   8) Ambivalence is when a person has an unreasonable fear of heights.

   9) Blocking is being able to cognitively stop having false beliefs.

   10) Agoraphobia is an extreme fear of living or working on a farm.

4. List at least three indicators of mental health.
5. List four indicators of mental disorder.
6. Name and briefly describe three psychiatric treatments for mental disorders.
7. Name at least four treatment settings for mental disorders.
8. State at least three occupational therapy goals for patients with mental disorders.

ANSWERS

1. The true statements are 1) and 2).
2. The true statements are 1), 4), 8), 9), and 10).
3. The true statements are 2), 3), 4), 5), 6), and 7).
4. The ability to withstand the stress of daily living, the ability to judge reality accurately, the ability to have lasting relationships with people, and the ability to love and accept love.
5. Mental disorder is dependent on many factors. Some symptoms do not necessarily indicate that a mental disorder exists. A change in the person's behavior and a lower level of functioning than existed previously may indicate the need for a psychiatric evaluation. Some indicators of mental disorder are hallucinations, delusions, and apparent changes in relationships, sleep habits, motor activity, thought processes, perception, sensorimotor activity, cognitive functioning, or other behaviors.
6.
   1) Pharmacotherapy: The patient is treated with drugs prescribed by the psychiatrist. These drugs affect the central nervous system and may be prescribed to elevate or depress the mood, to reduce excess motor activity, or for other behaviors.
   2) Behavior therapy: Principles of learning are used. Some techniques are aversion therapy, cognitive therapy, and systematic desensitization.
   3) Individual psychotherapy: A psychotherapist interacts with the patient in a prescribed manner believed to facilitate uncovering causes of certain undesired thoughts and behaviors.
7. Individuals with mental disorders can be treated as outpatients in the psychiatrist's office and in community day clinics and as inpatients in psychiatric units of general hospitals, in private psychiatric hospitals, and in state psychiatric hospitals.
8. Occupational therapy goals relate to activities of daily living, work, and leisure. Three goals of occupational therapy for patients with mental disorders may be as follows:
   1) to dress appropriately for a shopping trip in the community. This would relate to the activities of daily living that involve personal

hygiene, bathing, dressing, grooming, and all tasks involved in selecting appropriate clothes as a precursor to discharge to community living. An activity may be a simulated event in the treatment
setting.

2) to follow rules and participate actively in a selected group game.
This would relate to leisure activities that require social interaction,
such as communication skills and cognitive skills, including being
able to wait one's turn, responding appropriately when it is time to
participate, taking the appropriate time to respond, allowing another player to participate in the game, and accepting and giving
comments to others appropriately. Activities may be sedentary table
games, such as card or board games, or active games, such as volley
ball or other outdoor games.

3) to attend a meeting, on time and appropriately dressed and groomed.
This would relate to work activities. In addition to having specific
work skills needed for a particular job, the work situation usually
requires a certain type of dress, grooming, and behavior. Many work-
related skills can be learned in occupational therapy settings. An
activity can be to attend a scheduled meeting in the occupational
therapy area or the treatment setting in which a guest has been
invited to make a presentation to a small group, after which the
guest will meet with each individual for 3 to 5 minutes.

ADDITIONAL LEARNING ACTIVITIES

1. Make an appointment to visit a community mental health day program. Following orientation by the administrator or staff person, ask
permission to observe one of the activity programs. After your visit,
try to answer the following questions: How are individuals referred to
the program? What are the criteria qualifying a person to be in the
program? How is the program funded? Does each person have a goal
that is to be reached during attendance? What is the staff's role in
developing goals? Is each person required to attend a minimum number of days? Is there a maximum number of days each person can
attend? How is the decision made to terminate a patient's attendance?
What types of activity programs are available? Are progress reports
and records on each patient maintained? If so, how are the reports
used?

2. Make an appointment to visit or speak to someone in the service access and management unit for mental health/mental retardation in
your county. After your visit, try to answer the following questions:
When was the unit established? What are the goals of the unit? What
professional background do the staff members have? What is the relationship of the unit to state and federal psychiatric hospitals, mental

health units of general hospitals, and community day programs for individuals with psychosocial dysfunction?
3. If field visits are not part of your formal course, make appointments to visit occupational therapy departments in a mental health unit of a general hospital and of a state or federal hospital. Ask whether you may observe patients engaged in occupational therapy programs.

REFERENCES

Allen, C. K. (1985). *Occupational therapy for psychiatric diseases: Measurement and management of cognitive diseases.* Boston: Little, Brown Company.

American Psychiatric Association (1994). *Diagnostic and statistical manual of mental disorders* (4th ed.). Washington, DC: American Psychiatric Association.

Barris, R., Kielhofner, G., & Watts, J. H. (1983). *Psychosocial occupational therapy: Practice in a pluralistic arena.* Laurel, MD: RAMSCO Publishing Company.

Cohen, H. (1993). *Neuroscience for rehabilitation.* Philadelphia: J. B. Lippincott Company.

Corfman, E. (1979). *Depression, manic-depressive illness, and biological rhythms.* Rockville, MD: National Institute of Mental Health.

Cottrell, R. F. (Ed.). (1993). *Psychosocial occupational therapy: Proactive approaches.* Bethesda, MD: American Occupational Therapy Association, Inc.

Early, M. B. (1993). *Mental health concepts and techniques for the occupational therapy assistant* (2nd ed.). New York: Raven Press Books, Ltd.

Greben, S. E., Rakoff, V.M., & Voineskos, G. (Editorial Board). (1985). *A method of psychiatry* (2nd ed.). Philadelphia: Lea and Febiger.

Kaplan, H. I., & Sadock, B. J. (1988). *Synopsis of Psychiatry* (5th ed.). Baltimore: Williams and Wilkins.

Keith, S. L., & Mosher, L. R. (Editors-in-Chief). (1981). *Special report: Schizophrenia 1980.* Rockville, MD: National Institute of Mental Health.

King, L. J. (1985). Current schizophrenic research— implications for occupational therapy practice. *Mental Health Special Interest Section Newsletter, 7*(4), 14.

Mosey, A. C. (1973). *Activities therapy.* New York: Raven Press.

National Association of Private Psychiatric Hospitals. (1979). *Mental illness, its myths and truths.* Washington, DC: Author.

National Institute of Mental Health. (1972). *Mental illness and its treatment.* Rockville, MD, National Institute of Mental Health. .

National Institute of Mental Health. (1977). *Trends in mental health.* Washington, DC: Superintendent of Documents.

Pardes, H. (1981). *Schizophrenia: Is there an answer?* Rockville, MD: Centers for Studies of Schizophrenia, National Institute of Mental Health.

Rowe, C. J. (1984). *An outline of psychiatry.* Dubuque, IA: William C. Brown Company Publishers.

Sargent, M., & Swearingen, J. (1981). *Depressive disorders: Causes and treatment.* Rockville, MD: National Institute of Mental Health.

Thomas, C. L. (Ed.). (1993). *Taber's cyclopedic medical dictionary* (17th ed.). Philadelphia: F. A. Davis Company.

Yahraes, H. (1978). *Genes and mental health: The mechanisms of heredity in major mental illness.* Rockville, MD: National Institute of Mental Health.

SUGGESTED READINGS

Beck, M. A., & Callahan, D. K. (1980). Impact of institutionalization on the posture of chronic schizophrenic patients. *American Journal of Occupational Therapy, 34*(5), 332-335.

Engel, J. M. (1992). Relaxation training: A self-help approach for children with headaches. *American Journal of Occupational Therapy, 46*(7), 591-596.

Feil, N. (1989). *V/F, validation, the Feil method: How to help disoriented old-old* (rev. ed.). Cleveland: Edward Feil Productions.

Hasselkus, B. R. (1992). Meaning of activity: Day care for persons with Alzheimer disease. *American Journal of Occupational Therapy, 46*(3), 199-206.

Howe, M. C., Weaver, C. T., & Bulay, J. (1981). The development of a work oriented day center program. *American Journal of Occupational Therapy, 35*(11), 711-718.

Huebner, R. A. (1992). Autistic disorder: A neuro-psychological enigma. *American Journal of Occupational Therapy, 46*(6), 487-501.

Mace, N. L., & Rabins, P. V. (1991). *The 36-hour day: A family guide to caring for persons with Alzheimer's disease, related dementing illnesses, and memory loss in later life* (rev. ed.). Baltimore: Johns Hopkins University Press.

Wade, J. C. (1992). Socialization groups: Using *The book of questions* as a catalyst for interaction. *American Journal of Occupational Therapy, 46*(6), 541-545.

SUGGESTED LISTENING/VIEWING

Allen, C. K. (1991). *Why occupational therapists use crafts.* Bethesda, MD: American Occupational Therapy Association, Inc.

Morris, A., & Hunt, G. (1994). *A part of daily life: Alzheimer's caregivers simplify activities and the home.* Bethesda, MD: American Occupational

Therapy Association. (videocassette) (16 minutes).

Rabin, P. V. (1993). *The nursing home mental health series.* Baltimore: Video Press, University of Maryland (videocassette).

Agitation, aggression and violence. (20 minutes).

Confusion. (20 minutes).

Depression. (20 minutes).

Paranoia, suspiciousness and accusations. (20 minutes).

Positive approaches to difficult behaviors. (20 minutes).

Smith, L. (1978). *Evaluating functional skills in psychiatry.* Seattle: Division of Occupational Therapy, University of Washington (videocassette).

University of Southern California, Dept. of Psychiatry and Medical Education (1976). *Simulated psychiatric patient interviews.* Los Angeles: Author (videocassette).

Mrs. Bernard: Personality disorder (15 minutes).

Mr. Jordon: An organic brain syndrome with psychoses (10 minutes).

Mr. Paulin: Mental depression (10 minutes).

Mr. Ross: Neurosis: Phobia (17 minutes).

Mrs. Vail: Schizophrenia (16 minutes).

Mrs. Wiley: Manic-depressive (16 minutes).

26

EPILOGUE:
TRENDS IN HEALTH CARE

Some social, economic, technical, and health care trends likely to affect occupational therapy practice are highlighted.

LEARNING OBJECTIVES

At the end of this chapter, you should be able to:

1. Describe, in general, the future consumers of health care.
2. Discuss recent changes in delivery of health care.
3. State how social security benefits influence health care.
4. State how the method of payment of fees affects the delivery of health care.
5. Describe new products that afford the physically challenged individual greater independence in self-care tasks and productive and or leisure activities.
6. Discuss why occupational therapy research is needed.
7. Name at least three fundamental skills occupational therapy practitioners must have in order to provide effective service.

For a large part of the 20th century, most employees in the United States received complete health care coverage, including dependent care through plans provided by the employer. The average U.S. employee, still working or retired and on Social Security, expected com-plete, high-quality health care coverage throughout his or her life. In the last 2 decades, however, employees found themselves contributing more and more to the cost of their employer health care plan. Some employees found that greater participation in their own health care costs was not such a hardship, until they were suddenly unemployed, for one reason or another.

Health care is driven by the numbers and characteristics of those in need of services, the availability and qualifications of those who provide services, the funds available to pay for services, and many social and political issues related to the larger society. Some of the more recent issues in health care have to do with increased numbers of malpractice suits, which require health care providers to carry higher amounts of liability insurance; increased numbers of sophisticated evaluative procedures and consultations prior to and during medical procedures; older individuals who need services; services required for those who survive serious injury or disease; survivors of premature births; immigrants entering the country, the unemployed, and individuals in prisons, most of whom require some health care provided by state or federal funding; and complicated medical procedures that have arisen to replace or repair body parts. Additional issues pertain to decreased numbers of large corporations with jobs in certain sections of the country, decreasing amounts of federal and state funds available for health care, and limited numbers of health care professionals qualified to provide services.

TRENDS

A *trend* is either the general direction of occurrences or a bending from the current general direction. By being aware of trends, we can prepare ourselves to participate or not participate in them. Even if we are only partially prepared for a new trend, we are in a better position to help those who are in need of our services.

Because changes occur so rapidly in modern times, perhaps the best way to present the topic of trends in health care is to introduce some ideas related to the subject and request that the reader participate in gathering the most current information on health care that affects his or her community. You, as a reader, can actively participate by being alert to the topics presented in this chapter, by reading about these and related topics in newspapers, periodicals, and the electronic media, and by listening to radio and television shows that relate to the topics. Your up-to-date information will enable you to discuss the issues with others. You can then determine for yourself how the national trends in health care affect you, your community, and your profession. If you are using this chapter for a required course, and you maintain an active curiosity about what is happening in your community, your state, and your country, as well as about what is happening on earth and in space, you may find yourself filled with worthwhile information to share with your classmates and your instructor!

DEMOGRAPHICS

The demographics of the United States changed rapidly in the latter part of the 20th century. The baby boom that occurred after World War II was followed by a decline in the birth rate; however, more premature babies were saved. Previously, the word *prematurity* brought to mind a baby of approximately 7 months' gestation who was less than 5 pounds. The trend is for increasing numbers of much younger—down to 24 weeks' gestation—much smaller—weighing as little as a pound or even less— premature babies to survive. These infants bring with them unexplored and often complicated medical, psychological, social, economic, and educational needs. All professional services are forced to develop new protocols to help these infants grow and to assist their family members in managing both their own and their infants' lives.

Adults over age 65 continue to increase in number. Healthy and active life-styles, together with a focus on preventing illness and stress and formerly unheard-of medical advances, have allowed more and more adults to live many years beyond their retirement. At the end of the 20th century, older adults will account for approximately 12% of the population of the United States. By the third decade of the 21st century, adults aged 65 and older are expected to make up 20% of the population. The most rapidly increasing segment of the population is composed of persons over 85 years of age. By the second decade of the 21st century, an estimated 13 million persons will be over age 85 years (Shapiro, 1994).

Individuals aged 85 years and older will most likely continue to present health care professionals with new medical, economic, psychological, and sociological needs. Toward the end of the 20th century, an estimated 14% of men and 26% of women aged 85 years and older lived in homes with an adult child (Shapiro, 1994). As more older parents begin to live with an adult child, new issues will need to be resolved in order to make such living arrangements successful. Financial and legal concerns, as well as issues related to physical accommodations, the older parent's level of independence in self-care, ways to help the parent maintain a sense of productivity and self-worth, and satisfying leisure needs will require services from professionals. The psychological and physical well-being of the adult child caretaker and his or her family will be another important issue related to this trend.

The United States is struggling to develop a health care plan that will meet the needs of the country. Even with the current "information explosion" and rapid advances in technology, there is inadequate information on health care for the fast-increasing numbers of both people over 60 years of age and premature infants. A paucity of information also exists about new diseases, as well as conditions such as arthritis and heart disease that have been of concern for decades.

Although more Americans are taking responsibility for their health, the older adult group comprises more individuals with chronic conditions that can affect their mobility and independent performance of activities of daily living. Most older persons in need of health care usually require a greater number of services, more complicated services, and the use of those services over a longer period of time. The current debate about whether a person can choose to die when he or she has a terminal condition or a chronic, painful illness that precludes a reasonable quality of life rages on.

Medical science's growing ability to save lives following serious disease or injury has increased the number of adolescents and young adults with medical and physical conditions that require professional care. The number of young adults in need of health care has also increased due to sexually transmitted diseases, drug addiction, and a recurrence of tuberculosis that is resistant to previously effective medication.

The Americans with Disabilities Act of 1990, which went into effect in 1992 in order to ensure the inclusion of people with disabilities into society, has not significantly changed the 1986 numbers showing that two thirds of disabled persons are unemployed. A 1994 survey by Louis Harris and Associates revealed that 79% of disabled persons want to work, but are unemployed. The survey also found that only 26% of people with disabilities need special equipment in the workplace, at an average cost of $100 each. Occupational therapy practitioners will have to increase their efforts to advocate for the inclusion of qualified persons with disabilities into the economic, educational, social, and political fabric of society (Tressel & Pfaff, 1994).

Another group with expanding needs for health care is legal and illegal immigrants. Meeting the needs of individuals who differ culturally from the majority requires health care providers to deviate from their standard thinking and methods. The need to be alert to cultural diversity, as it relates to health care, will continue to grow with the increasing diversity of the inhabitants of the nation. The need to be sensitive to people who come from different countries and who differ dramatically from the mainstream population can be understood in terms of the need to be sensitive to such people who have been living in the United States for centuries—for example, the Amish.

The approximately 90 thousand U.S. Amish people live in rural farming areas in 23 states and Ontario, Canada. They are hardworking, family-oriented, religious people who live simply within their community. They use horse-drawn buggies and have no electricity, water, or gas lines coming into their community buildings in order to avoid permanent physical attachments to the outside world. They do not have telephones or televisions. They avoid anything they believe to be graven images and thus permit neither photographs to be taken of themselves nor voice transmission by audiotape (Hough & Kisseloff, 1994). The increasing numbers of people entering the United States from foreign countries with languages, past experiences, ways of life, beliefs, and values that differ from our own will require sensitivity and innovation in all aspects of intervention provided by occupational therapy practitioners.

FUNDING FOR HEALTH CARE

Less than 20 years after its inception, the Medicare program established by Congress in 1965 was reported to be in jeopardy, partly due to the increasing numbers of elderly persons and the rising cost of health care. A prospective payment system for health care was developed to resolve this problem.

On April 20, 1983, President Ronald Reagan signed into law the Social Security Amendments of 1983 (Health Care Financing Administration, 1983). According to these amendments, hospitals would receive payment for Medicare-eligible services based on a preset rate. The rate was dependent upon the type of medical diagnosis and the procedure performed, both related to criteria in the newly formulated *diagnosis-related group* (DRG). After a patient entered the hospital and received a primary diagnosis, the patient was assigned one of 468 identified DRGs. The DRG number covered a specific homogeneous grouping of medical diagnoses and procedures grounded in data compiled by the Yale University Center for Health Studies.

The hospital was to be paid a predetermined amount for each DRG, based on the average cost of treating that DRG in the past. With this *prospective payment system*, if the hospital services cost more than the Medicare payment, the hospital absorbed the extra cost. If the hospital services cost less than the Medicare payment, the hospital was allowed to keep the money as profit. The quality of treatment would be monitored by the Health Care Financing Administration, which administers Medicare (Health Care Financing Administration, 1983).

The prospective payment system required hospital administrators both to contain costs without financial loss and to provide needed services, which continued to increase in cost. In the 1980s, a trend toward for-profit hospitals became evident. For a hospital to remain profitable, every aspect of its operation needed to be scrutinized. Hospitals had to become cost effective if they expected to continue providing their services. Administrators scrutinized patients' lengths of stay, charges, and costs, the types of patients admitted by physicians, the services provided by hospital staff members, and the cost of those services (Wallace, 1983). All service providers had to document their evaluations, to furnish evidence that the patient was truly in need of the service to be rendered and to plan programs to achieve treatment goals in the most cost-effective way.

Despite problems with DRGs and prospective payment, most authorities agreed that the plan provided a more efficient record-keeping system than the previous Medicare plan, in which it was possible to submit bills to, and receive payments from, both the patient and the federal government.

Social Security and Medicare programs continue to be debated. In response to those who argue the need to cut Social Security and Medicare benefits because they are adding to the national deficit (Simpson, 1994), Moynihan (1994) states that the Social Security program is a social insurance program for which people establish their eligibility through their work and contributions, identified on their pay stubs as "FICA" (Federal Insurance Contributions Act). The argument that the cost of Social Security and Medicare is causing the federal deficit is untrue. Since the 1983 adjustments, the Social Security funds are ample, with a surplus of $100 billion expected by 1999. The Social Security Trust Funds reserve is expected to be nearly $3 trillion by 2020. To strengthen his statement that the Social Security funds are ample, Moynihan asserts that the most recent Social Security Board of Trustees' report indicates that the system will be solvent through 2029.

Managed care was introduced in the mid-1960s as a review process to determine whether Medicare funds were being spent only for medically necessary services. In the 1990's, "managed care" became a phrase to describe the changing health care delivery system. Managed care is a system to reduce the increasing cost of health care that resulted from fee-for-service reimbursement. Managed care has prepaid, capitated or case-rate reimbursement aimed at cost containment, quality medical outcomes, and increased productivity of service providers (Niemeyer & Foto, 1994b; Schwab, 1994). Occupational therapy practitioners are adapting to the changing delivery system just as they have adapted to other changes in the profession. Niemeyer and Foto (1994a) believe that the proactive, cooperative approach called "partnering," in which health care providers, insurers, and employers in the workers' compensation system share information on treating patients, with mutual goals of monitoring cost and quality of care to achieve the highest functional outcome possible in the shortest time, will improve the workers' compensation system.

Occupational therapy practitioners will be treating more patients with fewer resources and supervising more unlicensed personnel, at the same time maintaining the quality of their services with a focus on functional goals rather than reducing the effect of disabilities. They will also be increasingly responsible for the financial, as well as the clinical, aspects of treatment.

SETTINGS

The prospective payment system dramatically affected the delivery of health care services in the nation. Patients were discharged earlier from hospitals, and the need for home care increased (Carlson & Oriol, 1985). Almost half of the referrals for home health care were from hospitals.

The transition from acute care in hospitals to care in the home lowered the overall cost of health care. Nonprofessionals were able to provide 70% of the home care services. By 1994, there were more than 7,500 home health agencies. The need for qualified professional personnel to provide services in homes increased, as did the cost for services, with the estimated average cost for a home visit increasing by $25.00 from 1987 to 1994. Indications are that home health care will play a major role in the delivery of health care into the 21st century because of the increasing number of individuals aged 65 and older and children under the age of 5 who will need care at home.

Many patients who were discharged from the hospital while still in need of care could not return to their homes. The *subacute setting* was an alternative that met the needs of these patients. The 2,500 subacute settings that existed in 1994 will increase to 10,000 by 1999 in order to serve individuals who are unable either to return to their homes or to be placed in a long-term care facility or a rehabilitation center. The cost of caring for patients in subacute settings was estimated to be half of the cost in acute settings. Many acute care and rehabilitation hospitals developed their own separate subacute settings as a means of keeping patients within their purview when the patient needed to be discharged from their acute care setting (Munro, 1994).

The number of home health agencies and subacute care settings is expected to continue to increase during the 21st century. Existing hospitals will change their focus and seek ways to provide subacute care, long-term care, and community health services, in addition to acute care services, as the need for acute care beds decline. Hospice programs, either in a hospital or in a separate setting, are expected to grow to serve the needs of the dying and their families.

Long-term residential care will continue to be needed for the population 65 years of age and older. The increasing number of persons aged 85 or older with chronic conditions who will reside in long-term care settings will require innovative and alternative ways of delivering service to meet their needs and help them maintain as high a quality of life as possible. Since adult children, in concert with home health care agencies, will maintain many older persons in their homes for longer periods, the individuals admitted to long-term care facilities will likely be functioning at a much lower level of ability than those admitted in the past.

Because funding for technological research and physical rehabilitation services received priority during the 1980s, services to meet mental health needs declined. During the 1990s, many psychiatric hospitals were downsized or closed. Although the need for mental health services did not lessen, hospitals and corporations focused on services that generated income. Factors that may reverse the direction of mental health services in the next century are studies showing that persons aged 65 and older are not receiving needed psychiatric intervention and studies implicating stress in many conditions that affect health and productivity.

Human rights and the deinstitutionalization plan of the 1960s have influenced health care in the 20th century and continue to do so. Individuals were moved out of institutions and into communities, group homes, apartments, foster homes, or settings with their own families. In some cases, the community was burdened because it lacked appropriately trained personnel or community programs to meet the needs of these individuals.

The *independent living movement* began in the 1960s and early 1970s, when deinstitutionalization began. The first *independent living center* (ILC) was established in Berkeley, California, in 1972. In 1993, there were 240 ILCs that met the following criteria for such institutions: provision of core services, information and referral, peer counseling, training in independent living skills, and individual and systems advocacy for clients; provision of services for a constituency with various kinds of disabilities; and retention of a majority of persons with disabilities on governing boards and in decision-making and service delivery staff positions (Smith, Richards, Redd, & Frieden, 1994). Although ILCs were slow to develop, expanded services are anticipated because of the increasing need for alternative residential settings. Goals for the expansion are to include individuals with various disabilities, older persons, people with AIDS, persons with psychiatric problems, people with cognitive and learning disabilities, and persons with alternative life-styles. The ILC expansion movement will emphasize independence, inclusion, and empowerment in an effort to ensure that the quality of life of disabled people will improve (Heumann, 1994).

Over 11 million Americans living in rural areas of the United States have a chronic or permanent disability. Increasing the number of ILCs in these locations is hindered by a lack of resources. Occupational therapy professionals who work in these rural areas need to be resourceful, willing to travel to remote areas of the country, innovative, and able to use nontraditional methods to serve their clients' needs (Mathews, 1994). The health care needs of people living in rural America will require more attention in the future.

TECHNOLOGY IN HEALTH CARE

Advances in communication are not without potential problems. New legal and ethical concerns related to the confidentiality of information and the dissemination of misinformation have developed as more people have gained access to information transmitted by new technologies and as individuals have learned how to manipulate and falsify information.

Information can now be preserved more easily and in less space than ever before. Measurements and designs can be more accurate and refined. Materials used in the construction of equipment and devices are lighter in weight, stronger, more adaptable, and easier for the patient to wear or use than they were in the past.

Rehabilitation engineers working with therapists have developed seating and other equipment for patients who were previously unable to sit independently and use their upper extremities to perform functional activities of daily living. Wheelchairs and a variety of equipment are now available that enable the individual without strength in the lower extremities to stand in the chair and work at counter height or to participate in leisure activities (Pfaff, 1994; O'Reilly & Roshelli, 1994).

A variety of video display terminals and prosthetic devices for the upper extremities have been engineered to enable amputees to participate in a greater variety of leisure, self-care, and work activities (Celikyol, 1984). Bath products have been designed that enable greater independence in bathing and showering. Accessible bathtubs prevent transfer-related accidents and minimize the psychological and physical strain caretakers experience when bathing adults. Some such bathtubs have a door on the side of the tub that swings open like a car door. Others have a door that slides up and down on a wall-mounted track. The door is parallel to the ceiling, like a garage door, when open. When the door is closed, it becomes a wall of the bathtub. Still others have a door that rolls open like a shutter and is hidden beneath the floor of the tub when open. When the door is pulled up to close, it becomes a wall of the tub. All accessible bathtubs have safety features. Bath lifts help bathers get into and out of standard bathtubs. Accessible showers allow the person to take a shower while standing or while sitting in a chair (Mullick, 1994).

Computers enable permanently physically disabled individuals to engage in leisure, academic, and vocational pursuits. Computer environmental control systems allow severely physically disabled individuals to be more independent in daily living. Such systems enable persons with high-level quadriplegia, muscular dystrophy, and other disabling conditions to control lights, telephones, televisions, emergency alarms, doors, and many other household items (Lathem, Gregoria, & Garber, 1985).

A variety of environmental control system conform to the capabilities of the individual. Systems can be operated by voice recognition from as far as 6 feet away, for a person who cannot use a keyboard. Other environmental control systems are operated by one or more switches and are either voice or switch controlled. The switches, whether of the sip-and-puff or single, double, or multiswitch variety, can be matched to the person's motor and cognitive abilities (Marmer, 1993).

Computers are used to evaluate and monitor the patient's progress in treatment. Computer programs have been developed to provide visual stimulation and learning for developmentally delayed and physically handicapped children. The adaptability of switches enables the cognitively capable child, as well as the profoundly multiply handicapped child, to engage actively in both academic activities and computer games (Johann, 1994). Software programs allow therapists to help cognitively impaired patients increase their attention span, improve their memory, relearn the meanings of words, relearn number concepts, and develop other cognitive skills (Gracey, 1984). Computerized devices enable people with speech impairment to communicate. All of these systems can be adapted to the individual's intellectual and physical needs.

A new press-fit method of implanting joints that may last a lifetime has already been used. In the near future, radiographic techniques and three-dimensional computer graphic software will enable a patient's joint to be modeled on a video display terminal. The screen will show the ideal artificial knee installed. The components of the artificial knee will then be fabricated using machine tools controlled by the computer. Computer-generated electrical currents on implanted or surface electrodes can stimulate muscles of the hand to grasp an object. Similar currents on the legs and feet allow limited walking. Computer technology will enable orthotists and occupational therapy personnel to view an individual's surface geometry on the screen. Instead of the orthotist taking a cast of the surface, the computer will show high-pressure areas so that splints and braces can be fabricated more accurately and quickly (Tremblay, 1990).

Virtual reality (VR), which is a product of the National Aeronautics and Space Administration's effort to give astronauts a feeling of the environment of space while still on earth, is used in therapy. It will be possible to have a VR environment in the occupational therapy treatment area and change traditional types of activities. It will be possible to closely track the body part of concern as the patient engages in natural life activities. The patient's motivation to participate actively in the treatment is expected to increase. Driver training can safely be given in a VR environment after a stroke or brain injury, when vision is impaired, or when limitations arise due to physical injury or aging. Electric wheelchair training can be effective in a VR environment by setting up various obstacles the trainee is likely to encounter. It will be possible to engage in games and sports, such as archery, in which the player actually uses his or her upper extremities. Cooperative, multiplayer VR games are being used to help teach social behavior and academic skills to children with emotional disturbances or learning disabilities (Colan, 1994)

RESEARCH

Research in occupational therapy is crucial to the profession's continued acceptance as an effective and reimbursable treatment. Treatment given on a trial-and-error basis will no longer be acceptable, except in the most unusual cases.

Without research to validate what we believe to be effective treatment, we cannot state with conviction that a particular occupational therapy intervention, rather than some other factor, was responsible for the certain changes we observe. Increased numbers of occupational therapists are entering graduate programs (AOTA, 1995) and studying various aspects of occupational therapy practice. One example of research being conducted involves studying evaluation tools to find out whether the instruments we use are effective in evaluating what we need to know about a patient and in planning effective intervention programs; another examines whether a given evaluation is the most appropriate for the patient being evaluated (Letts et al., 1994). The effectiveness of specific treatment techniques is being studied as well (Neistadt, 1994). The effectiveness of items as basic as wheelchair cushions and methods as controversial as functional electrical stimulation needs to be researched objectively (Garber, 1985; Jaeger, 1994). The results of research will help occupational therapy practitioners base their decisions on scientific findings, rather than on personal biases and opinions.

THE ASSISTANT'S ROLE

Occupational therapists will continue to expand their involvement in research, education, program development, and consultation. Many will move into upper-level supervisory and management roles. Experienced certified occupational therapy assistants (COTAs) will need to be prepared to provide direct service to more patients in settings such as the patient's home, independent living centers, school systems, and other nonhospital settings. COTAs will be expected to travel during a day's time from one setting to another to treat patients. This will require 1) skills in time management in order to maintain a varied and often demanding schedule; 2) familiarity with the geographic location and traffic patterns in order to keep on schedule; 3) excellent communication skills to communicate with the supervising therapists, patients, and numerous individuals at different settings; and 4) the ability to document treatment in the style required by different supervising therapists, settings, and funding sources. The ability to use a computer for documentation will be a basic skill needed by the COTA. In general, the COTA will need to maintain his or her basic skills and gain additional specialized knowledge and skills appropriate to the particular work setting through continuing education.

The COTA will need supervisory skills for supervising less experienced COTAs, students, aides, and volunteers. COTAs have the opportunity to assume supervisory positions in retirement homes and other long-term care facilities, as activities directors planning daily activities for the residents.

The ability to read and use professional information will be an important skill for the COTA. Abstracts and summaries will help the COTA select articles to read in depth. The "information explosion" will continue, and the COTA will need to sort out the most pertinent information that relates to patients and to his or her professional growth and development.

Each work setting has specific knowledge and skill requirements. The COTA can be as effective as he or she desires by taking responsibility for acquiring the required knowledge and skills.

SUMMARY

Problems related to health care and the critical shortage of qualified health care personnel are frequently not given high priority by those faced with a huge list of national concerns. Nonetheless, as a health care profession that is concerned with the whole person, occupational therapy will continue to be an important service that can help meet the health care needs of many.

REVIEW QUESTIONS

1. What general groups of consumers will need health care in the future?
2. Discuss the changes that have come about within the last couple of decades in the delivery of health care.
3. How do Social Security benefits influence health care?
4. How does payment for health care services affect the delivery of those services?
5. Give some examples of new products, and show how they promote greater independence in the physically challenged individual in regard to self-maintenance tasks, work and productive activities, or leisure activities.
6. Discuss why occupational therapy research is needed.
7. Name at least three fundamental skills occupational therapy practitioners need in order to provide effective service.

In each of the following, circle the letter preceding the best ending that makes a complete and true statement:

8. Social Security:
   a. increased the number of adaptive devices available to patients.
   b. has an age requirement of 70 years or older for eligibility.

c. amendments established a prospective payment plan for medical care.

d. will be available only up to the year 2010.

9. Diagnosis-related groups (DRGs) were developed to:

a. control the number of admissions to particular hospitals.

b. help hospitals determine a patient's readiness for discharge.

c. help maintain the cost of medical care within reasonable limits.

d. help hospitals stay solvent by diagnosing patients prior to being admitted to the hospital.

10. The DRGs are one cause of the dramatic increase in occupational therapy services in:

a. state institutions.

b. private homes.

c. school systems.

d. psychiatric hospitals.

11. Environmental control units:

a. permit a person with a C1 to C4 spinal cord injury to control aspects of his or her self-care by using tongue or brow switches.

b. are Medicare-controlled living arrangements for the oldest of the old.

c. are state-regulated community living units for the developmentally delayed.

d. regulate the temperature, humidity, and bacterial count in hospital burn units.

12. Changes in the numbers and needs of the long-term care population:

a. indicate that more federal regulations are needed to contain the cost of care.

b. indicate that the quality of services and the quality of life cannot be priority issues.

c. require innovative and alternative ways of delivering service.

d. require increased numbers of direct care personnel in state and federal institutions.

13. A trend in hospitals has been:

a. an excessive number of acute care beds.

b. to increase the number of acute care beds.

c. to increase pediatric care units.

d. to build new acute care hospitals.

ANSWERS

1. Many will be over 80 years of age, frail, and with chronic problems and may have psychiatric problems. Many will be children with developmental delays—some severe—and in need of intervention in all performance areas.

2. The settings for the delivery of services have changed from acute care hospitals to the home and community. Therapists were more itinerant, traveling from one setting to another in a day. A greater accountability for establishing specific goals for treatment and for reaching those goals was expected. Reimbursable treatment and treatment for profit began to be emphasized in the last part of the 20th century.

3. An expected shortage of funds in the Social Security system prompted a plan to reduce the cost of health care. A change in the method of reimbursement by Medicare based on diagnosis-related groups resulted in shorter hospital stays, with discharged patients being sent home or to another facility while still needing medical care.

4. The delivery of health care services is grounded in principles of economics. Quality services can be delivered only when the costs of building and equipment, maintenance of equipment, the dissemination of information, personal salaries, and other expenses are paid for.

5. Among these products are accessible bathtubs; environmental control units with switches that remotely turn on appliances within the home by means of a motor, the voice, the breath, etc.; software programs for visual stimulation; games and educational activities; wheelchairs that allow the occupant to stand although muscle strength in the lower trunk and extremities is absent; and virtual reality environments that enable patients to learn how to maneuver their wheelchair, drive a car, and engage in archery or other activities.

6. There is need for objective studies which show that a particular occupational therapy intervention influenced a patient who has reached treatment goals, rather than that the result was due mostly to medication, the attention given by the therapist, or some other factor. Research provides information that can make occupational therapy intervention more predictable so that given treatment methods and protocols can be used to evaluate results that fall within given criteria. Finally, there will always be unique individual differences, but research will help the profession develop improved guidelines for evaluation and treatment.

7. Important for effective occupational therapy are communication skills, documentation skills, time management skills, and the ability to project a sincere interest in the patient and in the occupational therapy intervention to be given, in order to establish trust and confidence.

8 c

9. c

10. b

11. a

12. c

13. a

ADDITIONAL LEARNING ACTIVITIES

1. Ask an occupational therapy practitioner who has been practicing for 5 or more years to describe the changes he or she has observed in the types of patients, treatment methods, and settings.
2. Visit a subacute setting. Was the setting part of an acute hospital setting or rehabilitation center, or was it a separate setting? How did the subacute setting differ from an acute hospital, from a long-term care setting, and from a rehabilitation center?
3. Visit a retirement village. Ask your host or hostess when the village first opened. What are the ages of the residents? Has there been a change in the age of the persons who first apply to the village? How do the residents spend their days?
4. Watch for local newspaper articles or speak to local representatives to find out what plans your community has for programs for the over-65-year-old citizen.
5. Check the magazine section of your library. How many magazines are geared toward people over 60 years of age?
6. Ask occupational therapy practitioners who work with biomechanical engineers what devices and equipment they have developed.
7. Ask occupational therapy practitioners whether they are involved in research in their clinical practice. If so, what is the focus of their research?

REFERENCES

American Occupational Therapy Association, Inc. (1994). Listing of educational programs in occupational therapy. *American Journal of Occupational Therapy, 48*(11), 1060-1070.

American Occupational Therapy Association, Inc. (1995). *1995 education data survey final report: Survey of educational programs—1993-94 academic year.* Bethesda, MD: Author.

Carlson, E., & Oriol, W. (1985). Surviving Medicare's new obstacle course. *Modern Maturity, 28,* 25-27, 87-88, 94-103.

Celikyol, F. (1984). Prostheses, equipment, adapted performance: Reflections on these choices for the training of the amputee. *Occupational Therapy Strategies and Adaptations for Independent Daily Living, 1,* 89-115.

Colan, B. J. (September, 1994). VR technology will turn exercise into occupation. *ADVANCE for Occupational Therapists, 10*(38), 19.

Garber, S. L. (1985). Wheelchair cushions for spinal cord-injured individuals. *American Journal of Occupational Therapy, 39,* 722-725.

Gracey, S. (1984). Computer-assisted therapy for brain-injured patients: A team approach. *Physical Disabilities Special Interest Section Newsletter, 7*(2), 4.

Health Care Financing Administration (August, 1983). Medicare prospective payment. *HCFA Fact Sheet.* Washington, DC: Author.

Heumann, J. E. (Winter-Spring, 1994). The independent living movement. *OSERS: News in Print, 6*(2), 2.

Hough, S., & Kisseloff, L. (1994). Crossing cultures. *TeamRehab, 5*(3), 14-20.

Jaeger, R. J. (1994). Stimulating steps. *TeamRehab, 5*(7), 17-24.

Johann, C. M. (1994). Form and function. *TeamRehab, 5*(4), 14-16, 18.

Lathem, P. A., Gregoria, T. L., & Garber, S. L. (1985). High-level quadriplegia: An occupational therapy challenge. *American Journal of Occupational Therapy, 39,* 705-714.

Letts, L., Law, M., Rigby, P., Cooper, B., Stewart, D., & Strong, S. (1994). Person-environment assessments in occupational therapy. *American Journal of Occupational Therapy, 48*(7), 608-618.

Marmer, L. (July, 1993). ECUs: The next best thing to miracles. *ADVANCE for Occupational Therapists, 9*(29), 11.

Mathews, R. M. (1994). Best practices in rural independent living. *OSERS: News in Print, 6*(2), 23-29.

Moynihan, D. P. (1994). The case against entitlement cuts. *Modern Maturity, 37*(6), 13-14.

Mullick, A. (1994). Bathing easy. *TeamRehab, 5*(4),28-30.

Munro, D. (1994). Subacute subtleties. *Rehabilitation Today, 4*(1), 18-21.

Niemeyer, L. O., & Foto, M. (1994a). Partnering in workers' compensation. *Rehab Management, 7*(4), 138-139, 141.

Niemeyer, L. O., & Foto, M. (1994b). The workers' comp dilemma. *Rehab Management, 7*(2), 109-111, 115.

Neistadt, M. E. (1994). The effects of different treatment activities on functional fine motor coordination in adults with brain injury. *American Journal of Occupational Therapy, 48*(10), 877-882.

O'Reilly, K., & Roshelli, T. B. (1994) Just right. *TeamRehab, 5*(7), 14-17.

Pfaff, K. (1994). A model of accessibility. *TeamRehab, 5*(3), 22-26.

Schwab, A. (1994). Repositioning for managed care: The enlargement of clinical roles. *Rehab Management, 7*(2), 81, 83.

Shapiro, P. (November, 1994). My house is your house. *AARP Bulletin, 35*(10), 2.

Simpson, A. (1994). Why we need entitlement reform. *Modern Maturity, 37*(6), 12, 14.

Smith, Q., Richards, L., Redd, L. G., & Frieden, L. (1994). Improving management effectiveness in independent living centers through research training. *OSERS: News in Print, 6*(2), 30-36.

Tremblay, S. (1990). Capitalizing on technology: The adaptive equipment loan program. *RESNA '90 13th Annual Conference.* Washington, DC: June 15-20.

Tressel, P., & Pfaff, K. (1994). ADA hasn't changed employment numbers. *TeamRehab, 5*(7), 9, 38-39.

Wallace, C. (September, 1983). Managing along product lines is key to hospital profits under DRG system. *Modern Healthcare, 13,* 56.

SUGGESTED READINGS

ADVANCE for Occupational Therapists. This weekly news magazine provides easy-to-read current information on a variety of topics and is

OT Week. This weekly news magazine gives concise information on current research findings pertaining to medical, educational, and other topics related to occupational therapy. Reading *OT Week* will help you follow the direction being taken by your professional association. All members of the American Occupational Therapy Association receive *OT Week.*

APPENDIX:
STUDY GUIDE

W e each learn in our own unique fashion. We each study in our own way. Some of us study best alone, others study best in a small group. Some of us read, write information in a separate notebook (perhaps more than once), read related information in other books, and try to find more information in the library. Others can read the same information and remember the important points without further effort. This guide is for those who feel that they can use some ideas on how to study, or at least, how to study information that is quite foreign to them. Suggestions on studying, taking notes, and taking tests are included. Review questions test your retention of the information presented in each chapter.

WHY STUDY?

Select your response or responses to complete the following sentence:

I plan to study because I:

    _____ want to get through this course.
    _____ have a friend in the OTA Program.
    _____ want to graduate with a 4.0 GPA.
    _____ lost my job.
    _____ want to become an OTR.
    _____ believe that knowledge is power.
    _____ want to learn everything I can.
    _____ don't have anything more interesting to do.
    _____ want to get an A in this course.
    _____ don't know what I want to do in the future.
    _____ want to become a COTA.

Obviously, you have many reasons for studying, and your reasons may not be among the preceding choices. Most likely, you are reading this textbook because it is a required text in an introductory course in an occupational therapy assistant program. The topics may be entirely new to you, or your background may be such that you already have more information about some of the topics than is included in the chapters. For whatever reason you are reading this textbook, I hope it helps you achieve your goal.

EDUCATIONAL TAXONOMIES

You may find it helpful to review the educational level of the information you are studying and the purpose of that information. Benjamin Bloom (1956) and others formed taxonomies of objectives for all classifications of subject matter to be taught in educational settings. Among these objectives are cognitive, or intellectually based, objectives; affective, or emotionally based, objectives; and psychomotor objectives, which are a combination of physically and mentally based objectives.

Bloom's original text, as well as other literature, discusses his taxonomies in full. Only the cognitive domain will be discussed in this appendix.

The cognitive domain encompasses intellectual and other thought processes, including the following levels of cognition, ordered from lowest to highest:

1. *Recall.* The student recalls such information as facts, words, symbols, principles, and theories.
2. *Comprehension.* The student interprets information, translates information into another form, or uses information in various situations.
3. *Application.* The student applies knowledge to a new situation.
4. *Analysis.* The student decomposes a whole into parts and studies the parts and their relationships to each other.
5. *Synthesis.* The student puts small elements together and shows creativity in combining these elements.
6. *Evaluation.* The student uses well-defined criteria to judge the worth of a thing or idea.

You will probably recognize all of these levels of information as you take the courses required in your occupational therapy curriculum. You will want to reach the higher levels of the cognitive domain in order to become an excellent occupational therapy assistant.

Recalling facts, as is required in some basic courses such as this one, or remembering names of muscles in a gross anatomy course, is important, but may not be helpful if the factual information cannot be applied in a situation outside of the classroom. For example, in planning a dressing procedure for a person with a spinal cord injury, you will use all six levels of information. The following list shows how some of the information included in the occupational therapy curriculum can be matched to the six levels in the cognitive domain:

1. *Recall.* You are required only to recall and list on a test the three areas of occupational therapy performance skills: self-care, work, and play.

2. *Comprehension.* You comprehend the importance of activity analysis in occupational therapy as you recall the muscles and how they work together, how joints move, the body positions, the sensory processes, and all of the fine-motor and gross-motor skills needed to assemble a link belt.
3. *Application.* You recall information about anatomy, physiology, development, and activities, comprehend its relevance to occupational therapy, and are able to apply the knowledge to assess the effect of intervention on a person and the self-care, work, or leisure skills needed by the person.
4. *Analysis.* You can analyze the client's performance skills and objectives to determine specific areas in which occupational therapy intervention is required.
5. *Synthesis.* You are able to combine the various kinds of information studied (for example, the conditions for which patients are commonly referred for occupational therapy intervention, the analysis of different activities, and the different adaptive devices) and begin to relate information to specific clients in need of occupational therapy.
6. *Evaluation.* Finally, you develop a set of criteria to help determine whether the planned treatment program will be a reasonable one for a particular client.

HOW TO STUDY TO LEARN

To learn to be an occupational therapy assistant requires more than reading and remembering facts to pass an examination. Occupational therapy is an action-oriented profession. The student seeking to become an occupational therapy assistant should observe skilled professionals, practice under supervision, and expect to continue to study and learn. Learning requires motivation, concentration, reaction, organization, comprehension, and repetition.

1. *Motivation. You* need to want to learn. No one else can learn for you. Many factors influence your motivation. If it is lacking, try to find a reason for learning, and respond to that reason. A momentary lack of motivation may simply require a short walk or a nourishing snack. A generalized lack of motivation may suggest the need to talk to the campus counselor or some other trusted person.
2. *Concentration.* Study groups are helpful; however, you generally also need private time in familiar physical surroundings with few distractions. The cafeteria in the student center with loud music and students eating and talking is not the most conducive setting for concentrated study.
3. *Reaction.* Active involvement aids learning. When reading, create men-

tal images of the descriptions being read. Take notes, both while reading the assignments before class and during the class lecture. Reactions through visual, auditory, tactile, and kinesthetic channels increase the potential for learning.

4. *Organization*. When reading, it is helpful first to get a general picture of the whole (a *gestalt*) and then to look at the details. For example, when a few pages in a chapter are assigned, take time to scan the entire chapter. Read the abstract at the beginning or the summary at the end of the chapter first to learn what the chapter is generally about, and then study the assigned section.

MEMORY

Learning requires remembering. Learning researchers generally agree that memory can be divided into shortterm memory and long-term memory (Curtis, 1990; Staton, 1962). An example of short-term memory is remembering a phone number for 1 to 3 minutes after hearing it. Remembering a phone number used hours or years ago is an example of long-term memory.

Neuroscientists are uncertain exactly how short-term memory is converted to long-term memory or in what part of the brain long-term memory is located (Curtis, 1990). Some learning researchers (Algier & Algier, 1982) believe that information will reach long-term memory only if it is actively processed through the sensory store and through short-term memory. They hypothesize that some part of the brain takes raw data from the environment, processes it, and stores it for future use. The raw data taken from the environment does not necessarily provide meaningful information. The data are transformed into useable information through perception. These researchers state that the human information-processing system consists of three components: a sensory store, short-term memory, and long-term memory.

The function of the sensory store is to retain useful data long enough to perceive and interpret their content. Sensory stores exist for all of the senses. The visual sensory store is estimated to have a duration of one fourth of a second. The auditory sensory store can last for 3 to 4 seconds. An individual's ability to attend to available sensory data is limited by his or her attention. Appropriate attention enables individuals to filter out unnecessary and extraneous data and select only data that are important (Algier & Algier, 1982).

Although many serious students state that they are not able to attend to enough information, the occupational therapy student will learn that there can be a disadvantage in being able to attend to an excessive amount of sensory data. Therapists have spent decades searching for methods to help children who attend to excessive amounts of environmental stimuli.

Such children are unable to filter out relevant information needed to make an appropriate response.

Currently, two theories explain the limitation of attention to sensory data. One theory is that the data are limited, as when, for example, we hear something that has poor sound quality. The second theory is that our resources are limited—for example, we may not be physically close enough to the data presented.

In the early stage of processing data, the individual must be actively involved. The individual needs to feel that what is being perceived is of importance in order to pay sufficient attention. If the student attends to and perceives data within the duration of the sensory store, the data will be transferred to short-term memory. Without this processing, the data will be lost (Algier & Algier, 1982).

Short-term memory

If it survives the sensory component, information is transferred to short-term memory for further processing. Short-term memory, which has a duration of about 30 seconds, has two functions: storage and work. Short-term memory has a storage capacity for about seven pieces of information. Forgetting can be due to overloading the capacity or exceeding the duration of short-term memory. Rehearsal of information stored in short-term memory prevents forgetting. Learning researchers believe that there are two types of rehearsal. The first type, *repetition*, maintains information by recycling the information to short-term memory. The second type of rehearsal, which is done by organizing and relating information, prevents forgetting. This process of combining pieces of information into units is sometimes called *chunking* (Algier & Algier, 1982).

Long-term Memory

Large amounts of information can be permanently stored in long-term memory, which can be thought of as a vast network of memory traces that are organized and linked together. This network contains related and meaningful pieces of information that form concepts (semantic memory). Also tied into the network are memories of specific events or experiences (episodic memory) and images (visual memory) (Algier & Algier, 1982).

Working memory

Working memory is consciousness. That is, working memory controls what the individual is aware of at a given moment. Working memory is responsible for extracting information needed from long-term memory and for manipulating what is stored in short-term memory (Algier & Algier, 1982).

Forgetting

Forgetting in long-term memory is different from forgetting in short-term memory. In short-term memory, forgetting is caused by loss of information. In long-term memory, the information exists, but cannot be located. Some theorists believe that forgetting in long-term memory is due to either inappropriate storage or competition between memory traces (Algier & Algier, 1982).

Mnemonics

Mnemonics is an entertaining way of developing clues to aid remembering. It is a way of remembering by associating the information to be learned with something that has no direct relation to it. For example, to remember the names of all the planets, remember the sentence, "My very educated mother just served us nine pickles." The first letter of each word is the clue to the names of the planets (Mercury, Venus, Earth, Mars, Jupiter, Saturn, Uranus, Neptune, Pluto). A problem that some people who use mnemonics experience is that they forget what the clues are or what they mean.

Mnemonics can be a useful memory device. The process is considered a valid rehearsal technique by learning researchers (Staton, 1962).

TAKING NOTES

Organization is the key to effective listening and remembering. Taking notes is a way to organize thoughts, as well as to react through the kinesthetic, auditory, and visual channels. Organized notes help identify important ideas in a lecture and provide a permanent record that will aid in learning and remembering. It is important to attend classes, because the instructor usually gives information during lectures that is not available elsewhere, such as information on research studies that the instructor has read or heard about. This type of information enhances the information in the textbook, relating it to real situations. Also, during lectures, you can gain a sense of what the instructor considers important. It is helpful to remember that the instructor in an occupational therapy course will realize who is not attending classes. It is helpful to remember also that the instructor usually makes up the exams.

The following steps are recommended when you have reading assignments:

1. *Preview.* Read assignments before the lecture.
2. *Select.* Search for important ideas in the text and lecture.
3. *Question.* In class, ask for clarification of questions raised during reading.
4. *Organize.* Write notes in a logical form.

5. *Review.* Review notes as soon as possible after the lecture. Discussing the lecture with a classmate will also help you remember important information, as well as clarify certain points and raise questions that you can get clarified in the next lecture.

The following steps are recommended when you take notes in class:

1. Use a shorthand method and abbreviate words.
2. Use dashes for words missed.
3. Leave space to allow room to fill in information later.
4. Use symbols to call attention to important words. Develop your own special meaning for these symbols, be they underlines, capitals, circles, boxes, or other symbols.
5. When the instructor says, "This is important," write the words exactly as said, and mark them with a special symbol to indicate their importance. If possible, get another source for the same information. This may help clarify or help you to remember the information.
6. *Do not erase a mistake.* Draw a single line through it. This saves time, and the mistake may serve some useful purpose later.

Active Listening
To take useful notes and get the most from a lecture requires active listening and the following procedure:

1. Read the chapter before you attend the lecture.
2. Get to class on time.
3. Sit close enough to hear the instructor.
4. Sit in a position to see written information.
5. Look at the instructor and listen attentively.
6. Respond to the instructor with facial expressions and with body postures and movements to show your interest. (You can consider this practice for listening to your future patients.)
7. Ask relevant questions.
8. Contribute relevant information.

TAKING A TEST

The best preparation for taking a test is to want to learn, attend classes, listen, read, study, and follow instructions. If the instructor is willing to give information about the test, ask about the test in class. For example, is the test an objective test, an essay test, or a combination of both? Do certain questions count more than others? Is there a penalty for incorrect answers?

Some instructors will inform the class about the format of the test or quiz and review the sections to be covered. Other instructors will simply state that the student is responsible for anything and everything that was covered in class, in the reading assignments, and in audiovisual presentations. It is helpful to get to know the particular instructor's style of teaching and evaluating students.

The following are guidelines for taking objective tests:

1. Read the instructions, and follow them explicitly and completely. This is very important for electronically graded test forms.
2. Read the question and list of answers completely before answering. If the answer is supposed to be the *best* answer, make sure it is the best answer. If the answer is to be what is done *first*, make sure it is what is to be done first.
3. Do not confuse the test question by adding your own information to it.
4. Answer on the basis of the information given. If the question asks for an answer according to a specific reference (the guest speaker, the text), do not consider all the other information you have heard or read that contradicts the reference. Answer the question as it is stated.
5. Remember that the instructor is not trying to trick you. Do not think that the answer is so obvious that your answer must be wrong. Another text taker might not know what you know.
6. Do not change answers on mere doubt. Stay with your first choice, unless you have a very good reason to change it.
7. If there is no penalty for wrong answers, answer all of the questions, even if you feel that you do not know the exact answer. You may know more than you realize.

The following guidelines apply to taking essay tests:

1. Read the instructions carefully and follow them.
2. Read the question carefully. Then reread it.
3. Establish a priority as to what is most important, what needs elaboration, and how much elaboration is needed. List these in the margin or on the back of the paper to organize your thoughts. The time taken to decide what is most important, to set priorities, and to organize your thoughts will greatly increase your efficient use of the remaining writing time.
4. Avoid redundancy, but make certain that you provide enough information for the instructor to understand your statements.
5. Write with whatever instrument the instructions specify. If there are no specifications, use a good pen or a number 2 lead pencil so that the writing can be easily read.
6. Write legibly, and use correct spelling and proper grammar and punctuation.

7. Check your answers for clarity of thought, spelling, punctuation, and completeness.

QUESTIONS

The following questions are to help you review each chapter and test your memory. Answers are not given, but can quickly be found by referring back to the chapter. Before you look for any answers in the chapters, write out or state the information and the ideas that you believe best answer the question.

Chapter 1: Defining Occupational Therapy

1. What is the goal of occupational therapy?
2. What is common to all individuals referred for occupational therapy?
3. What is the basic characteristic of any therapeutic activity used in occupational therapy?
4. The definition of occupational therapy places individuals who can benefit from treatment into categories. Name at least five of these categories.
5. What are three major aims of occupational therapy?
6. List seven specific occupational therapy services.
7. How are services provided to occupational therapy patients?
8. In your own words, define occupational therapy.
9. Explain in your own words the difference between a person who is functional and one who is not.
10. How does the word "holistic" relate to occupational therapy?
11. What factors determines the therapeutic activity or activities selected for a particular patient?

Chapter 2: Philosophy of Occupational Therapy

1. What is meant by the phrase "philosophical base of occupational therapy"?
2. Why is it important to know the philosophical base of a profession?
3. Does a person's philosophy change as he or she matures?
4. Do all members of a profession have the same philosophical view?

Chapter 3: History of Occupational Therapy

1. Name two or three events or changes that were occurring in the United States which influenced the beginning of occupational therapy.
2. What were some patients' conditions that responded to early occupational therapy and captured the interest of physicians?
3. Who were the first supervisors of occupational therapy programs?
4. The first occupational therapy school within an academic institution began in 19____ and was located in _____.

5. It is interesting to compare the length of the early educational programs, such as the number of lecture and practice hours, to the current educational demands placed on occupational therapy students. What accounts for the differences?
6. How have changes in health care delivery influenced the delivery of occupational therapy services?
7. State the basic aims of the three early models of occupational therapy. Are these models consistent with the definition of occupational therapy given in Chapter 1 and with the philosophical base of occupational therapy given in Chapter 2?
8. What is meant by the medical model?
9. Is the medical model consistent with the philosophical base of occupational therapy? Justify your answer.

Chapter 4:
History of the Certified Occupational Therapy Assistant

1. State two situations or events occurring in the country and in the occupational therapy profession that influenced the creation of the occupational therapy assistant level within the profession.
2. List chronologically the main events in the development of the position of the COTA, beginning with the date of the proposal for such a position to the American Occupational Therapy Association (AOTA) Delegate Assembly and continuing on to the present time.
3. Explain how individuals become COTAs.
4. Discuss the range of employment possibilities for a person who is a COTA.
5. List ways in which a COTA can have input into AOTA.

Chapter 5: Occupational Therapy Settings

1. Name at least five different settings in which occupational therapy services are provided, and describe the type of patients generally treated in each.
2. How are treatment settings funded?
3. What effect does the source of funding have on the setting?
4. Why should the employed COTA know the organizational structure of the place of employment?

Chapter 6: The Assistant's Role

1. What is the difference between an entry-level COTA and an experienced COTA?
2. List and describe the six categories of COTA duties.
3. What factors determine what the COTA does in each of the six categories in any specific employment situation?
4 In what situations might a COTA be a supervisor?

5. State at least five ways that the COTA helps in the evaluation process.
6. In what ways might a COTA help during the process of discontinuing treatment of a patient?

Chapter 7: Interviewing Skills
1. When does a COTA conduct an interview with a patient?
2. In what types of interviews are closed questions most useful?
3. In what types of interviews are open-ended questions most useful?
4. Name important COTA behaviors in conducting any interview.
5. List and discuss precautions to observe during any interview.
6. List specific patient behaviors to which the COTA should be alert.

Chapter 8: Reports and Records
1. State four important reasons for reporting and recording a patient's treatment.
2. Why is it important to record objective information?
3. What factors make information objective?
4. What makes subjective information important?
5. What personal information should the COTA include in a written report?
6. What is meant by the data base in a patient's report?

Chapter 9: Evaluation
1. What is meant by evaluation in occupational therapy?
2. Explain the role of the occupational therapist (OTR) and the COTA in screening a patient.
3. Explain the role of the OTR and COTA in assessing a patient.
4. Explain the role of the COTA in the use of standardized tests to assess a patient.
5. State the steps in the process that begins with a patient being referred for occupational therapy and that ends with the patient's discharge from occupational therapy.

Chapter 10: Planning Treatment
1. Why is an occupational therapy treatment plan needed?
2. Who develops the treatment plan?
3. What roles do the COTA and patient play in the treatment plan?
4. What are five basic elements in most treatment plans?

Chapter 11: The Supervisory Function
1. What is meant by supervising?
2. Do COTAs do any supervising? If so, give some examples of their supervisory roles.
3. Name at least eight important attitudes of an effective supervisor.

4. Why is it important for a supervisor to have effective communication skills?
5. What are the important ingredients of effective communication?
6. Name at least 10 important, specific supervisory skills.
7. Why is it important for a supervisor to know and agree with the philosophy of the facility?

Chapter 12: Therapeutic Use of Self

1. How can a COTA, as a person, be a therapeutic tool?
2. Explain how Jerome Frank described the three selves in an individual.
3. Why is the acting self important in therapy?

Chapter 13: Analysis of Therapeutic Occupations

1. Recall the relationship of occupations to the definition and the philosophical base of occupational therapy.
2. State some important principles involved in the selection of occupations for a particular patient.
3. If an occupation is patient centered, is it appropriate to have the patient decide on the occupation to be used in therapy? Justify your answer.
4. List important factors to consider when deciding on the most appropriate therapeutic occupation to use with a particular patient.
5. What are some basic considerations involved in analyzing activities for their therapeutic value for a particular patient?

Chapter 14: Therapeutic Exercise and Therapeutic Activities

1. Define therapeutic exercise.
2. Are therapeutic occupations used as therapeutic exercise? Explain your answer.
3. Therapeutic exercises are usually prescribed to help patients achieve what general goals?
4. What relationship do progressive relaxation techniques have in occupational therapy for physical dysfunctions?
5. Why is endurance an important consideration in therapy?

Chapter 15: Therapeutic Equipment

1. What is the basic purpose for considering the use of therapeutic devices and equipment for a patient?
2. What might be determining factors for not using certain therapeutic devices or equipment?
3. Name a safety feature used when adapting clothing for a person in a wheelchair.
4. Name a safety feature used when adapting a wooden toy for a a spastic child with or a child with some other abnormal movement.

5. Name a safety feature used when adapting a kitchen or cooking uten-
   sil for a person who has the use of only one upper extremity.

Chapter 16: Splinting

1. What is a splint?
2. Discuss how the upper extremity and hand function.
3. What are the four phases of hand function? For each of the four
   phases, name a daily activity that is hindered when that phase is not
   possible.
4. Illustrate with your hand the seven prehension patterns.
5. What is meant by the functional position of the hand? Describe the
   position.
6. What is meant by the resting position of the hand? Describe the
   position.
7. What is the purpose of hand splinting?
8. Name at least six conditions in which hand splinting can be useful.
9. What are some advantages of using low-temperature plastic in
   splinting?
10. What are the main differences between static and dynamic splints?

Chapter 17: Developmental Disabilities

1. Name the law that defined developmental disabilities for eligibility
   for programs and funding in the nation.
2. List the seven areas of major life activities that are of concern in P.L.
   95-602.
3. How long can a person be considered developmentally disabled, according to P.L. 95-602?
4. Name the 1977 law that created a great shortage of OTRs and COTAs
   in the United States.
5. Explain the role of occupational therapy in the educational process of
   the student, according to the 1977 law.
6. What are the provisions of P.L. 102-119, the Individuals with Disabilities Education Act (IDEA).

Chapter 18: Mental Retardation

1. Define mental retardation.
2. What is meant by adaptive behavior?
3. Name some causes of mental retardation.
4. According to the definition, at what stage in life can an individual
   become mentally retarded?
5. What changes have occurred in the treatment of persons with mental
   retardation since the 1960s?

Chapter 19: Cerebral Palsy

1. What is meant by cerebral palsy?

2. What is meant by hemiplegia, quadriplegia, and diplegia, relative to cerebral palsy?
3. What is meant by athetosis and spasticity, relative to cerebral palsy?
4. What is meant by hypotonicity and hypertonicity, relative to cerebral palsy?
5. Do adults have cerebral palsy? Explain.
6. What are some causes of cerebral palsy?
7. Name symptoms seen in individuals with cerebral palsy.
8. How can COTAs assist in the treatment of individuals with cerebral palsy?

Chapter 20: Spinal Cord Injury

1. What is a spinal cord injury?
2. Why are some people with spinal cord injury able to walk, some able to participate in wheelchair sports, and some able to use computer keyboard only with adaptive devices for upper extremity function?
3. What is meant by paraplegia and quadriplegia relative to spinal cord injury?
4. What symptoms in a person with spinal cord injury suggest autonomic dysreflexia?
5. What action should be taken if the assistant sees the above symptoms?
6. What is meant by blood pooling in an individual with spinal cord injury. What is the procedure to follow when evidence of blood pooling is apparent?
7. List the general goals of occupational therapy for a patient with spinal cord injury.

Chapter 21: Geriatrics

1. Define geriatrics and gerontology.
2. What was the number-one cause of death for all ages in the United States in the 1990s?
3. What are four chronic conditions generally reported by noninstitutionalized persons 65 years and older?
4. Discuss the effect of the continuing increase in numbers of older persons on the occupational therapy profession.
5. Describe some of the nation's changes in advertising, clothing, food, and employment because of the increased numbers of older persons.

Chapter 22: Cerebrovascular Accident

1. State at least three possible causes of a CVA.
2. Describe some expected symptoms of a CVA.
3. Discuss the expected symptoms of a right CVA.
4. Discuss the expected symptoms of a left CVA.

5. Explain the reasons for the expected symptoms in a person with a right CVA, compared to a person with a left CVA.
6. Why can edema occur in a person with a CVA?

Chapter 23: Occupational Therapy in Adult Hemiplegia: Neurodevelopmental Approach

1. What are the underlying neurophysiological aims of neurodevelopmental treatment (NDT)?
2. Why is an entry-level occupational therapy assistant unprepared to provide NDT?
3. Do experienced COTAs participate in NDT? If so, what qualifies them to do so?
4. Describe examples of how experienced COTAs participate in NDT.

Chapter 24: Occupational Therapy for Arthritis

1. Explain why *arthritis* is an encompassing term.
2. Name an arthritic condition that is localized and another that is systemic, and explain why they are considered as such.
3. What arthritic condition affects more individuals than any others? Explain why so many people are affected.
4. What arthritic condition results in the most disability? Explain why it is considered the most disabling of the arthritic conditions.
5. What arthritic condition affects more older individuals? More teens and younger adults? More children? More men?

Chapter 25: Psychiatry

1. Define psychiatry.
2. What role did the early study of mental disorders have on the occupational therapy profession?
3. Discuss the early treatment of individuals with mental disorders.
4. List at least six indicators of mental health.
5. List at least six indicators of mental disorders, and tell what mental disorder each indicates.
6. Name two main classifications of mental disorders, and state generally how these differ.
7. Name symptoms of each of the mental disorders listed in Question 5.
8. Name at least five models of treatment for psychiatric disorders.
9. State the role occupational therapy can play in the treatment of mental disorders.

Chapter 26: Epilogue: Trends in Health Care

1. Why is it important to look at trends?
2. What are some general trends that help determine trends in health care?

3. Name at least two changes in the last decade that affected occupational therapy salaries?
4. Why is it important for occupational therapy personnel to be able to explain occupational therapy to the public and to legislators?
5. State at least two reasons why the American Occupational Therapy Association is strongly promoting graduate study for occupational therapists.
6. What is the reason for the change since the 1990s in the settings in which occupational therapy is provided?
7. How is the use of technology affecting the practice of occupational therapy?

Finally, as you try to learn new information and study for tests or prepare for experiences in actual occupational therapy settings, think about the following statement credited to Henry Ford:

> *If you think you can do a thing,*
> *or think you can't do a thing, you're right.*

(McWilliams & McWilliams, 1992, p. 115).

REFERENCES

Algier, A. S., & Algier, K. W. (Eds.). (1982). *Improving reading and study skills.* San Francisco: Jossey-Bass, Inc.

Bloom, B. S. (Ed.). (1956). *Taxonomy of educational objectives: Cognitive domain.* New York: David McKay.

Curtis, B. A. (1990). *Neurosciences: The basics.* Philadelphia: Lea & Febiger.

McWilliams, J.-R., & McWilliams, P. (1992). *The portable life 101.* Los Angeles: Prelude Press.

Staton, T. F. (1962). *How to Study* (rev. ed.). Montgomery, AL: Author.

GLOSSARY

[*Author's note.* The numbers in parentheses that follow each definition refer to the references at the end of this glossary.]

Activities of daily living (ADL). The self-care, communication, and mobility skills required for independence in everyday living. SYN: independent living skills, daily living skills (4). Self-maintenance tasks (1). See (1) for a list of tasks.

Activity analysis. A process used by occupational therapists to assess the psychosocial, psychodynamic, physical, or developmental characteristics of an activity in determining its utility as a therapeutic modality (4).

Acute. Having rapid onset, severe symptoms and a short course; not chronic (4).

Adaptation. Adjustment of an organism to a change in internal or external conditions or circumstances (4).

Adapted clothing. Garments designed with special features, such as Velcro closures, to permit independent dressing by persons with physical disabilities (4).

Adaptive device. Device specifically designed and fabricated with the purpose of permitting or assisting persons with disabilities to perform life tasks independently (4).

Adolescence. The period from the beginning of puberty until maturity. The onset of puberty and maturity is a gradual process and variable among individuals; thus it is not practical to set exact age or chronological limits in defining the adolescent period (4).

Adult foster care. Long-term care for elderly individuals in an adult foster care facility. Typically, such a facility resembles a residence rather than a nursing home, and thus might have fewer regulations than in a nursing home (4).

Afebrile. Without fever (4).

Affect. In psychology, the emotional reactions associated with an experience.
    a., blunted. Greatly diminished emotional response to a situation or condition. a., flat. Virtual absence of emotional response to a situation or condition (4).

Ageism. [Robert Butler, U. S. physician who coined the term in 1968]. Discrimination against aged persons (4).

Agnosia. Loss of comprehension of auditory, visual, or other sensations although the sensory sphere is intact.
    a., auditory. Mental inability to interpret sounds. a., finger. Inability to identify fingers of one's own hands or of others. a., optic. Mental inability to interpret images that are seen. a., tactile. Inability to distinguish objects by sense of touch (4).

Agraphia. Loss of the ability to write (4).

AIDS. Acquired Immune Deficiency Syndrome. The syndrome of opportunistic infections that occur as the final state of infection by human immunodeficiency virus (HIV) (4).

Alzheimer's disease. [Alois Alzheimer, Ger. neurologist, 1864-1915]. A chronic, organic mental disorder; a form of presenile dementia due to atrophy of frontal and occipital lobes. Onset is usually between ages 40 and 60 (4).

Ankylosis. Immobility of a joint (4).

Anopsia. Inability to use the vision, as in those confined in the dark, or from disuse of an eye in strabismus, or resulting from cataract, or in refractive errors (4).

Anorexia. Loss of appetite. *a. nervosa.* Occurs most commonly in females between the ages of 12 and 21 but may occur in older women and men (4). See (4) for diagnostic criteria.

Anxiety. A feeling of apprehension, worry, uneasiness, or dread, especially of the future (4).

Aphasia. Absence or impairment of the ability to communicate through speech, writing, or signs, due to dysfunction of brain centers. It is considered to be complete or total when both sensory and motor areas are involved.

  a., expressive, a., motor. Aphasia in which patients know what they want to say but cannot say it. Inability to coordinate muscles controlling speech. May be complete or partial. Broca's area is disordered or diseased.

  a., receptive, a., sensory. Inability to understand spoken words if auditory word center is involved (auditory aphasia) or the written word if visual word center is affected (visual aphasia). If both centers are involved, patient will not understand spoken or written words (4).

Arthritis. Inflammation of a joint, usually accompanied by pain, swelling, and, frequently, changes in structure.

  a., juvenile rheumatoid. Chronic, inflammatory, systemic disease which may cause joint or connective tissue damage and visceral lesions throughout the body. Affects juveniles with onset prior to age 16. Complete remission occurs in 75% of patients.

  a., osteo-. A chronic disease involving the joints, esp. those bearing weight. Characterized by degeneration of articular cartilage, overgrowth of bone with lipping and spur formation, and impaired function. SYN: *a., degenerative; a., hypertrophic; degenerative joint disease. a., rheumatoid.* A chronic systemic disease characterized by inflammatory changes in joints and related structures that result in crippling deformities (4).

Assessment. The use of skilled observation or evaluation by the administration and interpretation of standardized or nonstandardized tests and measurements to identify areas for occupational therapy services (1).

Astereognosis. Inability to recognize objects or forms by touch (4).

Ataxia. Defective muscular coordination, esp. that manifested when voluntary muscular movements are attempted (4).

Athetosis. A condition in which slow, irregular, twisting, snakelike movements occur in the upper extremities, esp. in the hands and fingers. These involuntary movements prevent sustaining the body, esp. the extremities, in one position. All four limbs may be affected or the involvement may be unilateral (4). See (4) for types of athetosis.

Atrophy. A wasting; a decrease in size of an organ or tissue (4).

Attention. Directing or concentrating one's consciousness on only one object or an internal or external stimulus (4).

Augmentative communication. The use

of technological systems, usually involving microcomputers, for improving or enabling disabled persons to have the ability to communicate (4).

Autism. Mental introversion in which the attention or interest is fastened upon the patient's own ego. A self-centered mental state from which reality tends to be excluded (4).

Autoimmune disease. A disease produced when the body's normal tolerance of its own antigenic markers on cells disappears (4). See (4) for listing of autoimmune diseases.

Behavior. 1. The manner in which one acts; the actions or reactions of individuals under specific circumstances. 2. Any response elicited from an organism (4).

Bipolar affective disorder. A disorder in which the patient exhibits both manic and depressive episodes (4).

Body image. The subjective image or picture people have of their physical appearance based on their own observations and the reactions of others (4).

Body mechanics. Application of kinesiology to use of the body in daily life activities and to the prevention and correction of problems related to posture and lifting (4).

Bulimia. Excessive and insatiable appetite (4).

Cerebral palsy. SEE: *palsy, cerebral* (4).

Cerebrovascular. Pertaining to the blood vessels of the brain, especially to pathological changes (4).

Cerebrovascular accident. A general term most commonly applied to cerebrovascular conditions that accompany either ischemic or hemorrhagic lesions. These conditions are usually secondary to atherosclerotic disease, hypertension, or a combi-nation of both. Also called apoplexy, stroke, or "a shock" (4).

Cervical. Of, pertaining to, or in the region of the neck (4).

Chromosome. A linear thread in the nucleus of a cell. It contains the DNA, which transmits genetic information (4). See (4) for more information.

Chronic. (2) Designating a disease showing little change or of slow progression. Opposite of acute (4).

Client. The patient of a health care professional (4).

Code. 1. A collection of rules and regulations or specifications. 3. A form of coded message used in transmitting information in a hospital, esp. when the information is broadcast over a public address system, e.g., "code blue" or "code 9" could be used to indicate a particular type of emergency to an emergency care team (4).

Cognition. Awareness with perception, reasoning, judgment, intuition, and memory; the mental process by which knowledge is acquired (4).

Cognitive integration and cognitive components. The ability to use higher brain functions (1). See (1) for components.

Confidentiality. Information the health care team obtains from or about a patient; i.e., laboratory data are considered to be privileged and thus cannot be disclosed to a third party without the patient's consent. In some instances when the information is important to public health, it may be illegal not to disclose those data (4).

Confusion. Not being aware of or oriented with respect to time, place, or self (6).

Congenital. Present at birth (4).

Contraction. A shortening or tightening, as that of a muscle, or reduction in size; a shrinking (4).

Contracture. Fibrosis of connective tissue in skin, fascia, muscle, or joint capsule that prevents normal mobility of the related tissue or joint (4).

Contraindication. Any symptom or circumstance indicating the inappropriateness of a form of treatment otherwise advisable (4).

Contralateral. Originating in, or affecting, the opposite side of the body. Opposed to homolateral and ipsilateral (4).

Contusion. An injury in which the skin is not broken; a bruise (4).

Convulsion. Paroxysms of involuntary muscular contractions and relaxations (4).

Coordination. Refers to skill and performance in gross motor activities using several muscle groups (1).

Cope. The ability to deal effectively with and handle the stresses to which one is subjected (4).

Decubitus. A bedsore (4).

Deformity. An alteration in the natural form of a part or organ. Distortion of any part or general disfigurement of the body. It may be acquired or congenital (4).

Delusion. A false belief brought about without appropriate external stimulation and inconsistent with the individual's own knowledge and experience. Seen most often in psychoses, in which patients cannot separate delusion from reality (4).

Dementia. A broad (global) impairment of intellectual function (cognition) that usually is progressive and that interferes with normal social and occupational activities. Patients with this condition have little insight into it and care for them is sought by their families or associates (4).

Depression. Mental state characterized by altered mood. An estimated 3% to 5% of the world's population experiences depression on any given date. There is loss of interest in all usually pleasurable outlets such as food, sex,, work, friends, hobbies, or entertainment.

d., bipolar. Depression in which disorders of both mood and elation are alternately present.

d., unipolar. Mental depression characterized by mind shifts from a normal baseline to a depressed state (4). See (4) for diagnostic criteria.

Developmental milestones. Those skills regarded as having special importance in the development of infants and toddlers and usually associated with a particular age range; e.g., sitting, crawling, walking (4).

Dexterity. Refers to skill and performance in tasks using small muscle groups (1).

Diagnose. To determine the cause and nature of a pathological condition; to recognize a disease (4).

Diagnosis related group (DRG). A system designed to attempt to standardize prospective payment for medical care. The reimbursement for treating all individuals within the same DRG is the same, regardless of actual cost to the health care facility. The facility may earn a profit if the patient's hospitalization is shorter than the specified average length of stay of that category of illness (4).

Diplegia. 1. Paralysis of similar parts on both sides of the body. 2. In cerebral palsy, usually refers to excessive stiffness in all limbs, but with greater stiffness in the legs than in the arms. (4).

Directionality. Ability to perceive one's position in relationship with the environment; sense of direction. Problems with directionality are frequently found in children with learning disabilities or suspected minimal brain dysfunction (4).

Disability. Any restriction or lack of

ability to perform an activity in the manner considered normal for a human being. d., developmental. Term used for conditions due to congenital abnormality, trauma, deprivation, or diseases that interrupt or delay the sequence and rate of normal growth, development, and maturation (4).

Discharge summary. A summary of the hospital or clinic record of a patient. Prepared after time of discharge (4).

Disease. Literally the lack of ease; a pathological condition of the body that presents a group of symptoms peculiar to it and that sets the condition apart as an abnormal entity, differing from other normal or pathological body states. d., acute. Disease having a rapid onset and of relatively short duration. d., chronic. Disease having a slow onset and lasting for a long period of time (4).

Disorientation. Inability to estimate direction or location, or to be cognizant of time or of persons (4).

Distractibility. A condition of mental wandering in which the thoughts are attracted by extraneous conditions or influenced by a dissociation of consciousness (4).

Echolalia. An involuntary parrotlike repetition of words spoken by others, often accompanied by twitching of muscles (4).

Elation. Joyful emotion. It is of pathological origin when out of accord with patient's actual circumstances (4).

Embolism. Obstruction of a blood vessel by foreign substances or a blood clot (4).

Embolus. A mass of undissolved matter present in a blood or lymphatic vessel brought there by the blood or lymph current. Emboli may be solid, liquid, or gaseous (4).

Exercise. Performed activity of the muscles, voluntary or otherwise, esp. to maintain fitness. e.g., range of motion. Movements of joints through their available range of motion. Can be used to prevent loss of motion (4). See (4) for range-of-motion and other types of exercise.

Extension. The movement by which both ends of any part are pulled apart. A movement that brings the members of a limb into or toward a straight condition. Opposite of flexion (4).

Family therapy. Treatment of the members of a family together, rather than an individual "patient"; the family unit is viewed as a social system important to all of its members (4).

Fine motor skills. Skills pertaining to the synergy of small muscles, primarily in the hand, and related to manual dexterity and coordination (4).

Flaccid. Relaxed, flabby, having defective or absent muscular tone (4).

Flight of ideas. Continuous but fragmentary stream of talk. The general train of thought can be followed but direction is frequently changed, often by chance stimuli from the environment. May be seen in acute manic states (4).

Function. 2. The act of carrying on or performing a special activity. Normal function is the normal action of an organ . . . . In humans, function can pertain to the manner in which the individual is able to successfully perform the tasks and roles required for everyday living (4).

Functional communication. Using equipment or systems to send and receive information, such as writing equipment, telephones, typewriters, computers, communication boards, call lights, emergency systems, Braille writers, telecommunication devices for the deaf, and augmentative communication systems (1).

Functional Independence Measure

(FIM). An objectively scored measure of functional independence used by rehabilitation practitioners. Includes items related to self-care, sphincter control, mobility, locomotion, communication, and social cognition (4).

Functional mobility. Moving from one position or place to another, such as in-bed mobility, wheelchair mobility, transfers (wheelchair, bed, car, tub, toilet, tub/shower, chair, floor). Performing functional ambulation and transporting objects (1).

Generalization. Applying previously learned concepts and behaviors to a variety of new situations (1).

Geriatrics. Branch of medicine concerned with the problems of aging. Included are all aspects of aging, including physiological, pathological, psychological, economic, and sociological problems (4).

Gerontology. Scientific study of the effects of aging and of age-related diseases on the human (4).

Goniometer. Apparatus to measure joint movements and angles (4).

Grandiose. In psychiatry, concerning one's unrealistic and exaggerated concept of self-worth, importance, wealth, and ability (4).

Gross motor skills. Skills pertaining to the synergy of large muscle groups, as in balancing, running, and throwing (4).

Group dynamics. In politics, sociology, and psychology, a study of the forces and conditions that influence the actions of the entire group as well as the relations of the individuals to each other in the group (4).

Guthrie test. Diagnostic test to detect phenylketonuria (PKU). Required by law in most states (4).

Habilitation. The process of educating or training persons with disadvantages or disabilities to improve their ability to function in society (4).

Hallucination. In psychology, a false perception having no relation to reality and not accounted for by any exterior stimuli. May be visual, auditory, or olfactory. Judgment may be impaired, and the patient will not be able to distinguish between the real and the imagined (4). See (4) for list of additional hallucinations.

Handicap. Disadvantage for a given individual, resulting from an impairment or a disability, that limits or prevents the fulfillment of a role that is normal, depending on age, sex, and social and cultural factors for that individual (4).

Heimlich maneuver. Technique for removing a foreign body from the trachea or pharynx, where it is preventing flow of air to the lungs. The obstruction usually is due to a bolus of food (4). See reference (4) for a description of the maneuver.

Hemianopia, Hemianopsia. Blindness for half the field of vision in one or both eyes (6).

Hemiplegia. Paralysis of only one side of the body (4).

Hemorrhage. Abnormal, severe internal or external discharge of blood. May be venous, arterial, or capillary from blood vessels into tissues, into or from the body. Venous blood is dark red; flow is continuous. Arterial blood is bright red; flows in spurts. Capillary blood is of a reddish color; exudes from tissue (4).

Home assessment. An evaluation of the home environment of persons with disability, usually by an occupational therapist for purposes of identifying architectural barriers and safety hazards and recommending modifications or devices for improving mobility, safety, and independent function (4).

Home care. The provision of equipment and services to the patient in the home for the purpose of restoring and maintaining maximal levels of comfort, function, and health of the individual (4).

Hypertension. 1. Tension or tonus that is greater than normal. 2. A condition in which the patient has a higher blood pressure than that judged to be normal (4).

Hypertonic. 2. Being in a state of greater than normal tension or of incomplete relaxation. Said of muscles (4).

Hypochondriasis. Abnormal anxiety about one's health; a frequent symptom in depressed patients (4).

Hypotonic. Pertaining to defective muscular tone or tension (4).

Illusion. Inaccurate perception; misinterpretation of sensory impressions, whereas a hallucination has no source in fact. Vague stimuli are conducive to the production of illusions, but essentially it is a disorder of ideation. If an illusion becomes fixed, it is said to be a delusion (4).

Image. 1. A mental picture representing a real object.

    i., body. The concept an individual has of his or her physical self. Many individuals have inappropriate self-images. For example, some obese individuals have the body image of a much less obese person (4).

Incidence. The frequency of occurrence of any event or condition over a period of time and in relation to the population in which it occurs, as incidence of a disease (4).

Incoordination. Inability to produce harmonious, rhythmic, muscular action that is not due to weakness (4).

Integration. The bringing together of various parts or functions so that they function as a harmonious whole (4).

Interpersonal. Concerning the relations and interactions between persons (4).

Intervention. Taking actions so as to modify an effect (4).

Joint protection. Techniques for minimizing stress on joints, including proper body mechanics and the avoidance of continuous weight-bearing or deforming postures (4).

Kinesthesia. The ability to perceive extent, distance or weight of movement (4).

Labile. Not fixed; unsteady; easily disarranged; rapidly shifting and changing emotions (4).

Lifestyle. The pattern of living and behavior of an individual, society, or culture, esp. as it distinguishes individuals concerned or included in the groups from other individuals or groups (4).

Mania. 2. A form of psychosis characterized by exalted feelings, delusions of grandeur, elevation of mood, psychomotor overactivity and overproduction of ideas (4).

Medical record. Transcript of information obtained from a patient, guardian, or professionals and presented in tabular, outline, or written form. It may contain history, diagnoses, treatment, prognosis, etc. Utilized by the school, place of employment, personal physician, hospital, etc. (4).

Medical record, problem-oriented. A technique of clinical record keeping described by Lawrence Weed, a contemporary U.S. physician. The patient's record is organized in a logical and efficient manner, including a list of problems and flowcharts determining diagnostic and therapeutic plans and indicating what has been done (4).

Medicare. Federal medical and hospital care program, in the U.S. for the elderly (6).

Medium. An agent through which an effect is obtained (4).

Mental retardation. Refers to significantly subaverage general intellectual functioning existing concurrently with deficits in adaptive behavior and manifested during the developmental period (3).

Method. The systematic manner, procedure, or technique in performing details of an operation, tests, treatment, or any act (4).

Mnemonics The art of improving or assisting memory. A device to help recall a series of related data, names, or anatomical terms (4).

Mobility. State or quality of being mobile; facility of movement (4).

Modality. 2. A method of application or the employment of any therapeutic agent; limited usually to physical agents and devices. 3. Any specific sensory stimulus such as taste, touch, vision, pressure, or hearing (4).

Mood. A pervasive and sustained emotion that may have a major influence on a person's perception of the world. Examples of mood include depression, joy, elation, anger, and anxiety (4).

Mood disorders. A group of disorders in which the disturbance of mood is accompanied by full or partial manic or depressive syndrome (4).

Motivation. The internal drive or externally arising stimulus to action or thought (4).

Movement. 1. Act of passing from place to place or changing position of body or its parts.

   m., active. Voluntary movement accomplished without external assistance.

   m., passive. Movement of the body or a part due to outside forces (4).

Nystagmus. Constant, involuntary, cyclical movement of the eyeball. Movement may be in any direction (4).

Occupational therapist. One who provides assessment and intervention to ameliorate physical and psychological deficits which interfere with the performance of activities and tasks of living (4). The certified *Occupational Therapist, Registered* (OTR) is one who has met all the AOTCB qualifications which include graduation from an accredited occupational therapy educational program, successful completion of all fieldwork requirements, and successful completion of the AOTCB examination (2).

Occupational therapy. See Chapter 1 of text.

Occupational therapy aide. An individual who has had on-the-job training or experience in occupational therapy who performs routine tasks under the direction of an occupational therapist (4).

Occupational therapy assistant. One who works under the supervision of an occupational therapist in evaluating clients and in planning and implementing programs designed to restore or develop a client's skills for self-care, work, play, or leisure time tasks. Although requiring supervision in conducting a remedial program, the assistant can function independently when conducting a maintenance program (4). The *Certified Occupational Therapy Assistant* (COTA) is one who has met all the AOTCB qualifications which include graduation from an accredited occupational therapy assistant educational program, successful completion of all fieldwork requirements, and successful completion of the AOTCB examination (2).

Ocular. 1. Concerning the eye or vision (4).

Orientation. Ability to comprehend and to adjust oneself in an environment with regard to time, location, and identity of persons. Partially or completely absent in some psychoses (4).

Orthotics. 1. The science pert. to mechanical appliances for orthopedic use (4).

Palsy, cerebral. A nonprogressive paralysis resulting from developmental defects in brain or trauma at birth (4).

Paralysis. Temporary suspension or permanent loss of function, especially loss of sensation or voluntary motion.

　p., flaccid. Paralysis in which there is loss of muscle tone, loss or reduction of tendon reflexes, atrophy and degeneration of muscles, and reaction of degeneration. Due to lesions of lower motor neurons of spinal cord.

　p., hysterical. Apparent loss of movement that may simulate any form of paralysis. There is no organic cause.

　p., spastic. Paralysis usually involving groups of muscles. Characterized by excessive tone and spasticity of muscles, exaggeration of tendon reflexes but loss of superficial reflexes, positive Babinski reflex, no atrophy or wasting except from prolonged disuse, and absence of reaction of degeneration. Due to lesion of upper motor neurons or cerebrum (4).

Paraplegia. Paralysis of lower portion of the body and of both legs (4).

Paresis. 1. Partial or incomplete paralysis (4).

Pediatric. Concerning the treatment of children (4).

Perception. 1. Process of being aware of objects; consciousness. 2. Process of receiving sensory impressions. 3. The elaboration of a sensory impression; the ideational association modifying, defining, and usually completing the primary impression or stimulus. Vague or inadequate association occurs in confused and depressed states (4).

Performance. The act of performing, i.e., the undertaking and completing of, either mental or physical work. Thus a person's performance is observed and measured in order to determine functional capability (4).

Performance areas. Broad categories of human activity that are typically part of daily life. They are activities of daily living, work and productive activities, and play or leisure activities (1).

Performance components. Fundamental human abilities that—to varying degrees and in differing combinations—are required for successful engagement in performance areas. These components are sensorimotor, cognitive, psychosocial, and psychological (1).

Performance contexts. Situations or factors that influence an individual's engagement in desired and/or required performance areas. Performance contexts consist of temporal aspects (chronological age, developmental age, place in the life cycle, and health status) and environmental aspects (physical, social, and cultural considerations) (1).

Perseveration. Continued repetition of a meaningless word or phrase, or repetition of answers that are not related to successive questions asked (4).

Personality. The unique organization of traits, characteristics, and modes of behavior of an individual, setting the individual apart from others and at the same time determining how others react to the individual. Personality refers to the mental aspects of an individual, in contrast to physique (4).

Phenylketonuria. 2. A recessive hereditary disease caused by the body's failure to oxidize an amino acid (phenylalanine) to tyrosine, because of a defective enzyme. If the disease is not treated early, brain damage may occur, causing severe mental retardation. Test for phenylketonuria should be made at birth; some states require it. The disease is seen equally in the sexes, and in the U.S., the incidence is approximately 1: 14,000 births (4).

Phobia. Any persistent and irrational fear of a specific object, activity, or situation that results in a compelling desire to avoid the feared or phobic stimulus. Phobias are classified into three types: agoraphobia, social phobia, or simple phobia (4).

Play. Involvement in a sport, amusement, or any form of recreation, esp. an activity other than that in which one is usually engaged as an occupation. What is play to one individual might be considered work to another. From the medical standpoint, it is important that the recreational activity be enjoyable and that participation in it be safe and satisfactory. From the medical aspect, the value of engaging in a sport or recreation that causes frustration, anger, or uncontrolled stress to the extent that the activity is no longer fun is questionable (4).

Play or leisure activities. Intrinsically motivating activities for amusement, relaxation, spontaneous enjoyment, or self-expression (1).

Positioning. In rehabilitation, a term used to refer to placing the body and extremities so as to aid treatment by inhibiting undesirable reflexes and preventing deformities. In treatment of children with developmental disabilities involving neuromotor function, the position of the body affects the presence of some primitive reflexes which can affect muscle tone. Alignment of the head, neck, and trunk is therefore thought to be important to reduce unnecessary influences on muscle tone, and the careful placement of the limbs is important to reduce or prevent contractions and deformities (4).

Postural alignment. Maintaining biomechanical integrity among body parts (1).

P.P.D. Purified protein derivative, substance used in intradermal test for tuberculosis (4).

Praxis. The ability to plan and execute coordinated movement (4).

Predisposition. The potential to develop a certain disease or condition in the presence of specific environmental stimuli (4).

Prevalence. The number of cases of a disease present in a specified population at a given time (4).

Preventive medicine. The branch of medicine concerned with preventing the occurrence of both mental and physical illness and disease (4).

Principle. 2. A fundamental truth. 3. An established role of action (4).

Problem-oriented medical record. (POMR). Method of establishing and maintaining the patient's medical record so that problems are clearly stated, usually in order of importance, and a rational plan for dealing with them is stated. These data are kept at the front of the chart and are evaluated as frequently as indicated with respect to recording changes in the patient's problems as well as progress made in solving the problems. Use of this system may bring a degree of comprehensiveness to total patient care that might not be possible with conventional medical records (4).

Professional liability. The obligation of health-care providers or their insurers to pay for damages resulting from the providers' acts of omission or commission in treating patients (4).

Professional Standards Review Organization (PSRO). Peer review at the local level required by Public Law 92-603 of the U.S. for the services provided under the Medicare, Medicaid, and maternal and child health programs funded by the federal government (4).

Prognosis. Prediction of course and end of disease, and the estimate of chance for recovery (4).

Progress notes. Notes made on the chart by those involved in caring for the patient. Physicians, nurses, consultants, and therapists may record their notes concerning the progress or lack of progress made by the patient in the interim between the previous note and the time of the most recent note. In patients who are not critically ill, a note concerning progress might be made daily or less frequently; in critical care situations, notes could be made hourly (4).

Progress report. The written or verbal account of a patient's present condition, esp. as compared to the previous state (4).

Projective technique. Any one of several forms of psychological assessment or evaluation. Using ambiguous activities and tasks which encourage self-expression, the products or results and the individual's verbalizations about them are evaluated and interpreted to determine indications of unconscious needs, thoughts or concerns (4).

Prone. 1. Lying horizontal with face downward. 2. Denoting the hand with the palm turned downward. Opposite of supine (4).

Proprioception. The awareness of posture, movement, and changes in equilibrium and the knowledge of position, weight, and resistance of objects in relation to the body (4).

Prospective payment system (PPS). A reimbursement method used in which a fixed, predetermined amount is allocated for treating patients with a specific diagnosis when an individual is hospitalized. Originally developed for use with Medi-

care recipients. Also referred to as payment-by-diagnosis (4).

Prosthetics. The branch of surgery dealing with replacement of missing parts (4).

Psychosis. A term formerly applied to any mental disorder, but now generally restricted to those disturbances of such magnitude that there is personality disintegration and loss of contact with reality. The disturbances are of psychogenic origin, or without clearly defined physical cause or structural change in the brain. They usually are characterized by delusions and hallucination, and hospitalization generally is required (4).

Psychosocial skills and psychological components. The ability to interact in society and to process emotions (1).

Quadriplegia. Paralysis of all four extremities and usually the trunk (4).

Quality assurance. Activities and programs designed to achieve a desired degree or grade of care in a defined medical, nursing, or health-care setting or program. The quality assurance program must include evaluation and educational components to identify and correct problems. Such programs are required for funding by the Public Health Act (4).

Quality of life. A concept that differs for each person and may vary for the same individual as that person's life situation changes. The holistic treatment of a patient requires that the health-care team assess what is most important to that individual. In some cases it is not possible to establish a situation in which there is complete freedom from the signs and symptoms of disease. In those cases, the goal is to have the quality of life be as good as possible despite the disease. Also, in persons who have suffered disabilities or loss of mental or physical skills, it is important to emphasize the positive features of their remaining capabilities rather than to dwell on the negative aspects of what has been lost (4).

Range of Motion. The range of movement of a joint (4).

Rapport. A relationship of mutual trust and understanding, esp. between the patient and physician, nurse, or other health care provider (4).

Reflex. An involuntary response to a stimulus; a reflex action. Reflexes are specific and predictable and are usually purposeful and adaptive. They depend upon an intact neural pathway between point of stimulation and responding organ (muscle or gland). This pathway is called reflex arc. In a simple reflex this includes a sensory receptor, afferent or sensory neuron, reflex center in brain or spinal cord, one or more efferent neurons, and an effector organ (muscle or gland) (4). See (4) for complete definition and list of reflexes.

Rehabilitation. The processes of treatment and education that lead the disabled individual to attainment of maximum function, a sense of well-being, and a personally satisfying level of independence (4). See (4) for a complete definition.

Sclerosis. 1. A hardening or induration of an organ or tissue, esp. that due to excessive growth of fibrous tissue. 3. Thickening and hardening of the layers in the wall of an artery (4). See (4) for complete listing.

Seizure. A sudden attack of pain, of a disease, or of certain symptoms (4). See (4) for listing of types of seizures.

Self-concept. An individual's perception of self in relation to others and the environment (4).

Self-esteem. One's personal evaluation or view of self, generally thought to influence feelings and behaviors.

One's personal successes, expectations, and appraisals of the views others hold toward oneself are thought to influence this personal appraisal (4).

Self-ranging. Patient administered passive range of motion following stroke. By using their unaffected arms and specific techniques, patients with hemiplegia can be taught to prevent contractures by moving their paralyzed extremities through full range of motion at the shoulder, elbow, wrist, and finger joints. Care should be exercised to prevent injury, especially at the shoulder (4).

Senility. Mental or physical weakness that may be associated with old age. *s., premature.* Onset of senile characteristics before old age, as early as 40 years (4).

Sensation. A feeling or awareness of conditions within or without the body resulting from the stimulation of sensory receptors (4).

Sensorimotor component. The ability to receive input, process information, and produce output (1).

Sensory integration. Skill and performance required in the development and coordination of sensory input, motor output, and sensory feedback. Includes sensory awareness, visual spatial awareness, body integration, balance, bilateral motor coordination, visual-motor integration, praxis, and other components (4).

Significant others. Persons with whom a patient or client has a close relationship. They may or may not include relatives or a spouse (4).

Signing. The use of sign language to communicate with hearing-impaired persons (4).

Somatic. 3. Pertaining to structures of the body wall, e.g., skeletal muscles (somatic musculature) in contrast to structures associated with the viscera, e.g. visceral muscles (splanchnic musculature) (4).

Space. 1. An area, region, or segment.

   s., personal. In psychiatry, an individual's personal area and the surrounding space. This space is important in interpersonal relations (4).

Spasticity. Increased tone or contractions of muscles causing stiff and awkward movements: the result of upper motor neuron lesion (4).

Spinal column. The vertebral column enclosing the spinal cord and consisting of 33 vertebrae: 7 cervical, 12 dorsal or thoracic, 5 lumbar, 5 sacral fused to form 1 bone and 4 in the coccyx fused to form 1 bone. The number is sometimes increased by additional vertebrae in one region, and sometimes one may be absent in another (4).

Spinal cord. An ovoid column of nervous tissue about 44 cm long, flattened anteroposteriorly, extending from the medulla to the second lumbar vertebra in the spinal canal. All nerves to the trunk and limbs are issued from the spinal cord, and it is the center of reflex action containing the conducting paths to and from the brain (4). See reference (4) for complete definition.

Spinal shock. Effects resulting from transverse section of the spinal cord and occurring in segments below level of section. Principal effects are anesthesia, paralysis, loss of muscle tone, and suppression of reflexes, both visceral and somatic (4).

Splint. An appliance made of bone, wood, metal and/or plaster of Paris, used for fixation, union, or protection of an injured part of the body.

   s., dynamic. A splint that assists in movements initiated by the patient (4). See (4) for listing of types of splints.

Splinting. Fixation of a dislocation or fracture with a splint. Splints are also used to help support weak joints, to actively assist with functional movement, to immobilize to promote healing, and to protect from injury and deformity (4).

Stereognosis. Ability to recognize form of solid objects by touch (4).

Strabismus. Disorder of eye in which optic axes cannot be directed to same objects (4).

Subluxation. A partial or incomplete dislocation (4).

Supine. 1. Lying on the back with the face upward. 2. Noting position of the hand or foot with the palm or foot facing upward. Opposite of prone (4).

Symmetry. Correspondence in shape, size, and relative position of parts on opposite sides of a body (4).

Symptom. Any perceptible change in the body or its functions that indicates disease or the kind or phases of disease. Symptoms may be classified as objective, subjective, cardinal, and sometimes as constitutional. However, another classification considers all symptoms as being subjective, with objective indications being called signs (4). See (4) for details.

Syndrome. A group of symptoms and signs of disordered function related to one another by means of some anatomic, physiologic, or biochemical peculiarity. This definition does not include a precise cause of an illness but does provide a framework of reference for investigating it (4).

Systemic. Pert. to a whole body rather than to one of its parts; somatic (4).

Systems theory. As used in clinical medicine, an approach that considers the human being as a whole as opposed to his parts. Human beings are considered open systems constantly exchanging information, matter, and energy with the environment. There are three levels of reference for systems: the system level, on which one is focusing, such as man; the suprasystems level above the focal system, such as man's family, the community, and the culture; and subsystems, the level below the focal system, such as the bodily systems and the cell. Those involved in health care must view persons as being affected constantly by supra- and subsystems. Health care, in the systems approach, transcends the idea of treating illness and addresses the larger issue of attaining and maintaining health through assessment and treatment of the total person (4).

Tactile. Perceptible to the touch (4).

Tactile defensiveness. A defense reaction due to sensitivity to being touched (4).

Theory. A supposition or an assumption based on certain evidence or observations but lacking scientific proof. When a theory becomes generally accepted and firmly established, it is called a doctrine or principle (4).

Therapeutic exercise. Scientific supervision of exercise for the purpose of preventing muscular atrophy, restoring joint and muscle function, increasing muscular strength, and improving efficiency of cardiovascular and pulmonary function (4).

Therapy. Treatment of a disease or pathological condition (4).

Thoracic. Pertaining to the chest or thorax (4).

Thrombosis. The formation, development, or existence of a blood clot or thrombus within the vascular system (4). See (4) for complete definition.

Thrombus. A blood clot that obstructs a blood vessel of a cavity of the heart (4).

Tone. 1. That state of a body or any of its organs or parts in which the functions are healthy and normal. In a more restricted sense, the resistance of muscles to passive elongation or stretch.

t., muscular. Condition in which a muscle is in a steady state of contraction; the ability of a muscle to resist a force for a considerable period of time without change in length (4).

Transferring. The act of moving a person with limited function from one location to another. May be accomplished by the patient or with assistance (4).

Ulcer. An open sore or lesion of the skin or mucous membrane accompanied by sloughing of inflamed necrotic tissue.

u., decubitus. Ischemic necrosis and ulceration of tissue, esp. over a bony prominence. Due to pressure from prolonged confinement in bed or from a cast or splint (4). See (4) for complete definition and listing of types of ulcers.

Vestibular nerve. A main division of the auditory nerve. Arises in the vestibular ganglion and is concerned with equilibrium (4).

Visual field. The area within which objects may be seen when the eye is fixed (4).

Visual function. The process of receiving stimuli transmitted to the eye and then to the brain and translating those stimuli into images. There are three aspects of visual function: form sense, color sense, and light sense (4). See (4) for complete definition.

Work and productive activities. Purposeful activities for self-development, social contribution, and livelihood (1).

REFERENCES

(1) American Occupational Therapy Association, Inc. (1994). Uniform terminology for occupational therapy. *American Journal of Occupational Therapy,* *48*(12), 1047-1054.

(2) American Occupational Therapy Certification Board, Inc. (1991). *Questions most frequently asked by students about certification.* Gaithersburg, MD: Author.

(3) Grossman, H. J. (Ed.). (1983). *Classification in mental retardation.* Washington, DC: American Association on Mental Deficiency.

(4) Thomas, C. L. (Ed.). (1993). *Taber's cyclopedic medical dictionary* (17th ed.). Philadelphia: F. A. Davis Company. (with permission from F. A. Davis Company).

INDEX

ABOUT THE AUTHOR

Haru Hirama, Ed.D., O.T.R/L, FAOTA, is developing a professional-level occupational therapy program at Alvernia College in Reading, Pennsylvania. She was the founder and director of the occupational therapy assistant (OTA) program at the Pennsylvania State University and professor and director of the OTA program at Lehigh Carbon (PA) Community College. She was the director of occupational therapy at Hamburg (PA) Center, Allentown (PA) State Hospital, and the National Jewish Hospital, Denver, Colorado. She was a commissioned Army officer and the assistant chief of occupational therapy at the U.S. Army Hospital, Fort Carson, Colorado, and staff therapist at Fitzsimons Army Hospital, Denver. She holds degrees in occupational therapy and in home economics from Colorado State University. She received her master's degree in educational counseling and her doctorate in special education from Lehigh University, Bethlehem, Pennsylvania.

Dr. Hirama has published numerous articles in professional journals. She is author of *Self-injurious Behavior: A Somatosensory Treatment Approach* and *Activity Analysis: A Primer,* also published by CHESS Publications.